Handbook of Experimental Pharmacology

Volume 134

Springer
Berlin
Heidelberg
New York
Barcelona
Budapest
Hong Kong
London
Milan
Paris
Singapore
Tokyo

Neurotrophic Factors

Contributors

P. Aebischer, Y.-A. Barde, S. Boyce, E. Escandon, S. Harper, F. Hefti, R.G. Hill, A.F. Hottinger, C.F. Ibáñez, D.N. Ishii, K. Krieglstein, J.M.A. Laird, K. Nikolics, S. Pollack, S-F Pu, C.A. Rask, N.M.J. Rupniak, M. Sendtner, R. Smith, C. Suter-Crazzolara, C. Swain, K. Unsicker

Editor

Franz Hefti

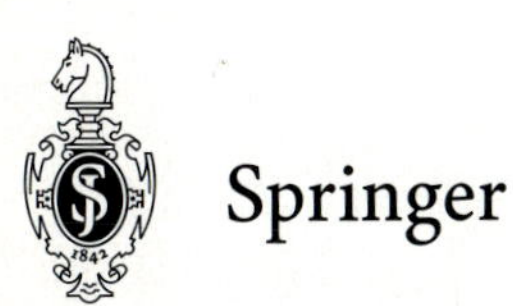

Springer

Professor
Franz Hefti, Ph.D.
Merck Sharp & Dohme
Neuroscience Research Centre
Terlings Park
Harlow, Essex CM20 2QR
United Kingdom

With 28 Figures and 12 Tables

ISBN 3-540-64614-0 Springer-Verlag Berlin Heidelberg New York

Library of Congress Cataloging-in-Publication Data

Neurotrophic factors / contributors, P. Aebischer . . . [et al.]; editor, Franz Hefti.
p. cm.—(Handbook of experimental pharmacology; v. 134)
Includes bibliographical references and index.
ISBN 3-540-64614-0 (hardcover: alk. paper)
1. Neurotrophic functions. 2. Nerve growth factor. 3. Nervous system—Diseases.
I. Aebischer, P. (Patrick) II. Hefti, Franz. III. Series.
[DNLM: 1. Nerve Growth Factors—pharmacology. 2. Nerve Growth Factors—therapeutic use. 3. Nervous System Diseases—therapy.
W1HA51L v. 134 1998]
RC350.G75N48 1998
[QP905.H3]
615′.1 s—dc21
[615′.78]
DNLM/DLC
for Library of Congress 98-27067
CIP

Printed in Germany

Cover design: *design & production* GmbH, Heidelberg

Typesetting: Best-set Typesetter Ltd., Hong Kong

Production Editor: Angélique Gcouta

SPIN: 10565573 27/3020 – 5 4 3 2 1 0 – Printed on acid-free paper

Preface

The pharmacology of neurotrophic factors is part of the general field called *neuroprotection* or *neurodegeneration*, which has emerged during the past two decades. This new broad research area has identified molecular mechanisms that regulate the morphological plasticity of the nervous system and, in consequence, discovered novel pharmacological approaches to manipulate these processes in disease states. The new, structural neuropharmacology as described in this volume attempts to regulate the anatomic aspects of the nervous system and is perhaps comparable to hardware manipulation in computer systems. In contrast, classical neuropharmacology identified multiple ways to modify the function of existing synapses or ion channels in the nervous system, comparable to software manipulations in the computer field. The pharmacology of neurotrophic factor is at an early stage and has not produced any major drugs yet. However, the first quintessential clinical trials have been carried out in the past two years or are currently in progress. Rapid further advances can be expected.

The discovery of nerve growth factor (NGF), the first protein known to promote survival and growth of nerve cells, led to the discovery of a family of related proteins, the *neurotrophins* and their receptors. This concept was generalized to incorporate many other protein families that are included in the functional definition of *neurotrophic factors*, i.e., proteins able to regulate survival and differentiation of neurons. Aside from being important in nervous system physiology, some of these proteins are efficacious pharmacologically, in conditions of experimental degeneration and regeneration of the central and peripheral nervous system. The publication of this volume is timely, since it coincides with the first attempts to use the pharmacological effects of neurotrophic factors for human therapy. Initial efforts focused on diseases of the peripheral nervous system, where systemic administration of neurotrophic factors is possible. While the first two trials, with ciliary neurotrophic factor and brain-derived neurotrophic factor in amyotrophic lateral sclerosis, resulted in failure, the clinical study with NGF in neuropathies of the peripheral sensory nervous system reported a positive outcome. For degenerative diseases of the brain, the need to administer the proteins directly into the brain complicates the use of neurotrophic factors. An initial attempt with NGF in Alzheimer's disease revealed not only beneficial effects but also adverse ones associated with the intracerebroventricular route of administration. The difficulties posed by the pharmacokinetic properties of proteins and their inability to pass the blood–brain barrier triggered many attempts towards alternative administration strategies, including cellular delivery and gene therapy. Several animal models of human diseases have demonstrated the efficacy of these approaches and it continues to be evaluated. Finally, many researchers in academic institutions and in industry endeavor to replace the therapeutic proteins with small molecule mimetics. A broad array of molecules has been disclosed, some of which are near clinical development.

This volume provides an introduction into the biology of neurotrophic factors and a synopsis of their pharmacology. The book is organized to reflect the progression from protein therapeutics to alternative administration strategies and the development of small molecule mimetics: in other words, it attempts to cover all forms of *neurotrophics*. Hopefully, the volume reflects the general promise of the field, helps quickly acquaint newcomers with its essential features and problems, and provides a source of reference for those actively engaged in this new area.

FRANZ HEFTI

List of Contributors

AEBISCHER, P., Gene Therapy Center and Surgical Research Division, Centre Hospitalier Universitaire Vaudois, Lausanne University Medical School, 1011 Lausanne-CHUV, Switzerland

BARDE, Y.-A., Max Planck Institute of Neurobiology, Department of Neurobiochemistry, D-82152 Planegg-Martinsried, Germany

BOYCE, S., Merck Sharp and Dohme Research Laboratories, Neuroscience Research Centre, Terlings Park, Eastwick Road, Harlow, Essex CM20 2QR, UK

ESCANDON, E., Genentech, Inc. One DNA Way, South San Francisco, CA 94080, USA

HARPER, S., Neuroscience Research Centre, Merck Sharp & Dohme Research Laboratories, Harlow, Essex, CM20 2QR, UK

HEFTI, F., Neuroscience Research Centre, Merck Sharp & Dohme Research Laboratories, Harlow, Essex, CM20 2QR, UK

HILL, R.G., Merck Sharp and Dohme Research Laboratories, Neuroscience Research Centre, Terlings Park, Eastwick Road, Harlow, Essex CM20 2QR, UK

HOTTINGER, A.F., Gene Therapy Center and Surgical Research Division, Centre Hospitalier Universitaire Vaudois, Lausanne University Medical School, 1011 Lausanne-CHUV, Switzerland

IBÁÑEZ, C.F., Division of Molecular Neurobiology, Department of Neuroscience, Karolinska Institute, 17177 Stockholm, Sweden

ISHII, D.N., Department of Physiology, and Department of Biochemistry and Molecular Biology, Colorado State University, Fort Collins, CO 80523, USA

Krieglstein, K., Neuroanatomy, Department of Anatomy and Cell Biology, The University of Heidelberg, Im Neuenheimer Feld 307, D-69120 Heidelberg, Germany

Laird, J.M.A., Departamento de Fisiologia y Farmacologia, Facultad de Medicina, Universidad de Alcala de Henares, 28871 Madrid, Spain

Nikolics, K., AGY Therapeutics, Inc., One Corporate Drive, South San Francisco, CA 94080, USA

Pollack, S., Neuroscience Research Centre, Merck Sharp & Dohme Research Laboratories, Harlow, Essex, CM20 2QR, UK

Pu, S.-F., Department of Physiology, and Department of Biochemistry and Molecular Biology, Colorado State University, Fort Collins, CO 80523, USA

Rask, C.A., Genentech, Inc. One DNA Way, South San Francisco, CA 94080, USA

Rupniak, N.M.J., Merck Sharp and Dohme Research Laboratories, Neuroscience Research Centre, Terlings Park, Eastwick Road, Harlow, Essex CM20 2QR, UK

Sendtner, M., Klinische Forschergruppe Neuroregeneration, University of Würzburg, Josef-Schneider-Str.11, D-97080 Würzburg, Germany

Smith, R., Department of Biochemistry & Physiology, Merck and Co., PO Box 2000 Rahway, NJ 07065-0900, USA

Suter-Crazzolara, C., Neuroanatomy, Department of Anatomy and Cell Biology, The University of Heidelberg, Im Neuenheimer Feld 307, D-69120 Heidelberg, Germany

Swain, C., Neuroscience Research Centre, Merck Sharp & Dohme Research Laboratories, Harlow, Essex, CM20 2QR, UK

Unsicker, K., Neuroanatomy, Department of Anatomy and Cell Biology, The University of Heidelberg, Im Neuenheimer Feld 307, D-69120 Heidelberg, Germany

Contents

CHAPTER 10

Strategies for Administering Neurotrophic Factors to the Central Nervous System

CHAPTER 11

Neurotrophic Factor Mimetics

CHAPTER 1

Biological Roles of Neurotrophins

Y.-A. BARDE

A. Introduction

Neurotrophins are proteins that are structurally related and exert profound effects on cells of the nervous system. Four distinct neurotrophin genes have been identified in mice and in humans that encode for small dimeric, secretory proteins named nerve growth factor (NGF), brain-derived neurotrophic factor (BDNF), neurotrophin-3 (NT3) and neurotrophin-4/5 (NT4/5).

Two classes of receptors have been identified on neurotrophin-responsive cells: one class consists of three related tyrosine kinase receptors, belonging to the *trk* family (for review, see BARBACID 1994) and the other consists of the neurotrophin receptor p75 ($p75^{NTR}$) (for reviews, see MEAKIN and SHOOTER 1992; MCDONALD and CHAO 1995). While all neurotrophins bind to $p75^{NTR}$ with at least nanomolar affinity, they bind with significant selectivity to the *trk* receptors. NGF binds to *trk*A, BDNF and NT4/5 to *trk*B, and NT3 preferentially to *trk*C receptors (for review, see BARBACID 1994).

The activation of the *trk* family members seems to account for essentially all the trophic effects of neurotrophins described to-date. In some instances (see below), BDNF and NT4/5 have been shown to elicit distinct biological responses. This may be explained, in part, by the co-receptor role of $p75^{NTR}$ that seems to be more significant for the binding of NT4/5 to *trk*B than of BDNF (CURTIS et al. 1995; RYDÉN et al. 1995). Also, a splice variant of *trk*B has been described that has a higher selectivity for BDNF than for NT4/5 (STROHMAIER et al. 1996).

The co-expression of $p75^{NTR}$ and *trk*A on cells expressing both receptors somehow increases the affinity of NGF binding (MAHADEO et al. 1994), and there is evidence that this is of relevance in vivo, given the presumed limiting concentrations of NGF in many tissues (LEE et al. 1992; DAVIES et al. 1993b; LEE et al. 1994; RYDÉN et al. 1997).

The main focus of this chapter is on the in vivo effects of the neurotrophins, both in the developing and in the adult vertebrate nervous system. Work with cultured cells is sparsely referred to, even though it has been of critical importance in the identification of the first two neurotrophins and of major classes of responsive neuronal populations.

Neurotrophins exert numerous effects on cells of the nervous system. This pleiotropy seems to be the result both of receptor activation by neurotrophins, in neurons at different stages of differentiation, from the genesis of these cells to the stage when they are highly differentiated, and of receptor localization in specific neuronal compartments, such as dendrites. Also, the activation by neurotrophins of two different receptor systems and signaling pathways further expands the repertoire of their biological activities, an extreme in vivo example being the promotion of cell death or of cell survival (see below).

B. Neurotrophins in Different Species

The identification of NGF was the key discovery in the neurotrophin field and, indeed, in the entire area of "growth factors", defined as extracellular proteins affecting cell fate (Bueker 1948; Levi-Montalcini and Hamburger 1953; Cohen 1960; Levi-Montalcini and Booker 1960). For reasons that are still not understood, approximately 1% of the soluble proteins in extracts of the submandibular gland of the male adult mouse consist of NGF. This made the isolation of the protein possible, including the crucial in vivo demonstration that the lack of NGF prevents the development of parts of the peripheral nervous system (PNS) (Cohen 1960; Levi-Montalcini and Booker 1960). The mouse salivary gland also represented a convenient source, allowing the isolation of a reasonably pure reagent for about two decades (but see Levi-Montalcini 1980), before the availability of recombinant proteins. Like the netrins (Serafini et al. 1994), NGF was purified using a fiber outgrowth assay, whereby, in the case of NGF, explants of chick dorsal root ganglia (DRG) were used (Levi-Montalcini et al. 1954; Cohen 1960). The second neurotrophin, BDNF, was purified from pig brain using its ability to prevent the death of a sub-population of DRG neurons (Barde et al. 1982).

The realization that the amino-acid sequences of BDNF and NGF were related (Leibrock et al. 1989) greatly facilitated the subsequent isolation of NT3 and NT4/5, on the basis of their sequence relatedness, and not of their biological properties (Ernfors et al. 1990a; Hohn et al. 1990; Jones and Reichardt 1990; Rosenthal et al. 1990). NT3 was also identified in a human-glioma cDNA library on the basis of its sequence relatedness to NGF alone (Kaisho et al. 1990).

NT4 was first discovered using a *Xenopus laevis* DNA template (Hallböök et al. 1991), while NT5 was later found in human (Berkemeier et al. 1991). The sequence divergence between amphibian NT4 and human NT5 is high compared with the sequences of the other three neurotrophins. However, subsequent work (Ip et al. 1992) indicated that recombinant NT4 and NT5 share many biological properties and may be functionally equivalent, hence the designation NT4/5. Of note is the fact that *Xenopus* NT4, unlike human NT5, does not support the survival of chick neurons (Davies et al. 1993a). In addition, no NT4/5 sequence has been identified in the chick genome so far, and not much work has been performed in amphibia with NT4. The designation NT4/5 reflects these uncertainties and will be used throughout the chapter.

A gene designated as neurotrophin-6 (NT6) has been identified in the genome of *Xiphophorus* (GÖTZ et al. 1994), but so far no mammalian equivalent has been found. In vitro assays suggest that NT6 has NGF-like properties, though it is clear that the NT6 gene co-exists with a bona fide NGF gene in *Xiphophorus* (GÖTZ et al. 1992). The respective in vivo targets of NGF and NT6 have not been identified at this stage. More generally, the overwhelming part of the work dealing with the biological properties of neurotrophins has been performed in birds and rodents, and still very little is known in lower vertebrates such as teleost fishes in particular. Several neurotrophin and receptor genes have been identified in the zebrafish *Danio rerio* by conventional means (MARTIN et al. 1995), but it is not known, at this stage, whether mutants have been identified in the projects of large-scale chemical mutagenesis in this species (DRIEVER et al. 1996; HAFFTER et al. 1996).

So far, no sequence even remotely related to those of the neurotrophins has been isolated in the invertebrates, such *Caenorhabditis elegans* or *Drosophila melanogaster*, commonly used by geneticists. This is in contrast to other growth factor families, including members of the transforming growth factor β (TGFβ) super family in particular. In drosophila, it appears likely that the products of the genes *spaetzle*, *trunk* and *beaten path* (MORISATO and ANDERSON 1994; CASANOVA et al. 1995; FAMBROUGH and GOODMAN 1996; BAZAN and GOODMAN 1997) encode proteins forming a "cystine knot", a three-dimensional, structural hallmark of the neurotrophins, TGF-βs and platelet-derived growth factors A and B (MCDONALD and HENDRICKSON 1993). However, at present, there is no evidence that these proteins bind to neurotrophin receptors.

C. Trophic Roles of Neurotrophins in the Peripheral Nervous System

The most thoroughly studied property of the neurotrophins is their ability to prevent the death of PNS neurons during development. Detailed in vitro studies with isolated neurons and in vivo histological investigations of birds and rodents indicate that all neurotrophins are essential to prevent the death of specific sub-populations of neurons. This action can be explained by assuming that the death program, particularly sensitive to modulation by extracellular signals when neuroblasts exit the cell cycle, can be blocked by the neurotrophins, following activation of the *trk* receptors. There is evidence to indicate that vertebrate neurons die using components of the intracellular death pathway found in cells of a variety of organisms (for review, see GARCIA et al. 1992; GAGLIARDINI et al. 1994; HORVITZ et al. 1994; MARTINOU et al. 1994).

It should be noted, however, that some neurons in the PNS do not require neurotrophins for survival, as perhaps best illustrated with the cholinergic neurons forming the ciliary ganglion. Intriguingly, their death cannot be prevented by the intracellular injection of bcl-2, a manipulation that typically prevents the death of neurotrophin-dependent neurons (Allsop et al. 1993). In addition, the vast population of neurons in the digestive tract does not seem to be dependent on neurotrophins for survival in vivo, as no striking defects have been reported in the gut plexi of mice carrying null mutations in neurotrophin genes (they are absent in mice carrying a deletion in the gene coding for glial cell line-derived neurotrophic factor, GDNF).

I. Sensory Neurons

All neurotrophins act on neuronal sub-populations contained in sensory ganglia. Culture studies indicated that in neural crest-derived sensory ganglia, the survival effects of NGF and BDNF were additive (Barde et al. 1982). Also, neural crest-derived, but not placode-derived sensory neurons, were shown to respond to NGF (Davies and Lindsay 1985), with the exception of the neurons comprising the trigeminal mesencephalic nucleus (Davies et al. 1986). These neurons are located in the central nervous system (CNS), but are derived from the neural crest, and respond to BDNF and NT3, but not to NGF (Davies 1986; Hohn et al. 1990). Avian embryos have been especially useful in delineating the spectrum of action of neurotrophins on sensory neurons, both as a result of the accessibility of various populations of sensory neurons for culture experiments and the establishment of their embryonic origin in quail-chick chimera experiments (Le Douarin 1980).

In mammals, work with transgenic mice carrying deletions in the neurotrophin genes or in their tyrosine kinase receptors has greatly contributed to expanding our understanding of the in vivo role of the neurotrophins in the developing PNS (for review, see Snider 1994). With regard to peripheral innervation, the most comprehensive analyses have been performed in the whisker pad of the mouse (Rice et al. 1997), a structure that is richly innervated by a variety of sensory endings with a precise and predictable topology, especially with regard to the innervation of the whisker follicles.

1. Nerve Growth Factor

Antibody-deprivation experiments (Johnson et al. 1980; Pearson et al. 1983), later confirmed in *ngf* and *trkA* gene-targeting experiments (Crowley et al. 1994; Smeyne et al. 1994), showed that 70%–80% of sensory neurons in the DRG and the trigeminal ganglion (the medial portion of this ganglion being neural crest-derived) are dependent on NGF during development. In contrast, mature sensory neurons do not seem to require exogenous NGF for survival, not even in culture (Lindsay 1988). This allowed the unambiguous demonstration that the action of NGF is not limited to only the prevention of death of these neurons during development, but is also involved in the modulation of neuropeptide found in NGF-responsive sensory neurons, such as calcitonin gene-related peptide (CGRP) and substance P (Lindsay and Harmar 1989), in line with previous experiments which have shown that injections of NGF or its antibodies in vivo dramatically regulate the levels of peptides in sensory neurons (for review, see OTTEN 1984). Functionally, there is a large body of evidence to suggest that NGF-dependent neurons are involved in the detection of painful stimuli. Thus, for example in the adult, the administration of NGF markedly decreases the pain threshold in both rats and humans (LEWIN et al. 1993; PETTY et al. 1994). Conversely, the administration of antibodies to NGF blocks hyperalgesia following tissue inflammation (for reviews, see LEWIN and MENDELL 1993a; WOOLF 1996).

In the mouse whisker pad, nine sets of unmyelinated and thinly myelinated sensory and autonomic axons can be distinguished, and all but one (absent in *nt3* −/− animals) are eliminated in mice carrying deletions in the *ngf* or *trk*A genes (RICE et al. 1997). Conversely, NGF overexpression in transgenic mice leads to enhanced axonal, as opposed to terminal, growth. (RICE et al. 1997). Medium-size myelinated afferents are also lost in the *ngf* and *trk*A animals, affecting, in particular, reticular and lanceolate endings (FUNDIN et al. 1997).

2. Brain-Derived Neurotrophic Factor

During development, exogenous BDNF has long been known to prevent the death of placode-derived, NGF-insensitive neurons in vivo (HOFER and BARDE 1988). Also, the death of some cells forming the DRG that is observed in vivo, when a membrane is inserted between the neural tube and the DRG anlage, can be prevented when such membranes are coated with BDNF and laminin (KALCHEIM et al. 1987). In the dorsal root and nodose ganglia of *bdnf* −/− mice, about 35% of the neurons are lost (ERNFORS et al. 1994a; JONES et al. 1994).

The development of the innervation of the inner ear provides a useful model to study the role of BDNF and NT3 (reviewed in FRITZSCH et al. 1997). Mice lacking the *bdnf* gene lose all innervation of the semicircular canals, have reduced innervation of the outer hair cells in the cochlea, and the number of vestibular ganglia neurons is reduced by more than 80%. Similar observations were made with *trk*B −/− animals, suggesting that BDNF (not NT4/5) is the important ligand in this system. This was directly confirmed in a study comparing the effects of mutation in the *bdnf* and *nt4/5* genes (BIANCHI et al. 1996). Related observations with *nt3* −/− or *trk*C animals revealed that the number of neurons in the cochlear ganglion is reduced by more than 80%. In mice lacking both BDNF and NT3 (or *trk*B and *trk*C), there is a complete loss of innervation of the inner ear (ERNFORS et al. 1995; SCHIMMANG et al. 1995). The selective expression patterns of the neurotrophins in various structures of the inner ear provide a good example of the selective target localization of these essential factors (illustrated in FRITZSCH et al. 1997).

Analysis of visceral afferents in the nodose-petrosum ganglia of *bdnf*−/− animals revealed that they lack a subset of afferents involved in ventilatory control. These animals exhibit severe respiratory abnormalities characterized by depressed and irregular breathing and reduced chemosensory drive (Erickson et al. 1996). BDNF is therefore required for expression of normal respiratory behavior in newborn animals, and this may be one of the reasons why the life-span of these animals is limited (see Table 1).

In the DRG, work using *bdnf* +/− animals has been useful in delineating the physiological properties of BDNF-responsive DRG neurons. Using electrophysiological recordings from cutaneous nerves, specific functional impairments have been observed in slowly adapting, cutaneous afferents innervating touch domes in the skin: the threshold of response to mechanical stimuli was massively elevated, while the other stimuli remained equally effective. This phenotype could be rescued by injections of BDNF (Lewin and Koltzenburg 1997).

The majority of sensory neurons that are NGF-responsive express the BDNF gene, and its expression is up-regulated by NGF (Ernfors and Persson 1991; Apfel et al. 1996; Cho et al. 1997; Michael et al. 1997). There is clear evidence that BDNF is transported anterogradely from the DRG cell bodies into the spinal cord, in the projection fields of NGF-sensitive neurons (Zhou and Rush 1996; Michael et al. 1997). This is functionally relevant as BDNF, localized to the dense core vesicles of some sensory afferents in the spinal cord (Michael et al. 1997), appears to be a crucial mediator of the phenomenon of "central sensitization" (C.J. Woolf, personal communication). Indeed, this hypersensitization, caused by activation of peripheral fibers by chemical irritants, disappears following intra-thecal injection of *trk*B fusion proteins (C. Woolf, personal communication), and there is evidence indicating that inflammation increases NGF levels, which in turn increases BDNF levels in NGF-responsive neurons (Cho et al. 1997).

The central sensitization caused by BDNF may be a result of the phosphorylation of NMDA receptor subunits of post-synaptic receptors in the spinal cord (Suen et al. 1997). In the whisker pad, the lack of BDNF clearly affects the Ruffini endings, which are severely reduced in numbers in *bdnf*−/−, and absent in *trkB* −/− animals (Fundin et al. 1997). These endings are normal in *nt4/5* −/− animals.

3. Neurotrophin-3

NT3 is a major, early survival factor for many peripheral sensory neurons. The number of neurons in sensory ganglia of quail embryos treated with NT3-blocking antibodies is markedly reduced early, both in placode-derived and neural crest-derived ganglia (Gaese et al. 1994). Parallel experiments with NGF antibodies indicate that NGF is required later than NT3 as a survival factor in DRG development, and that the effects of both antibodies combined are not additive (Gaese et al. 1994).

The suggestion that NGF-dependent sensory neurons first depend on NT3 for survival is in line with studies carried out using *nt3* −/− animals,

Table 1. Some characteristics of neurotrophin *null* mutant mice

	Nerve Growth Factor	Brain-Derived Neurotrophic Factor	Neurotrophin-3	Neurotrophin-4/5
Lifespan	Some survive until weaning	Most die by 3 weeks of age	Most die during the first postnatal days	Survive until adulthood and breed
Sympathetic ganglia	Absence of sympathetic neurons in paravertebral ganglia	No cell loss	About 50% cell loss in the superior cervical ganglion	No cell loss
Sensory ganglia (DRGs)	70–80% Cell loss	Modest cell loss (30%?)	About 65% cell loss	Marginal cell loss
	Loss of small neurons with unmyelinated C fibers and of thinly myelinated Aδ fibers. Loss of nociception	Reduced mechanical sensitivity of slowly adapting mechanoreceptors.	Probably some loss of neurons in all classes (early effect of the mutation). Selective and complete loss of muscle spindle and tendon afferents of slowly adapting mechanoreceptors and of D-hair (thinly myelinated) afferents and of Merkel cells.	Loss of D-hair afferents

indicating that the number of DRG neurons is already markedly reduced early during sensory gangliogenesis, before target innervation (ElShamy and Ernfors 1996; Fariñas et al. 1996). Most classes of DRG neurons are severely depleted in *nt3* −/− mice (Airaksinen and Meyer 1996). Expression of *trk*C is widespread early during the formation of the DRG, to become more restricted later in development, mostly to large proprioceptive neurons (Tessarollo et al. 1993). NT3 may be an essential survival factor for dividing sensory neuroblasts (ElShamy and Ernfors 1996), but using the same approach, no evidence was found to support this possibility (Fariñas et al. 1996). The explanation offered instead was that NT3 would function as an essential mitogen for dividing sensory neuroblasts (Fariñas et al. 1996).

The possibility that increased levels of NT3 would increase the number of sensory neurons in peripheral ganglia has been tested using avian embryos (Ockel et al. 1996). Unexpectedly, the early, but not late, administration of NT3 to quail embryos decreased the number of sensory neurons, both in the nodose and DRG. While this seems to contradict the results of NT3 antibody administration, they can be explained if NT3 is an essential survival factor for those neuroblasts that have been taken out of the cell cycle by the action of NT3. This interpretation is in line with the conclusions of the study by ElShamy and Ernfors, but is opposite to that reached by Fariñas et al. It thus appears that the exact in vivo role of NT3 on sensory neuroblasts is unclear, though there is agreement that it is essential.

*Trk*C−/− animals show smaller losses of sensory neurons in peripheral ganglia than *nt3*−/− animals, and this has been convincingly explained by the demonstration that NT3 can use *trk*A or *trk*B in the absence of *trk*C (Davies et al. 1995).

In the DRG, NT3 specifically supports the survival of muscle-innervating sensory neurons (Hory-Lee et al. 1993; LoPresti and Scott 1994; Oakley et al. 1995), and in *nt3* −/− mice, muscle spindle afferents and Golgi tendon organ afferents are missing (Ernfors et al. 1994b; Fariñas et al. 1994). Amongst the cutaneous afferents, D-hair receptors and slowly adapting mechanoreceptors are selectively affected in *nt3* +/− animals, and Merkel cells (the end organ of slowly adapting mechanoreceptors, allowing fine tactile discrimination) are reduced in numbers (Airaksinen et al. 1996): they are absent in *nt3* −/− animals. In contrast to the muscle spindles, which never form in such animals, the loss of Merkel cells and of their innervation occurs postnatally (Airaksinen et al. 1996). A marked reduction has already been noted at birth in the mouse whisker pad (Fundin et al. 1997).

Detailed analyses of the whisker pads of mice carrying deletions in the *nt3* and *trkC* genes (Fundin et al. 1997) confirmed two important points resulting from analyses of the sensory ganglia and involving cell counts. First, the absence of NT3 has a depleting effect on all NGF-dependent endings. This can be best explained by the switch from NT3 to NGF dependency for survival of most peripheral sensory neurons. Second, the effects of the *trk*C mutation are much less severe than those of the NT3 mutation, again suggesting that, in the absence of *trk*C, NT3 uses *trk*A and *trk*B (RICE et al. 1997).

4. Neurotrophin-4/5

Gene targeting has been the only way to appreciate the significance of NT4/5 in vivo. Unlike with *bdnf−/−* animals, the *nt4/5* mutants are viable (see Table 1) even though severe reductions in cell numbers were found in some cranial ganglia. Cell losses in the trigeminal and DRG were not significant (CONOVER et al. 1995; LIU et al. 1995).

Like BDNF, NT4/5 is required for the survival of primary somatic and visceral sensory neurons, including those of the nodose-petrosal ganglion complex. Analysis of newborn transgenic mice lacking *bdnf* or *nt4/5*, or both, revealed that survival of many afferents is proportional to the number of functional *bdnf* alleles, whereas only one functional *nt4/5* allele is required to support survival of all *nt4*-dependent neurons. In addition, sub-population analysis revealed that BDNF and NT4/5 can compensate for the loss of the other to support a subset of dopaminergic ganglion cells (ERICKSON et al. 1996).

Skin afferents of *nt4/5 −/−* animals show no difference in slow-adapting mechanoreceptors (in contrast to *bdnf −/−* mutant animals). However, the thinly myelinated D-hair afferents are virtually absent in *nt4/5 −/−* animals, and this is accompanied by an overrepresentation of the A-fiber mechano-nociceptors (which are also thinly myelinated axons) (STUCKY et al. 1996). It thus appears that NT4/5 is responsible for the development of D-hair receptors, but not for the survival of other types of cutaneous mechano-sensitive neurons.

In the epidermis of the whisker pad, NT4/5 appears to be involved in suppressing the development of the NGF-dependent sensory endings (RICE et al. 1997). Increased innervation is observed in *nt4/5−/−* animals. While this is also the case with *bdnf−/−* animals, the effects are more pronounced with *nt4/5−/−*, in line with the epidermal expression of NT4/5 in the epidermis (both BDNF and NT4/5 are expressed in the dermis). *TrkB−/−* and $p75^{ntr}$ *−/−* animals show a similar phenotype, and over-expression of BDNF under a keratin promoter severely reduces the development of NGF-dependent sensory endings in the dermis and epidermis (RICE et al. 1997). These surprising results indicate that neurotrophins also negatively regulate the growth of endings, though the mechanisms are not clear at this stage.

In summary, neurotrophins now have a well-documented, physiological role as intrinsic factors acting on specific populations of peripheral sensory neurons. This specificity can be used to select out sub-populations and to compare their patterns of gene expression, such as those involved in nociception and proprioception (FRIEDEL et al. 1997).

II. Sympathetic Neurons

NGF is known to be required for the development of the sympathetic paravertebral chain, as demonstrated in the seminal experiments of Cohen and Levi-Montalcini using newborn mice treated with rabbit NGF antibodies (Cohen 1960; Levi-Montalcini and Booker 1960). Virtually all sympathetic neurons disappear in the superior cervical ganglion following antibody injection at birth, a finding confirmed in more recent studies of animals lacking functional *ngf* or *trkA* genes (Crowley et al. 1994; Smeyne et al. 1994).

For a long time, NGF has also been known to promote fiber outgrowth from DRG and sympathetic ganglia in vitro (Levi-Montalcini et al. 1954). Until recently, it remained unclear whether de novo axonal outgrowth, as opposed to regeneration, also represented a significant part of NGF's physiological role in vivo. Detailed analyses of the superior cervical ganglia of *trkA* −/− mice at different developmental stages revealed that these ganglia form normally, and that the time course of neuronal death in the mutant animals follows that of normally occurring cell death (Fagan et al. 1996). Initial axonal outgrowth was also not distinguishable from that seen in wild-type animals, suggesting that this is an NGF-independent process (Fagan et al. 1996). This finding agrees well with the results of previous experiments with sensory ganglia explanted at a time preceding axonal outgrowth in vivo (Lumsden and Davies 1983). It was also noted that the sympathetic axons did not reach the distal targets, either as a result of cell death (assuming that NGF is required for survival of neurons innervating distal targets before their innervation), or because NGF is required for axonal elongation over long distances (Fagan et al. 1996).

In vitro experiments have demonstrated that much like NGF-responsive sensory neurons, many sympathetic neurons first go through a phase of NT3 dependence (Birren et al. 1993; Dechant et al. 1993) and express *trk*C mRNA (Fagan et al. 1996; Wyatt et al. 1997). With neurons isolated from thoracolumbar sympathetic ganglia of the rat, it has been suggested that NT3 induces the expression of *trk*A (Verdi and Anderson 1994). However, in the superior cervical ganglion of *trk*C −/− animals, the temporal and extent of expression of *trk*A is indistinguishable from that seen in wild-type, and no losses of neurons are observed (Fagan et al. 1996). In *nt3*−/− animals, approximately 50% of the neurons are missing in the superior cervical ganglion (Ernfors et al. 1994b; Fariñas et al. 1994), indicating that NT3 *is* required as a survival factor by developing sympathetic neurons.

The apparently discordant results between neuronal counts in the superior cervical ganglion of *trk*C and *nt3* −/− animals can be explained by the ability of NT3 to activate *trk*A and, in contrast to sensory ganglia, it appears that, in vivo, NT3 is not required before NGF, but together with it for the survival of these neurons (Wyatt et al. 1997). In addition, antibody-induced NT3 deprivation experiments performed post-natally in rats cause a marked reduction in cell numbers in superior cervical, stellate and superior mesenteric ganglia, indicating a postnatal dependency on NT3 for survival (Zhou and

RUSH 1995). It thus appears that many peripheral sympathetic neurons require both NT3 and NGF for survival during the same developmental period, and a report indicating early cell loss in sympathetic ganglia of *nt3* −/− animals (ELSHAMY et al. 1996) could not be confirmed in later studies (WYATT et al. 1997).

In the adult, sympathetic (unlike sensory) neurons still require NGF, and possibly also NT3, for survival (GORIN and JOHNSON 1980; see discussion in ZHOU and RUSH 1995).

Beyond its survival function for sympathetic neurons, NGF also modulates the size of neuronal cell bodies and dendritic arbors in the superior cervical ganglion (RUIT et al. 1990) and prevents the loss of functional synaptic connections made by pre-ganglionic efferents onto sympathetic neurons after their axons were cut (PURVES and NJA 1976; for review, see PURVES 1988).

The size of the sympathetic neurons has long been known to regulate the number of pre-ganglionic axons, as demonstrated with newborn rats treated with NGF (SCHÄFER et al. 1983). This treatment results in massive hypertrophy of the sympathetic neurons and of the pre-ganglionic trunks, as well as of synaptic neurons on sympathetic cell bodies. In this context, it is interesting to note that over-expression of BDNF in sympathetic neurons (using the promoter of the dopamine-β hydroxylase gene) causes the hypertrophy of preganglionic cell bodies and axons (CAUSING et al. 1997). However, it is unclear whether NGF up-regulates BDNF levels in sympathetic neurons as it does in sensory neurons.

D. Trophic Roles of Neurotrophins in the Central Nervous System

I. Prevention of Cell Death

Cell death can be readily observed during CNS development and, just as in the PNS, it can be increased by separating neuronal cell bodies from their target tissues (for review, see OPPENHEIM 1991). Several examples document the fact that the administration of neurotrophins can prevent axotomy-induced death, for example, of motoneurons in the spinal cord or the facial nucleus (SENDTNER et al. 1992; YAN et al. 1992; KOLIATSOS et al. 1993) or of retinal ganglion cells (MANSOUR-ROBAEY et al. 1994). Also, the death of locus coeruleus neurons induced by 6-hydroxydopamine in adult rats can be prevented by NT3 (ARENAS and PERSSON 1994). However, during the period of target innervation, the neurotrophins appear not to be essential survival factors, unlike in the CNS. Populations that can be readily studied in this context are facial or spinal cord motoneurons and retinal ganglion cells. No motoneurons seem to be missing in animals with null mutations in both the *bdnf* and *nt4/5* genes (CONOVER et al. 1995; LIU et al. 1995), and the number of retinal ganglion cell axons is not decreased in *bdnf* −/− animals (CELLERINO et al. 1997).

In *nt3* −/− animals, fewer gamma motoneurons have been observed, but this is likely to be secondary to the absence of muscle spindles (KUCERA et al.

1995). Nevertheless, a series of recent experiments has clearly demonstrated that neurotrophins are essential survival factors for CNS neurons in situations not related to target innervation. Thus, detailed investigations of the brains of mice carrying mutations in the *trkB* gene have revealed massive and widespread effects in the first weeks after birth (ALCÁNTARA et al. 1997). Especially during the second and third week (beyond which the animals die), increased cell death has been observed in the hippocampus (especially the dentate gyrus), cortical layers II-V, the thalamus and the striatum (ALCÁNTARA et al. 1997).

Neuronal cell bodies are markedly reduced in size, as measured on Nissl-stained sections of the hilar region of the hippocampus or in layer V of the somato-sensory cortex (ALCÁNTARA et al. 1997). The hippocampus and cerebellum of mice with mutations in the three *trk* genes have also been investigated (MINICHIELLO and KLEIN 1996) and cell loss was found to be particularly dramatic in mice carrying mutations in both *trk*B and *trk*C (−/−; +/− or +/−; −/−). Thus, for example, during the second post-natal week, up to seven times more dying cells were observed in the external granule cell layer of the cerebellum in animals with combined mutations than in animals with single homozygote mutations (MINICHIELLO and KLEIN 1996).

In *bdnf−/−* mice, the optic nerve was found to contain normal numbers of axons until 3 weeks after birth. However, myelination was markedly compromised, and the diameter of the axons was reduced (CELLERINO et al. 1997). CNS myelin markers were expressed at substantially lower levels in the hippocampus and the cerebral cortex, but not in the cerebellum. This result is in line with the smaller size of many CNS neurons observed in the *trkB −/−* animals, whereby it is unclear whether this is a cause or a consequence of abnormal myelination. Myelination of the facial nerve was normal, suggesting that these motoneurons are less dependent on BDNF than other populations of CNS neurons for myelination (CELLERINO et al. 1997). However, fewer (27%) of these neurons survive axotomy (at P5) when compared with control animals (53%) (ALCÁNTRA et al. 1997).

Recently, the post-natal cerebella of *bdnf−/−* mice have been examined in detail and many aspects of cerebellar development were found to be abnormal, including defects in the rostro-caudal foliation pattern, stunted growth of Purkinje cell dendrites and increased death of granule cells, which also appear to be present in smaller numbers (SCHWARTZ et al. 1997). While all these studies establish that neurotrophins are essential in supporting the survival of CNS neurons, it is unclear at this stage whether some of these effects are direct or indirect consequences of the mutation. Indeed, *bdnf−/−* animals are markedly reduced in size, and it is conceivable that CNS defects may be secondary to other defects taking place earlier in the PNS. The selective deletion of the neurotrophin or neurotrophin receptor gene post-natally, and only in the CNS, would greatly help in trying to answer this question.

In the chick, increased levels of BDNF prevent cell death early during the formation of the retina (FRADE et al. 1997), and the administration of NT3 antibodies severely compromises its development (BOVOLENTA et al. 1996). As these effects were observed early in development, before any substantial connection between the retina and the rest of the CNS occurred, it appears likely that they are not due to peripheral effects of the neurotrophins. However, in both *bdnf* and *nt3* −/− mice, the retina appears to be normal, suggesting significant species differences. Compared with mammals, the much more rapid and massive development of the avian retina may render it more susceptible to acute changes in neurotrophin levels.

Amongst the non-neuronal targets of neurotrophins, rat oligodendrocytes have been shown to respond to NT3, which, in vitro, is one of the numerous agents supporting the survival and division of these cells (BARRES et al. 1994). In the rat optic nerve, NT3 is a significant contributor to the development of these cells, as the acute administration of NT3 antibodies markedly reduces the number of oligodendrocytes that can be isolated from the nerves (BARRES et al. 1994). However, in the few *nt3* −/− mice surviving as long as 13 days after birth, myelination does not seem to be grossly affected (CELLERINO et al. 1997).

II. Other Trophic Actions

1. Regulation of Gene Expression

The activation of the *trk* receptors by neurotrophins in the CNS is typically followed by changes in transcriptional activity, as observed, for example, by increased levels of c-fos (IP et al. 1993). In addition, specific changes have been observed in expression levels of genes directly related to neuronal function. Thus, in the rodent septo-hippocampal system, injections of NGF prevent the down-regulation of genes expressed by basal cholinergic forebrain neurons following axotomy, as reflected by the levels of choline acetyl transferase and of $p75^{NTR}$, and neuronal atrophy is also prevented (HEFTI 1986; HAGG et al. 1988). In the rat, axotomy of these neurons and loss of contact with their distal targets may not cause the death of these neurons (see NAUMANN et al. 1992), but most importantly, NGF reverses their atrophy, as observed after lesion or in aging rats, and improves their behavioral performance (FISCHER et al. 1987).

These results point to a role of NGF as a factor important for maintaining the functional state of these neurons in the adult (see also GAROFALO et al. 1992). In line with this, recent results indicate that *ngf*−/+ mice have atrophic cholinergic neurons (presumably as a result of decreased activation of *trk*A + neurons) and memory deficits (CHEN et al. 1997). In *trkA* −/− animals, marked reductions of acetylcholinesterase levels have been noted (SMEYNE et al. 1994).

Injections of BDNF and NGF into the cortex and hippocampus of adult rats revealed that BDNF, but not NGF, increases the levels of neuropeptide Y, cholecystokinin, and somatostatin (the latter only in the cortex), but decreased the levels of dynorphin in the hippocampus (CROLL et al. 1994), suggesting that

BDNF potentially affects the functional states of a variety of neuronal populations, in agreement with the widespread expression of its catalytic receptor *trk*B (KLEIN et al. 1989).

2. Functional and Morphological Effects on the Developing Cortex and Motoneurons

While the four neurotrophin genes are expressed in the cerebral cortex of all mammals that have been examined, the functional consequences of their regulated expression (see below) took some time to be appreciated. Elegant studies with slices prepared from the visual cortex of 2-week old ferrets have impressively demonstrated that neurotrophins regulate the morphology of dendritic arbors. Transfection of the slices with plasmids coding for a marker allowing the visualization of these neurons and of their processes (LO et al. 1994) demonstrated that increased levels of neurotrophins affect the growth of basal dendrites in a neurotrophin and layer-specific manner. BDNF was most effective in stimulating the growth of basal dendrites of neurons located in layer IV, whereas NT3 and NT4/5 were essentially inactive and NGF moderately so (MCALLISTER et al. 1995). With cell bodies located in layers V and VI, NT4/5 was the most effective growth stimulating neurotrophin (MCALLISTER et al. 1995).

These results demonstrate that, in a situation where much of the complexity of the cerebral tissue architecture is preserved, marked growth-stimulating actions of the neurotrophins can be observed. Currently, this is the most direct demonstration that neurotrophins may regulate in vivo the density of post-synaptic sites during development of the cerebral cortex. Using the same methodology, neurotrophins were also demonstrated to participate in regressive events.

Morphological changes induced by neurotrophins, of the sort observed in slices, are very likely to also take place in vivo. Indeed, monocular deprivation in ferrets leads to atrophy of neurons in the lateral geniculate, presumably as a result of a competition for factors present in the visual cortex taken up by the input corresponding to the non-deprived eye. The local delivery of NT4/5 in the cortex, together with a retrograde tracer allowing the identification of the neurons exposed to this neurotrophin, largely prevented the effects of the monocular deprivation (RIDDLE et al. 1995). The suggestion that *trk*B ligands, such has NT4/5, may be important factors participating in afferent competition in the visual cortex is supported by experiments using agents inhibiting their actions. The formation of ocular dominance patches in layer IV of the cat visual cortex is blocked by the infusion of *trk*B-fusion proteins. *Trk*A- or *trk*C fusion proteins remain without effects. These results suggest that an endogenous *trk*B ligand (the experiment does not allow the distinction between BDNF or NT4/5) may be present in limited amounts within the visual cortex and is necessary for the selective growth and remodeling of lateral geniculate axons into eye-specific patches (CABELLI et al. 1997; see also CABELLI et al. 1995).

NGF also participates in the development of the visual cortex. In particular, NGF antibodies indicated that neurons in the visual cortex have a reduced acuity, i.e., larger receptive fields (BERARDI et al. 1994). Furthermore, the developmental critical period over which ocular dominance plasticity could be elicited was extended (DOMINICI et al. 1994; for review, see CELLERINO and MAFFEI 1996).

Morphological changes induced by neurotrophins are not limited to the developing mammalian CNS. In amphibia, the accessibility of the developing CNS allowed the important demonstration that injections of BDNF into the tectum of live tadpoles increased the branching and complexity of optic axons' terminal arbor, whereas BDNF-antibodies caused the opposite result (COHEN-CORY and SCOTT 1995).

Like all neurotrophins, NT4/5 is also expressed in numerous tissues outside the nervous system, including skeletal muscle. Blockade of neuromuscular transmission in adult rats with alpha bungarotoxin decreased NT4/5 mRNA levels, while electrical stimulation of the denervated muscle increased them (FUNAKOSHI et al. 1995). In addition, the intra-muscular administration of NT4/5 increases sprouting at the intact neuromuscular junction, indicating that this neurotrophin may regulate nerve branching and be a signal regulated in an activity-dependent fashion (FUNAKOSHI et al. 1995).

E. Synaptic Transmission

Neurotrophins directly affect synaptic transmission, as first shown in experiments with the developing amphibian neuromuscular junction. The application of NT3 and BDNF increased spontaneous and stimulus-evoked release of acetylcholine (LOHOF et al. 1993). Similar conclusions were reached using cultured hippocampal neurons (LESSMANN et al. 1994), in which BDNF or NT3 were shown to rapidly increase intracellular calcium (BERNINGER et al. 1993). NT3 has also been reported to increase the activity of these neurons, possibly by decreasing GABAergic transmission (KIM et al. 1994), and BDNF to rapidly increase synaptic transmission (by *trk*-dependent mechanisms) in dissociated cells of the hippocampus (LEVINE et al. 1995).

When synaptic transmission is examined in slices at synapses between the Schaffer collaterals and CA1 pyramidal neurons, both BDNF and NT3 (but not NGF) elicit a marked and prolonged enhancement of synaptic transmission (KANG and SCHUMAN 1995). This enhancement develops after 10 min, or so, and can be blocked by inhibitors of protein synthesis (KANG and SCHUMAN 1996). This requirement is also evident when the neuropil is separated from the cell bodies, indicating that neurotrophins locally control the synthesis of proteins (presumably in dendrites of CA1 neurons) required for the induction of synaptic enhancement (KANG and SCHUMAN 1996).

It appears very likely that neurotrophins are also involved in the regulation of synaptic transmission in vivo. Indeed, in *bdnf* −/− animals, two studies have demonstrated compromised LTP in the CA1 sub-field, the incidence and the amplitude of the potentiation seen after stimulation of the so-called Schaffer collaterals being reduced by about 70% (Korte et al. 1995; Patterson et al. 1996). About the same reduction was observed in both heterozygous and homozygous animals, suggesting that the levels of BDNF in the CNS are normally present in limiting amounts, and that decreases of BDNF levels lead to impairments in synaptic function. This is also important in the context of indirect or development-related effects resulting from the complete lack of BDNF. In particular, the growth curves of wild type and *bdnf* −/+ are indistinguishable, whereas those of *bdnf* −/− are markedly different with most animals dying beyond the third week after birth (Conover et al. 1995).

The impairment in LTP induction could be reversed by the re-addition of BDNF to the slices isolated from *bdnf* mutant animals, either as a recombinant protein or delivered in the CA1 region by adenoviruses carrying BDNF (Korte et al. 1996; Patterson et al. 1996). In the context of LTP, it is also interesting to note that stimuli leading to long-term potentiation in the CA1 or CA3 regions of the hippocampus increase BDNF gene expression (Patterson et al. 1992).

F. Modulation of Transcription of Neurotrophin Genes

The first clear indication that activity controls neurotrophin gene expression in the CNS was in the hippocampus: limbic seizures were shown to lead to increased NGF mRNA expression by hippocampal neurons (Gall and Isackson 1989). This was a crucial finding, as it not only confirmed that this neurotrophin gene (as later shown for the others) is primarily expressed in neurons in the adult CNS, but also that its expression can be dramatically and quickly up-regulated as a function of increased activity. Subsequently, excitatory neurotransmitters were shown to up-regulate BDNF and NGF mRNA levels in cultured hippocampal neurons (Zafra et al. 1990). There is a wealth of evidence (for review, see Lindholm et al. 1994) that the steady-state levels of BDNF mRNAs are regulated in an activity-dependent fashion, both during development and in the adult.

In the chick tectum, BDNF mRNA levels increase during the period of innervation by the retinal ganglion cells, and this increase is regulated by the activity of the retinal afferents at the time of the first contact between the axons of the retinal ganglion cells, as demonstrated by the unilateral injection of tetrodotoxin or section of the optic stalk (Herzog et al. 1994). Previous experiments in the visual cortex of the adult rats had demonstrated that BDNF (but not NGF) mRNA levels were down-regulated when animals were maintained in darkness and were restored to normal levels after 1 h of exposure to light (Castrén et al. 1992). As in the developing chick, tetrodotoxin decreased the levels of BDNF mRNA in the contra-lateral visual cortex within hours of re-exposure to light (CASTRÉN et al. 1992). These results indicate that BDNF levels are regulated in a pathway-specific manner from the earliest stages of development of the visual system.

The activity-dependent regulation of BDNF mRNA levels has been demonstrated in numerous other ways. For example, stimuli-rich environments increased mRNA levels in the rat hippocampus (FALKENBERG et al. 1992), as did physical exercise in several brain areas (NEEPER et al. 1995). Also, numerous studies showed that both NGF and BDNF mRNA levels were dramatically up-regulated by hippocampal seizure activity induced by chemical and electrical stimuli (for review, see LINDHOLM et al. 1994) and that the time-course, the distribution and the extent of mRNA induction differed for BDNF and NGF (see in particular ISACKSON et al. 1991). Blocking neurotransmission has also been useful to demonstrate that on going-activity regulates neurotrophin mRNA levels (ZAFRA et al. 1991). Thus, the administration of MK-801, benzodiazepine or muscimol all affect steady-state levels of NGF and BDNF mRNA levels in adult rats, indicating that the major excitatory and inhibitory neurotransmitter systems in the CNS participate in this regulation (ZAFRA et al. 1991).

It seems that changes in NGF and BDNF mRNA levels result in increases in proteins levels (see e.g., ZAFRA et al. 1991; NAWA et al. 1995). While virtually nothing is known about the biosynthetic pathway followed by neurotrophins in neurons, it appears likely that their precursor is glycosylated and subsequently cleaved by a furin-like enzyme in the Golgi apparatus and packed in vesicles, the exact nature of which is unknown. BDNF-immunoreactivity has been localized to dendrites (GOODMAN et al. 1996) where BDNF mRNA has also been seen in some studies (see DUGICH-DJORDJEVIC et al. 1992). But whether or not local synthesis of bioactive BDNF occurs is unclear, given the apparent necessity for the BDNF precursor to travel through the Golgi apparatus.

The secretion of both NGF and BDNF has been demonstrated in slices and cultures of hippocampal neurons, and is clearly activity-dependent (BLÖCHL and THOENEN 1995; GOODMAN et al. 1996). Interestingly, this release is less dependent on the mobilization of extracellular calcium than the release of neurotransmitter, and intracellular calcium can substitute (see BLÖCHL and THOENEN 1995, 1996). This fits with the notion that, like peptide neurotransmitters, BDNF may be packed in dense core vesicles (MICHAEL et al. 1997). In line with the neurotransmitter-like characteristics of neurotrophins, there is good evidence for anterograde transport of neurotrophins in neurons expressing neurotrophin genes, both in the PNS (see Sect. C.I.2) and in the CNS (VON BARTHELD et al. 1996; ALTAR et al. 1997). Thus, for example, the bulk of BDNF in the rat striatum is derived from anterogradely transported BDNF, and this transport is functionally relevant for gene expression in postsynaptic cells (ALTAR et al. 1997).

Hormones, including steroid hormones, have been shown to regulate the levels of NGF and BDNF transcripts. Injection of corticosteroids decreased

NGF mRNA levels in the brain (LINDHOLM et al. 1990) and adrenalectomy increased BDNF mRNA in the hippocampus and the cortex, both in resting conditions and after seizure (LAUTERBORN et al. 1995). With regard to thyroid hormone, T3 increases NT3 mRNA levels in the cerebellum, while hypothyroidism decreases these levels (LINDHOLM et al. 1993), as do BDNF mRNA levels (NEVEU and ARENAS 1996). Cell death in the cerebellum can be prevented by the implantation of cells secreting NT3 or BDNF (NEVEU and ARENAS 1996).

In the intact CNS, while the neurotrophin genes are primary expressed in neurons, there is also evidence that microglial cells express the *nt3* gene in a region- and differentiation-specific manner. Very recently, NGF was also localized in microglial cells in the developing chick retina, and these cells seem to be the major source of NGF in its pro-apoptotic function (FRADE and BARDE 1998, and see below). In addition, both BDNF and NT3 increase the incorporation of thymidine in cultured microglial cells, and NT3 induces phagocytic activity (ELKABES et al. 1996).

G. Regressive Events and Neurotrophins

The fact that neurotrophins bind to two unrelated receptors raised the possibility that different signal-transduction pathways may be activated (for review, see DECHANT and BARDE 1997). Still very little is known in neurons with regard to the ability of $p75^{NTR}$ to transduce biochemical responses following neurotrophin binding. In primary cultures of rat Schwann cells which express $p75^{NTR}$, but not catalytic *trk*s, the unexpected observation has been made that only NGF, and not BDNF or NT3, was able to activate $p75^{NTR}$, as reflected by the translocation of NF-kB (CARTER et al. 1996). In vivo, a consequence of $p75^{NTR}$ activation by NGF is cell death: NGF antibodies led to a marked decrease in normally occurring cell death in the developing chick retina (FRADE et al. 1996). This apparently paradoxical result was obtained early during neurogenesis, before axons leave the retina to form the optic nerve. Many cells, including essentially all dying neurons, express $p75^{NTR}$, and injection of antibodies blocking the binding of NGF to $p75^{NTR}$ also caused a reduction in cell death. Similar results were recently obtained in the developing mouse retina using $p75^{NTR}$ deficient mice (FRADE, personal communication).

Cell death mediated by $p75^{NTR}$ is not limited to the retina. In the basal forebrain of rodents, 30%–50% of cholinergic neurons express $p75^{NTR}$ and not *trk*A (VAN DER ZEE et al. 1996), and in $p75^{ntr}$ −/− animals, these neurons do not die post-natally (VAN DER ZEE et al. 1996). The activation of $p75^{NTR}$ is likely to be caused by the binding of endogenous NGF, since the injection of a NGF peptide, corresponding to its $p75^{NTR}$ binding loop (IBÁÑEZ et al. 1992), also led to the prevention of cell death in wild-type mice. In addition, cholinergic neurons in the basal forebrain of $p75^{ntr}$ −/− mutant mice were found to be larger than in controls and to have increased levels of choline acetyltransferase

(YEO et al. 1997). Also, cholinergic innervation of the hippocampus was found to be increased in *p75 −/−* animals (YEO et al. 1997).

In recent experiments aimed at testing the cell-killing potential of the cytoplasmic domain of $p75^{NTR}$, large neuronal losses were observed in both the PNS and CNS of mice expressing the cytoplasmic domain of $p75^{NTR}$ under the control of a tubulin promoter (MAJDAN et al. 1997). This result reinforces the idea that activation of $p75^{NTR}$ has the potential to cause cell death in vivo in a variety of neuronal populations, first suggested with serum-deprived cultured cells transfected with $p75^{NTR}$ (RABIZADEH et al. 1993).

In vivo, there is still no convincing evidence that only NGF activates $p75^{NTR}$ to cause cell death. Primary cultures of rat oligodendrocytes have been useful to directly demonstrate that NGF can cause cell death that is accompanied by the activation of *jun* kinase (CASACCIA-BONNEFIL et al. 1996). Neither BDNF nor NT3 were able to do so, but it remains unclear whether a concomitant activation of *trk*B and *trk*C (the latter known to be expressed by these cells) may have counteracted any death-promoting action of these ligands. In general, it has been difficult, so far, to find suitable in vitro systems to study the death-promoting action of NGF. Presumably, this is due to the non-catalytic nature of this receptor, which may need to recruit a variety of cytoplasmic components to exert its action.

$p75^{NTR}$ shares similar structural features with FAS/Apo-1/CD95 and TNFR1 (two receptors that can be activated by ligands to cause cell death; for review, see NAGATA 1997). This is particularly obvious in the extracellular domains which have cysteine-rich domains that are similarly organized, a feature that has been used to group the various members of this still-growing family of receptors. Recently, the similarities have been extended to the cytoplasmic domains in nuclear magnetic resonance studies, with the delineation of six alpha helices in what is thought to be the effector domain of FAS and $p75^{NTR}$ (HUANG et al. 1996; LIEPINSH et al. 1997).

Microglial cells have been shown in the retina both to represent the cellular source of NGF and to use NGF to kill cells in development (FRADE and BARDE 1998). As tumor necrosis factor is typically found in activated macrophages, this result further strengthens, at the cellular level, parallels between $p75^{NTR}$ and other receptors of this family.

At present, still very little is known about other in vivo actions of NGF mediated by $p75^{NTR}$. In explants of sciatic nerves, the migration of Schwann cells (which express $p75^{NTR}$ during development or after nerve lesion) is enhanced by a $p75^{NTR}$–NGF-mediated action (ANTON et al. 1994). Also, there is an intriguing possibility that increased sphingomyelin hydrolysis, which leads to the production of ceramide, may negatively modulate axonal extension or dendrite arborization. Indeed, activation of $p75^{NTR}$ by neurotrophins in cell lines has been shown to trigger sphingomyelin hydrolysis and ceramide release (DOBROWSKY et al. 1994, 1995), and ceramide has been shown to inhibit neurite outgrowth in cultured rat sympathetic neurons (DE CHAVES et al. 1997). The hypothesis has been put forward that this may be a mechanism used to regulate neurite outgrowth (De Chaves et al. 1997). In this model, growth promoting action would be mediated by the activation of *trk*A, and growth inhibition by the activation of $p75^{NTR}$.

In cortical slices of ferrets, surprising results have been obtained using BDNF and NT3. While in some instances (see Sect. D.II.2), growth of dendrites was promoted by these neurotrophins, in others, clear negative effects were observed. Thus for example, in layer IV, both endogenous and exogenous NT3 inhibited the dendritic growth stimulated by BDNF. In contrast, in layer VI, both endogenous and exogenous BDNF inhibit dendritic growth stimulated by NT3 (McAllister et al. 1997). In addition, such mechanisms may normally be operating in vivo, as the addition of antibody-like reagents caused enhanced growth (McAllister et al. 1997). At present, the molecular explanation for these observations are unclear, but the important point is that endogenous neurotrophins can influence the growth of dendrite in both a positive and negative fashion, and in a layer-specific manner. Possibly, neurotrophins are required continuously to prevent retraction, and competition for binding at neurotrophin receptors on dendrites may cause retraction. Alternatively, neurotrophins may also cause the release of substances locally, preventing dendritic growth.

H. Conclusions and Perspectives

The neurotrophins have remained a small family of only four genes in higher vertebrates, and over the last few years, novel aspects of their biological action have been revealed. In particular, it has become apparent that NGF can negatively regulate the number of neurons during development, and that other neurotrophins seem to be involved in "anti-trophic" effects as well. Their more traditional anti-cell death function can be now illustrated in vivo with at least a few examples for each of the neurotrophins.

The old notion, well-documented with NGF, that neurotrophins do more than control neuronal survival during development has been considerably enlarged to include novel phenomena, and it now appears that, in some respects, neurotrophins resemble neurotransmitters: in the nervous system, their genes are expressed mostly in neurons, their expression is regulated by electrical activity and they seem to be contained in vesicles, transported anterogradely and released as a function of synaptic activity.

In the CNS, the target specificity of neurotrophins is much broader than in the PNS and, in the adult, BDNF and its tyrosine kinase receptor *trk*B are expressed in a wide variety of neuronal populations. Work in the developing visual system has revealed that the availability of neurotrophins affects neuronal shape and, given their activity-dependent synthesis and release, the neurotrophins seem to represent, at this stage, the most convincing group of growth factors controlled by activity and affecting brain architecture in vertebrates.

Still very little is known about the precise localization of neurotrophin receptors in differentiated neurons, and what kind of signals they generate in dendrites in particular. Some of the regressive biological effects reported recently cannot be clearly accounted for, on the basis of our present knowledge, and it will be necessary to better understand the biological consequences of receptor activation in neurons, as opposed to tumor cells. For example, when rat or chick *trk*B is expressed in cell lines, Xenopus and human NT4/5 are equally effective with regard to tyrosine phosphorylation, but only Xenopus NT4/5 and not human NT4/5 will support the survival of avian neurons. And the activation of the receptor $p75^{NTR}$, which like other receptors of this family needs cytoplasmic interactors to signal, is entirely dependent on the cellular context in which it is expressed.

Perhaps the major concern in the field is that, so far, neurotrophins have failed to show clear beneficial effects in several clinical tests. However, NGF seems to be efficacious in the treatment of peripheral sensory neuropathies (Apfel et al. 1997) and its clinical development continues, as does that of BDNF and NT3 in a variety of clinical conditions. Unfortunately, as yet, too little is known about the molecular basis of the conditions in which neurotrophins are assumed to play a useful role, and delivering these comparatively large, very basic and hydrophobic molecules to the desired site of action remains a considerable problem. It can only be hoped that the wealth of information obtained over the last few years on the remarkably diverse biological roles of neurotrophins will help to better target their use in pathological situations.

References

Airaksinen MS, Meyer M (1996) Most classes of dorsal root ganglion neurons are severely depleted but not absent in mice lacking neurotrophin-3. Neuroscience 73:907–911

Airaksinen MS, Koltzenburg M, Lewin GR, Masu Y, Helbig C, Wolf E, Brem G, Toyka KV, Thoenen H, Meyer M (1996) Specific subtypes of cutaneous mechanoreceptors require neurotrophin-3 following peripheral target innervation. Neuron 16:287–295

Alcántara S, Frisén J, Del Río JA, Soriano E, Barbacid M, Silos-Santiago I (1997) TrkB signaling is required for postnatal survival of CNS neurons and protects hippocampal and motor neurons from axotomy-induced cell death. J Neurosci 17:3623–3633

Allsopp TE, Wyatt S, Paterson HF, Davies AM (1993) The proto-oncogene bcl-2 can selectively rescue neurotrophic factor-dependent neurons from apoptosis. Cell 73:295–307

Altar CA, Cai N, Bliven T, Juhasz M, Conner JM, Acheson AL, Lindsay RM, Wiegand SJ (1997) Anterograde transport of brain-derived neurotrophic factor and its role in the brain. Nature 389:856–860

Anton ES, Weskamp G, Reichardt LF, Matthew WD (1994) Nerve growth factor and its low-affinity receptor promote Schwann cell migration. Proc Natl Acad Sci USA 91:2795–2799

Apfel SC, Kessler JA, Adornato BT, Litchy WJ, Sanders C, Rask CA (1998) Recombinant human nerve growth factor in the treatment of diabetic polyneuropathy(in press)

Apfel SC, Wright DE, Wiideman AM, Dormia C, Snider WD, Kessler JA (1996) Nerve growth factor regulates the expression of brain-derived neurotrophic factor mRNA in the peripheral nervous system. Mol Cell Neurosci 7:134–142

Arenas E, Persson H (1994) Neurotrophin-3 prevents the death of adult central noradrenergic neurons in vivo. Nature 367:368–371

Barbacid M (1994) The trk family of neurotrophin receptors. J Neurobiol 25:1386–1403

Barde YA, Edgar D, Thoenen H (1982) Purification of a new neurotrophic factor from mammalian brain. EMBO J 1:549–553

Barres BA, Raff MC, Gaese F, Bartke I, Dechant G, Barde YA (1994) A crucial role for neurotrophin-3 in oligodendrocyte development. Nature 367:371–375

Bazan JF, Goodman CS (1997) Modular structure of the drosophila beat protein. Curr Biol 7:R338–339

Berardi N, Cellerino A, Domenici L, Fagiolini M, Pizzorusso T, Cattaneo A, Maffei L (1994) Monoclonal antibodies to nerve growth factor affect the postnatal development of the visual system. Proc Natl Acad Sci USA 91:684–688

Berkemeier LR, Winslow JW, Kaplan DR, Nikolics K, Goeddel DV, Rosenthal A (1991) Neurotrophin-5: A novel neurotrophic factor that activates trk and trkB. Neuron 7:857–866

Berninger B, Garcia DE, Inagaki N, Hahnel C, Lindholm D (1993) BDNF and NT-3 induce intracellular Ca^{2+} elevation in hippocampal neurones. Neuroreport 4:1303–1306

Bianchi LM, Conover JC, Fritzsch B, DeChiara T, Lindsay RM, Yancopoulos GD (1996) Degeneration of vestibular neurons in late embryogenesis of both heterozygous and homozygous BDNF null mutant mice. Development 122:1965–1973

Birren SJ, Lo L, Anderson DJ (1993) Sympathetic neuroblasts undergo a developmental switch in trophic dependence. Development 119:597–610

Blöchl A, Thoenen H (1995) Characterization of nerve growth factor (NGF) release from hippocampal neurons: Evidence for a constitutive and an unconventional sodium-dependent regulated pathway. Eur J Neurosci 7:1220–1228

Blöchl A, Thoenen H (1996) Localization of cellular storage compartments and sites of constitutive and activity-dependent release of nerve growth factor (NGF) in primary cultures of hippocampal neurons. Mol Cell Neurosci 7:173–190

Bovolenta P, Frade JM, Martí E, Rodríguez-Peña MA, Barde YA, Rodríguez-Tébar A (1996) Neurotrophin-3 antibodies disrupt the normal development of the chick retina. J Neurosci 16(14):4402–4410

Bueker ED (1948) Implantation of tumors in the hind limb field of the embryonic chick and the developmental response of the lumbosacral nervous system. Anat Rec 102:369–390

Cabelli RJ, Hohn A, Shatz CJ (1995) Inhibition of ocular dominance column formation by infusion of NT-4/5 or BDNF. Science 267:1662–1666

Cabelli RJ, Shelton DL, Segal RA, Shatz CJ (1997) Blockade of endogenous ligands of trkB inhibits formation of ocular dominance columns. Neuron 19:63–76

Carter BD, Kaltschmidt C, Kaltschmidt B, Offenhäuser N, Böhm-Matthaei R, Baeuerle PA, Barde YA (1996) Selective activation of NF-kappaB by nerve growth factor through the neurotrophin receptor p75. Science 272:542–545

Casaccia-Bonnefil P, Carter BD, Dobrowsky RT, Chao MV (1996) Death of oligodendrocytes mediated by the interaction of nerve growth factor with its receptor p75. Nature 383:716–719

Casanova J, Furriols M, McCormick A, Struhl G (1995) Similarities between trunk and spätzle, putative extracellular ligands specifying body pattern in Drosophila. Genes Dev 9:2539–2544

Castrén E, Zafra F, Thoenen H, Lindholm D (1992) Light regulates expression of brain-derived neurotrophic factor mRNA in rat visual cortex. Proc Natl Acad Sci USA 89:9444–9448

Causing CG, Gloster A, Aloyz R, Bamji SX, Chang E, Fawcett J, Kuchel G, Miller FD (1997) Synaptic innervation density is regulated by neuron-derived BDNF. Neuron 18:257–267

Cellerino A, Maffei L (1996) The action of neurotrophins in the development of the visual system. Prog Neurobiol 49:53–71

Cellerino A, Carroll P, Thoenen H, Barde YA (1997) Reduced size of retinal ganglion cell axons and hypomyelination in mice lacking brain-derived neurotrophic factor. Mol Cell Neurosci 9:397–408

Chen KS, Nishimura MC, Armanini MP, Crowley C, Spencer SD, Phillips HS (1997) Disruption of a single allele of the nerve growth factor gene results in atrophy of basal forebrain cholinergic neurons and memory deficits. J Neurosci 17:7288–7296

Cho HJ, Kim SY, Park MJ, Kim DS, Kim JK, Chu MY (1997) Expression of mRNA for brain-derived neurotrophic factor in the dorsal root ganglion following peripheral inflammation. Brain Res 749:358–362

Cohen S (1960) Purification of a nerve-growth promoting protein from the mouse salivary gland and its neuro-cytotoxic antiserum. Proc Natl Acad Sci USA 46:302–311

Cohen-Cory S, Fraser SE (1995) Effects of brain-derived neurotrophic factor on optic axon branching and remodelling in vivo. Nature 378:192–196

Conover JC, Erickson JT, Katz DM, Bianchi LM, Poueymirou WT, McClain J, Pan L, Helgren M, Ip NY, Boland P, Friedman B, Wiegand S, Vejsada R, Kato AC, DeChiara TM, Yancopoulos GD (1995) Neuronal deficits, not involving motor neurons, in mice lacking BDNF and/or NT4. Nature 375:235–238

Croll SD, Wiegand SJ, Anderson KD, Lindsay RM, Nawa H (1994) Regulation of neuropeptides in adult rat forebrain by the neurotrophins BDNF and NGF. Eur J Neurosci 6:1343–1353

Crowley C, Spencer SD, Nishimura MC, Chen KS, Pitts-Meek S, Armanini MP, Ling LH, McMahon SB, Shelton DL, Levinson AD, Phillips HS (1994) Mice lacking nerve growth factor display perinatal loss of sensory and sympathetic neurons yet develop basal forebrain cholinergic neurons. Cell 76:1001–1011

Curtis R, Adryan KM, Stark JL, Park JS, Compton DL, Weskamp G, Huber LJ, Chao MV, Jaenisch R, Lee KF, Lindsay RM, Distefano PS (1995) Differential role of the low affinity neurotrophin receptor (p75) in retrograde axonal transport of the neurotrophins. Neuron 14:1201–1211

Davies AM (1986) The survival and growth of embryonic proprioceptive neurons is promoted by a factor present in skeletal muscle. Dev Biol 115:55–67

Davies AM, Lindsay RM (1985) The cranial sensory ganglia in culture: differences in the response of placode-derived and neural crest-derived neurons to nerve growth factor. Dev Biol 111:62–72

Davies AM, Thoenen H, Barde YA (1986) Different factors from the central nervous system and periphery regulate the survival of sensory neurones. Nature 319:497–499

Davies AM, Horton A, Burton LE, Schmelzer C, Vandlen R, Rosenthal A (1993a) Neurotrophin-4/5 is a mammalian-specific survival factor for distinct populations of sensory neurons. J Neurosci 13:4961–4967

Davies AM, Lee KF, Jaenisch R (1993b) p75-deficient trigeminal sensory neurons have an altered response to NGF but not to other neurotrophins. Neuron 11:565–574

Davies AM, Minichiello L, Klein R (1995) Developmental changes in NT3 signalling via TrkA and TrkB in embryonic neurons. EMBO J 14:4482–4489

De Chaves EIP, Bussière M, Vance DE, Campenot RB, Vance JE (1997) Elevation of ceramide within distal neurites inhibits neurite growth in cultured rat sympathetic neurons. J Biol Chem 272:3028–3035

Dechant G, Barde YA (1997) Signalling through the neurotrophin receptor $p75^{NTR}$. Curr Opin Neurobiol 7:413–418

Dechant G, Rodríguez-Tébar A, Kolbeck R, Barde YA (1993) Specific high-affinity receptors for neurotrophin-3 on sympathetic neurons. J Neurosci 13:2610–2616

Dobrowsky RT, Werner MH, Castellino AM, Chao MV, Hannun YA (1994) Activation of the sphingomyelin cycle through the low-affinity neurotrophin receptor. Science 265:1596–1599

Dobrowsky RT, Jenkins GM, Hannun YA (1995) Neurotrophins induce sphingomyelin hydrolysis – Modulation by Co-expression of p75^{NTR} with Trk receptors. J Biol Chem 270:22135–22142

Domenici L, Cellerino A, Berardi N, Cattaneo A, Maffei L (1994) Antibodies to nerve growth factor (NGF) prolong the sensitive period for monocular deprivation in the rat. Neuroreport 5:2041–2044

Driever W, Solnica-Krezel L, Schier AF, Neuhauss SCF, Malicki J, Stemple DL, Stainier DYR, Zwartkruis F, Abdelilah S, Rangini Z, Belak J, Boggs C (1996) A genetic screen for mutations affecting embryogenesis in zebrafish. Development 123:37–46

Dugich-Djordjevic MM, Tocco G, Lapchak PA, Pasinetti GM, Najm I, Baudry M, Hefti F (1992) Regionally specific and rapid increases in brain-derived neurotrophic factor messenger RNA in the adult rat brain following seizures induced by systemic administration of kainic acid. Neuroscience 47:303–315

Elkabes S, DiCicco-Bloom EM, Black IB (1996) Brain microglia macrophages express neurotrophins that selectively regulate microglial proliferation and function. J Neurosci 16:2508–2521

ElShamy WM, Ernfors P (1996) A local action of neurotrophin-3 prevents the death of proliferating sensory neuron precursor cells. Neuron 16:963–972

ElShamy WM, Linnarsson S, Lee KF, Jaenisch R, Ernfors P (1996) Prenatal and postnatal requirements of NT-3 for sympathetic neuroblast survival and innervation of specific targets. Development 122:491–500

Erickson JT, Conover JC, Borday V, Champagnat J, Barbacid M, Yancopoulos G, Katz DM (1996) Mice lacking brain-derived neurotrophic factor exhibit visceral sensory neuron losses distinct from mice lacking NT4 and display a severe developmental deficit in control of breathing. J Neurosci 16:5361–5371

Ernfors P, Persson H (1991) Developmentally regulated expression of HDNF/NT-3 mRNA in rat spinal cord motoneurons and expression of BDNF mRNA in embryonic dorsal root ganglion. Eur J Neurosci 3:953–961

Ernfors P, Ibáñez CF, Ebendal T, Olson L, Persson H (1990a) Molecular cloning and neurotrophic activities of a protein with structural similarities to nerve growth factor: Developmental and topographical expression in the brain. Proc Natl Acad Sci USA 87:5454–5458

Ernfors P, Wetmore C, Olson L, Persson H (1990b) Identification of cells in rat brain and peripheral tissues expressing mRNA for members of the nerve growth factor family. Neuron 5:511–526

Ernfors P, Lee KF, Jaenisch R (1994a) Mice lacking brain-derived neurotrophic factor develop with sensory deficits. Nature 368:147–150

Ernfors P, Lee KF, Kucera J, Jaenisch R (1994b) Lack of neurotrophin-3 leads to deficiencies in the peripheral nervous system and loss of limb proprioceptive afferents. Cell 77:503–512

Ernfors P, Van de Water T, Loring J, Jaenisch R (1995) Complementary roles of BDNF and NT-3 in vestibular and auditory development. Neuron 14:1153–1164

Fagan AM, Zhang H, Landis S, Smeyne RJ, Silos-Santiago I, Barbacid M (1996) TrkA, but not TrkC, receptors are essential for survival of sympathetic neurons in vivo. J Neurosci 16:6208–6218

Falkenberg T, Mohammed AK, Henriksson B, Persson H, Winblad B, Lindefors N (1992) Increased expression of brain-derived neurotrophic factor mRNA in rat hippocampus is associated with improved spatial memory and enriched environment. Neurosci Lett 138:153–156

Fambrough D, Goodman CS (1996) The Drosophila beaten path gene encodes a novel secreted protein that regulates defasciculation at motor axon choice points. Cell 87:1049–1058

Fariñas I, Jones KR, Backus C, Wang X-Y, Reichardt LF (1994) Severe sensory and sympathetic deficits in mice lacking neurotrophin-3. Nature 369:658–661

Fariñas I, Yoshida CK, Backus C, Reichardt LF (1996) Lack of neurotrophin-3 results in death of spinal sensory neurons and premature differentiation of their precursors. Neuron 17:1065–1078

Fischer W, Wictorin K, Bjoerklund A, Williams LR, Varon S, Gage FH (1987) Amelioration of cholinergic neuron atrophy and spatial memory impairment in aged rats by nerve growth factor. Nature 329:65–68

Frade JM, Barde YA (1998) Microglia-derived nerve growth factor causes cell death in the developing retina. Neuron 20:35–41

Frade JM, Rodríguez-Tébar A, Barde YA (1996) Induction of cell death by endogenous nerve growth factor through its p75 receptor. Nature 383:166–168

Frade JM, Bovolenta P, Martínez-Morales JR, Arribas A, Barbas JA, Rodríguez-Tébar A (1997) Control of early cell death by BDNF in the chick retina. Development 124:3313–3320

Friedel RH, Schnürch H, Stubbusch J, Barde YA (1997) Identification of genes differentially expressed by nerve growth factor- and neurotrophin-3-dependent sensory neurons. Proc Natl Acad Sci USA 94:12670–12675

Fritzsch B, Silos-Santiago I, Bianchi LM, Fariñas I (1997) The role of neurotrophic factors in regulating the development of inner ear innervation. TINS 20:159–164

Funakoshi H, Belluardo N, Arenas E, Yamamoto Y, Casabona A, Persson H, Ibáñez CF (1995) Muscle-derived neurotrophin-4 as an activity-dependent trophic signal for adult motor neurons. Science 268:1495–1499

Fundin BT, Silos-Santiago I, Ernfors P, Fagan AM, Aldskogius H, DeChiara TM, Phillips HS, Barbacid M, Yancopoulos GD, Rice FL (1997) Differential dependency of cutaneous mechanoreceptors on neurotrophins, trk receptors, and p75 LNGFR. Dev Biol 190:94–116

Gaese F, Kolbeck R, Barde YA (1994) Sensory ganglia require neurotrophin-3 early in development. Development 120:1613–1619

Gagliardini V, Fernandez P-A, Lee RKK, Drexler HCA, Rotello RJ, Fishman MC, Yuan J (1994) Prevention of vertebrate neuronal death by the crmA gene. Science 263:826–828

Gall CM, Isackson PJ (1989) Limbic seizures increase neuronal production of messenger RNA for nerve growth factor. Science 245:758–761

Garcia I, Martinou I, Tsujimoto Y, Martinou J-C (1992) Prevention of programmed cell death of sympathetic neurons by the bcl-2 proto-oncogene. Science 258:302–304

Garofalo L, Ribeiro-da-Silva A, Cuello AC (1992) Nerve growth factor-induced synaptogenesis and hypertrophy of cortical cholinergic terminals. Proc Natl Acad Sci USA 89:2639–2643

Goodman LJ, Valverde J, Lim F, Geschwind MD, Federoff HJ, Geller AI, Hefti F (1996) Regulated release and polarized localization of brain-derived neurotrophic factor in hippocampal neurons. Mol Cell Neurosci 7:222–238

Gorin PD, Johnson EM (1980) Effects of long-term nerve growth factor deprivation on the nervous system of the adult rat: an autoimmune approach. Brain Res 198:27–42

Götz R, Raulf F, Schartl M (1992) Brain-derived neurotrophic factor is more highly conserved in structure and function than nerve growth factor during vertebrate evolution. J Neurochem 59:432–442

Götz R, Köster R, Winkler C, Raulf F, Lottspeich F, Schartl M, Thoenen H (1994) Neurotrophin-6 is a new member of the nerve growth factor family. Nature 372:266–269

Haffter P, Granato M, Brand M, Mullins MC, Hammerschmidt M, Kane DA, Odenthal J, Van Eeden FJM, Jiang YJ, Heisenberg CP, Kelsh RN, Furutani-Seiki M, Vogelsang E, Beuchle D, Schach U, Fabian C, Nüsslein-Volhard C (1996) The identification of genes with unique and essential functions in the development of the zebrafish, Danio rerio. Development 123:1–36

Hagg T, Manthorpe M, Vahlsing HL, Varon S (1988) Delayed treatment with nerve growth factor reverses the apparent loss of cholinergic neurons after acute brain damage. Exp Neurol 101:303–312

Hallböök F, Ibáñez CF, Persson H (1991) Evolutionary studies of the nerve growth factor family reveal a novel member abundantly expressed in Xenopus ovary. Neuron 6:1–20

Hefti F (1986) Nerve growth factor promotes survival of septal cholinergic neurons after fimbrial transections. J Neurosci 6:2155–2162

Herzog KH, Bailey K, Barde YA (1994) Expression of the BDNF gene in the developing visual system of the chick. Development 120:1643–1649

Hofer MM, Barde YA (1988) Brain-derived neurotrophic factor prevents neuronal death in vivo. Nature 331:261–262

Hohn A, Leibrock J, Bailey K, Barde YA (1990) Identification and characterization of a novel member of the nerve growth factor/brain-derived neurotrophic factor family. Nature 344:339–341

Horvitz HR, Shaham S, Hengartner MO (1994) The genetics of programmed cell death in the nematode Caenorhabditis elegans. Cold Spring Harb Symp Quant Biol 59:377–386

Hory-Lee F, Russell M, Lindsay RM, Frank E (1993) Neurotrophin 3 supports the survival of developing muscle sensory neurons in culture. Proc Natl Acad Sci USA 90:2613–2617

Huang B, Eberstadt M, Olejniczak ET, Meadows RP, Fesik SW (1996) NMR structure and mutagenesis of the FAS (APO-1/CD95) death domain. Nature 384:638–641

Ibáñez CF, Ebendal T, Barbany G, Murray-Rust J, Blundell TL, Persson H (1992) Disruption of the low affinity receptor-binding site in NGF allows neuronal survival and differentiation by binding to trk gene product. Cell 69:329–341

Ip NY, Ibáñez CF, Nye SH, McClain J, Jones PF, Gies DR, Belluscio L, Le Beau MM, Espinosa III R, Squinto SP, Persson H, Yancopoulos GD (1992) Mammalian neurotrophin-4: structure, chromosomal localization, tissue distribution, and receptor specificity. Proc Natl Acad Sci USA 89:3060–3064

Ip NY, Li Y, Yancopoulos GD, Lindsay RM (1993) Cultured hippocampal neurons show responses to BDNF, NT-3, and NT-4, but not NGF. J Neurosci 13:3394–3405

Isackson PJ, Huntsman MM, Murray KD, Gall CM (1991) BDNF mRNA expression is increased in adult rat forebrain after limbic seizures: Temporal patterns of induction distinct from NGF. Neuron 6:937–948

Johnson EM, Gorin PD, Brandeis LD, Pearson J (1980) Dorsal root ganglion neurons are destroyed by exposure in utero to maternal antibodies to nerve growth factor. Science 210:916–918

Jones KR, Reichardt LF (1990) Molecular cloning of a human gene that is a member of the nerve growth factor family. Proc Natl Acad Sci USA 87:8060–8064

Jones KR, Fariñas I, Backus C, Reichardt LF (1994) Targeted disruption of the BDNF gene perturbs brain and sensory neuron development but not motor neuron development. Cell 76:989–999

Kaisho Y, Yoshimura K, Nakahama K (1990) Cloning and expression of a cDNA encoding a novel human neurotrophic factor. FEBS Lett 266:187–191

Kalcheim C, Barde YA, Thoenen H, Le Douarin NM (1987) In vivo effect of brain-derived neurotrophic factor on the survival of developing dorsal root ganglion cells. EMBO J 6:2871–2873

Kang H, Schuman EM (1995) Long-lasting neurotrophin-induced enhancement of synaptic transmission in the adult hippocampus. Science 267:1658–1662

Kang HJ, Schuman EM (1996) A requirement for local protein synthesis in neurotrophin-induced hippocampal synaptic plasticity. Science 273:1402–1406

Kim HG, Wang T, Olafsson P, Lu B (1994) Neurotrophin 3 potentiates neuronal activity and inhibits gamma-aminobutyratergic synaptic transmission in cortical neurons. Proc Natl Acad Sci USA 91:12341–12345

Klein R, Parada LF, Coulier F, Barbacid M (1989) trkB, a novel tyrosine protein kinase receptor expressed during mouse neural development. EMBO J 8:3701–3709

Koliatsos VE, Clatterbuck RE, Winslow JW, Cayouette MH, Price DL (1993) Evidence that brain-derived neurotrophic factor is a trophic factor for motor neurons in vivo. Neuron 10:359–367

Korte M, Carroll P, Wolf E, Brem G, Thoenen H, Bonhoeffer T. (1995) Hippocampal long-term potentiation is impaired in mice lacking brain-derived neurotrophic factor. Proc Natl Acad Sci USA 92:8856–8860

Korte M, Griesbeck O, Gravel C, Carroll P, Staiger V, Thoenen H, Bonhoeffer T (1996) Virus-mediated gene transfer into hippocampal CA1 region restores long-term potentiation in brain-derived neurotrophic factor mutant mice. Proc Natl Acad Sci USA 93:12547–12552

Kucera J, Ernfors P, Walro J, Jaenisch R (1995) Reduction in the number of spinal motor neurons in neurotrophin-3-deficient mice. Neuroscience 69:321–330

Lauterborn J, Berschauer R, Gall C (1995) Cell-specific modulation of basal and seizure-induced neurotrophin expression by adrenalectomy. Neuroscience 68:363–378

Le Douarin NM (1980) The ontogeny of the neural crest in chick embryo chimaeras. Nature 286:663–669

Lee KF, Li E, Huber LJ, Landis SC, Sharpe AH, Chao MV, Jaenisch R (1992) Targeted mutation of the p75 low affinity NGF receptor gene leads to deficits in the peripheral sensory nervous system. Cell 69:737–749

Lee KF, Davies AM, Jaenisch R (1994) p75-deficient embryonic dorsal root sensory and neonatal sympathetic neurons display a decreased sensitivity to NGF. Development 120:1027–1033

Leibrock J, Lottspeich F, Hohn A, Hofer M, Hengerer B, Masiakowski P, Thoenen H, Barde YA (1989) Molecular cloning and expression of brain-derived neurotrophic factor. Nature 341:149–152

Lessmann V, Gottmann K, Heumann R (1994) BDNF and NT-4/5 enhance glutamatergic synaptic transmission in cultured hippocampal neurones. Neuroreport 6:21–25

Levi-Montalcini R (1980) Polydipsia after intracranial injections – a property of NGF or a contaminant? Nature 284:577

Levi-Montalcini R, Booker B (1960) Destruction of the sympathetic ganglia in mammals by an antiserum to a nerve growth protein. Proc Natl Acad Sci USA 46:384–391

Levi-Montalcini R, Hamburger V (1953) A diffusible agent of mouse sarcoma producing hyperplasia of sympathetic ganglia and hyperneurotization of viscera in the chick embryo. J Exp Zool 123:233–278

Levi-Montalcini R, Meyer H, Hamburger V (1954) In vitro experiments on the effects of mouse sarcomas 180 and 37 on the spinal and sympathetic ganglia of the chick embryo. Cancer Res 14:49–57

Levine ES, Dreyfus CF, Black IB, Plummer MR (1995) Brain-derived neurotrophic factor rapidly enhances synaptic transmission in hippocampal neurons via postsynaptic tyrosine kinase receptors. Proc Natl Acad Sci USA 92:8074–8077

Lewin GR, Koltzenburg M (1997) Rescue of cutaneous sensory neuron function in BDNF deficient mice by exogenous BDNF. Neuroscience Abstracts 667.12:1703

Lewin GR, Mendell LM (1993) Nerve growth factor and nociception. Trends Neurosci 16:353–359

Lewin GR, Ritter AM, Mendell LM (1993) Nerve growth factor-induced hyperalgesia in the neonatal and adult rat. J Neurosci 13:2136–2148

Liepinsh E, Ilag LL, Otting G, Ibáñez CF (1997) NMR structure of the death domain of the p75 neurotrophin receptor. EMBO J 16:4999–5005

Lindholm D, Hengerer B, Heumann R, Carroll P, Thoenen H (1990) Glucocorticoid hormones negatively regulate nerve growth factor expression in vivo and in cultured rat fibroblasts. Eur J Neurosci 2:795–801

Lindholm D, Castrén E, Tsoulfas P, Kolbeck R, Da Penha Berzaghi M, Leingärtner A, Heisenberg CP, Tesarollo L, Parada LF, Thoenen H (1993) Neurotrophin-3 induced by tri-iodothyronine in cerebellar granule cells promotes Purkinje cell differentiation. J Cell Biol 122:443–450

Lindholm D, Castrén E, Berzaghi MP, Blöchl A, Thoenen H (1994) Activity-dependent and hormonal regulation of neurotrophin mRNA levels in the brain – implications for neuronal plasticity. J Neurobiol 25:1362–1372

Lindsay RM (1988) Nerve growth factors (NGF, BDNF) enhance axonal regeneration but are not required for survival of adult sensory neurons. J Neurosci 8:2394–2405

Lindsay RM, Harmar AJ (1989) Nerve growth factor regulates expression of neuropeptide genes in adult sensory neurons. Nature 337:362–364

Liu X, Ernfors P, Wu H, Jaenisch R (1995) Sensory but not motor neuron deficits in mice lacking NT4 and BDNF. Nature 375:238–241

Lo DC, McAllister AK, Katz LC (1994) Neuronal transfection in brain slices using particle-mediated gene transfer. Neuron 13:1263–1268

Lohof AM, Ip NY, Poo M (1993) Potentiation of developing neuromuscular synapses by the neurotrophins NT-3 and BDNF. Nature 363:350–353

LoPresti P, Scott SA (1994) Target specificity and size of avian sensory neurons supported in vitro by nerve growth factor, brain-derived neurotrophic factor, and neurotrophin-3. J Neurobiol 25:1613–1624

Lumsden AGS, Davies AM (1983) Earliest sensory nerve fibers are guided to peripheral targets by attractants other than nerve growth factor. Nature 306:786–788

Mahadeo D, Kaplan L, Chao MV, Hempstead BL (1994) High affinity nerve growth factor binding displays a faster rate of association than $p140^{trk}$ binding. Implications for multi-subunit polypeptide receptors. J Biol Chem 269:6884–6891

Majdan M, Lachance C, Gloster A, Aloyz R, Zeindler C, Bamji S, Bhakar A, Belliveau D, Fawcett J, Miller FD, Barker PA (1997) Transgenic mice expressing the intracellular domain of the p75 neurotrophin receptor undergo neuronal apoptosis. J Neurosci 17:6988–6998

Mansour-Robaey S, Clarke DB, Wang Y-C, Bray GM, Aguayo AJ (1994) Effects of ocular injury and administration of brain-derived neurotrophic factor on survival and regrowth of axotomized retinal ganglion cells. Proc Natl Acad Sci USA 91:1632–1636

Martin SC, Marazzi G, Sandell JH, Heinrich G (1995) Five Trk receptors in the zebrafish. Dev Biol 169:745–758

Martinou JC, Dubois-Dauphin M, Staple JK, Rodriguez I, Frankowski H, Missotten M, Albertini P, Talabot D, Catsicas S, Pietra C, Huarte J (1994) Overexpression of BCL-2 in transgenic mice protects neurons from naturally occurring cell death and experimental ischemia. Neuron 13:1017–1030

McAllister AK, Lo DC, Katz LC (1995) Neurotrophins regulate dendritic growth in developing visual cortex. Neuron 15:791–803

McAllister AK, Katz LC, Lo DC (1997) Opposing roles for endogenous BDNF and NT-3 in regulating cortical dendritic growth. Neuron 18:767–778

McDonald NQ, Chao MV (1995) Structural determinants of neurotrophin action. J Biol Chem 270:19669–19672

McDonald NQ, Hendrickson WA (1993) A structural superfamily of growth factors containing a cystine knot motif. Cell 73:421–424

Meakin SO, Shooter EM (1992) The nerve growth factor family of receptors. TINS 15:323–331

Michael GJ, Averill S, Nitkunan A, Rattray M, Bennett DLH, Yan Q, Priestley JV (1997) Nerve growth factor treatment increases brain-derived neurotrophic factor selectively in tyrosine kinase A-expressing dorsal root ganglion cells and in their central terminations within the spinal cord. J Neurosci 17:8476–8490

Minichiello L, Klein R (1996) TrkB and TrkC neurotrophin receptors cooperate in promoting survival of hippocampal and cerebellar granule neurons. Genes Dev 10:2849–2858

Morisato D, Anderson KV (1994) The spätzle gene encodes a component of the extracellular signaling pathway establishing the dorso-ventral pattern of the Drosophila embryo. Cell:677–688

Nagata S (1997) Apoptosis by death factor. Cell 88:355–365

Naumann T, Peterson GM, Frotscher M (1992) Fine structure of rat septohippocampal neurons:II. A time course analysis following axotomy. J Comp Neurol 325:219–242

Nawa H, Carnahan J, Gall C (1995) BDNF protein measured by a novel enzyme immunoassay in normal brain and after seizure: Partial disagreement with mRNA levels. Eur J Neurosci 7:1527–1535

Neeper SA, Gómez-Pinilla F, Choi J, Cotman C (1995) Exercise and brain neurotrophins. Nature 373:109

Neveu I, Arenas E (1996) Neurotrophins promote the survival and development of neurons in the cerebellum of hypothyroid rats in vivo. J Cell Biol 133:631–646

Oakley RA, Garner AS, Large TH, Frank E (1995) Muscle sensory neurons require neurotrophin-3 from peripheral tissues during the period of normal cell death. Development 121:1341–1350

Ockel M, Lewin GR, Barde YA (1996) In vivo effects of neurotrophin-3 during sensory neurogenesis. Development 122:301–307

Oppenheim RW (1991) Cell death during development of the nervous system. Annu Rev Neurosci 14:453–501

Otten U (1984) Nerve growth factor and the peptidergic sensory neurons. Trends Pharmacol Sci 5:307–310

Patterson SL, Grover LM, Schwartzkroin PA, Bothwell M (1992) Neurotrophin expression in rat hippocampal slices: A stimulus paradigm inducing LTP in CA1 evokes increases in BDNF and NT-3 mRNAs. Neuron 9:1081–1088

Patterson SL, Abel T, Deuel TAS, MArtin KC, Rose JC, Kandel ER (1996) Recombinant BDNF rescues deficits in basal synaptic transmission and hippocampal LTP in BDNF knockout mice. Neuron 16:1137–1145

Pearson J, Johnson EM, Brandeis L (1983) Effects of antibodies to nerve growth factor on intrauterine development of derivatives of cranial neural crest and placode in the guinea pig. Dev Biol 96:32–36

Petty BG, Cornblath DR, Adornato BT, Chaudhry V, Flexner C, Wachsman M, Sinicropi D, Burton LE, Peroutka SJ (1994) The effect of systemically administered recombinant human nerve growth factor in healthy human subjects. Ann Neurol 36:244–246

Purves D (1988) Body and brain. A trophic theory of neural connections. Harvard University Press, Cambridge, Massachusetts

Purves D, Nja A (1976) Effect of nerve growth factor on synaptic depression after axotomy. Nature 260:535–536

Rabizadeh S, Oh J, Zhong L, Yang J, Bitler CM, Butcher LL, Bredesen DE (1993) Induction of apoptosis by the low-affinity NGF receptor. Science 261:345–348

Rice FL, Albers KM, Davis BM, Silos-Santiago I, Wilkinson GA, LeMaster AM, Ernfors P, Smeyne RJ, Aldskogius H, Phillips HS, Barbacid M, DeChiara TM, Yancopoulos GD, Fundin BT (1998). Differential dependency of unmyelinated and Aδ epidermal and upper dermal innervation on neurotrophins, trk receptors and $p75^{LNGFR}$. Dev Biol (in press)

Riddle DR, Lo DC, Katz LC (1995) NT-4-mediated rescue of lateral geniculate neurons from effects of monocular deprivation. Nature 378:189–191

Rosenthal A, Goeddel DV, Nguyen T, Lewis M, Shih A, Laramee GR, Nikolics K, Winslow JW (1990) Primary structure and biological activity of a novel human neurotrophic factor. Neuron 4:767–773

Ruit, KG, Osborne PA, Schmidt RE, Johnson EM jr, Snider WD (1990) Nerve growth factor regulates sympathetic ganglion cell morphology and survival in the adult mouse. J Neurosci 10:2412–2419

Rydén M, Murray-Rust J, Glass D, Ilag LL, Trupp M, Yancopoulos GD, McDonald NQ, Ibáñez CF (1995) Functional analysis of mutant neurotrophins deficient in low-affinity binding reveals a role for p75^{LNGFR} in NT-4 signalling. EMBO J 14:1979–1990

Rydén M, Hempstead B, Ibáñez CF (1997) Differential modulation of neuron survival during development by nerve growth factor binding to the p75 neurotrophin receptor. J Biol Chem 272:16322–16328

Schäfer T, Schwab ME, Thoenen H (1983) Increased formation of preganglionic synapses and axons due to a retrograde trans-synaptic action of nerve growth factor in the rat sympathetic nervous system. J Neurosci 3:1501–1520

Schimmang T, Minichiello L, Vazquez E, Jose IS, Giraldez F, Klein R, Represa J (1995) Developing inner ear sensory neurons require TrkB and TrkC receptors for innervation of their peripheral targets. Development 121:3381–3391

Schwartz PM, Borghesani PR, Levy RL, Pomeroy SL, Segal RA (1997) Abnormal cerebellar development and foliation in BDNF−/− mice reveals a role for neurotrophins in CNS patterning. Neuron 19:269–281

Sendtner M, Holtmann B, Kolbeck R, Thoenen H, Barde YA (1992) Brain-derived neurotrophic factor prevents the death of motoneurons in newborn rats after nerve section. Nature 360:757–759

Serafini T, Kennedy TE, Galko MJ, Mirzayan C, Jessell TM, Tessier-Lavigne M (1994) The netrins define a family of axon outgrowth-promoting proteins homologous to C. elegans UNC-6. Cell 78:409–424

Smeyne RJ, Klein R, Schnapp A, Long LK, Bryant S, Lewin A, Lira SA, Barbacid M (1994) Severe sensory and sympathetic neuropathies in mice carrying a disrupted Trk/NGF receptor gene. Nature 368:246–249

Snider WD (1994) Functions of the neurotrophins during nervous system development: What the knockouts are teaching us. Cell 77:627–638

Strohmaier C, Carter BD, Urfer R, Barde YA, Dechant G (1996) A splice variant of the neurotrophin receptor trkB with increased specificity for brain-derived neurotrophic factor. EMBO J 15:3332–3337

Stucky CL, Koltzenburg M, Lindsay RM, Yancopoulos GD (1996) Neurotrophin-4 (NT-4) is required for the development of a subclass of cutaneous sensory neurons. Neuroscience Abstracts 396.5:992

Suen PC, Wu K, Levine ES, Mount HTJ, Xu JL, Lin SY, Black IB (1997) Brain-derived neurotrophic factor rapidly enhances phosphorylation of the postsynaptic N-methyl-D-aspartate receptor subunit 1. Proc Natl Acad Sci USA 94:8191–8195

Tessarollo L, Tsoulfas P, Martin-Zanca D, Gilbert DJ, Jenkins NA, Copeland NG, Parada LF (1993) trkC, a receptor for neurotrophin-3, is widely expressed in the developing nervous system and in non-neuronal tissues. Development 118:463–475

Van der Zee CEEM, Ross GM, Riopelle RJ, Hagg T (1996) Survival of cholinergic forebrain neurons in developing p75^{NGFR}-deficient mice. Science 274:1729–1732

Verdi JM, Anderson DJ (1994) Neurotrophins regulate sequential changes in neurotrophin receptor expression by sympathetic neuroblasts. Neuron 13:1359–1372

von Bartheld CS, Byers MR, Williams R, Bothwell M (1996). Anterograde transport of neurotrophins and axodendritic transfer in the developing visual system. Nature 379:830–833

Woolf CJ (1996) Phenotypic modification of primary sensory neurons: the role of nerve growth factor in the production of persistent pain. Philos Trans R Soc Lond B Biol Sci 351:441–448

Wyatt S, Piñón LGP, Ernfors P, Davies AM (1997) Sympathetic neuron survival and TrkA expression in NT3-deficient mouse embryos. EMBO J 16:3115–3123

Yan Q, Elliott J, Snider WD (1992) Brain-derived neurotrophic factor rescues spinal motor neurons from axotomy-induced cell death. Nature 360:753–755

Yeo TT, Chua-Couzens J, Butcher LL, Bredesen DE, Cooper JD, Valletta JS, Mobley WC, Longo FM (1997) Absence of p75NTR causes increased basal forebrain cholinergic neuron size, choline acetyltransferase activity, and target innervation. J Neurosci 17:7594–7605

Zafra F, Hengerer B, Leibrock J, Thoenen H, Lindholm D (1990) Activity dependent regulation of BDNF and NGF mRNAs in the rat hippocampus is mediated by non-NMDA glutamate receptors. EMBO J 9:3545–3550

Zafra F, Castrén E, Thoenen H, Lindholm D (1991) Interplay between glutamate and gamma-aminobutyric acid transmitter systems in the physiological regulation of brain-derived neurotrophic factor and nerve growth factor synthesis in hippocampal neurons. Proc Natl Acad Sci USA 88:10037–10041

Zhou XF, Rush RA (1995) Sympathetic neurons in neonatal rats require endogenous neurotrophin-3 for survival. J Neurosci 15:6521–6530

Zhou XF, Rush RA (1996) Endogenous brain-derived neurotrophic factor is anterogradely transported in primary sensory neurons. Neurosci 74:945–953

CHAPTER 2

Molecular Anatomy of Neurotrophic Factors

C.F. IBÁÑEZ

A. Multi-Component Receptors, Specificity and Cross-Talk

Neurotrophic factors, like all polypeptide hormones, deliver their message to the cell interior via interaction with cell-surface receptors. More often than not, neurotrophic factors interact with multi-component receptors consisting of several distinct protein subunits. In some cases, such as the receptor complexes for ciliary neurotrophic factor (CNTF) and glial cell line-derived neurotrophic factor (GDNF), the tasks of ligand binding and downstream signaling are segregated among the different subunits (IP et al. 1992; DAVIS et al. 1993b; JING et al. 1996; TREANOR et al. 1996) (Fig. 1).

In a simplified model of receptor activation, a ligand-binding component, the "alpha" subunit, first associates with the hormone. This complex is subsequently recognized by the signaling receptor, the "beta" subunit, which thereby becomes activated. A number of variations of this basic model are known to exist. The alpha subunits of the GDNF and CNTF receptor complexes are shed to some extent after cleavage of their glycosylphosphatidyl inositol (GPI) anchors. Soluble forms of alpha-receptor components are believed to capture the ligand from the extracellular environment for subsequent assembly into a functional receptor complex on the membrane of cells carrying signaling subunits (DAVIS et al. 1993a; TREANOR et al. 1996; TRUPP et al. 1997a). In the case of GDNF, crosslinking studies indicate that GDNF contacts both the alpha subunit (GDNFR-α, herein called GFRα-1) and the signaling subunit, the receptor tyrosine kinase RET (TRUPP et al. 1996). In addition, GFRα-1 has some intrinsic affinity for RET in the absence of ligand (SANICOLA et al. 1997), suggesting that pre-formed complexes of alpha and beta subunits are also present at the cell surface.

For other neurotrophic factors, however, ligand binding and signaling are not segregated into different receptor polypeptide chains. The neurotrophin nerve growth factor (NGF) binds to two different receptors, the p75 neurotrophin receptor ($p75^{NTR}$) and the receptor tyrosine kinase TrkA, each with distinct signaling capabilities (BARBACID 1994; CHAO 1994; DECHANT and BARDE 1997) (Fig. 1). Although multimeric receptor complexes and functional interactions between both receptors have been observed, it is clear that NGF

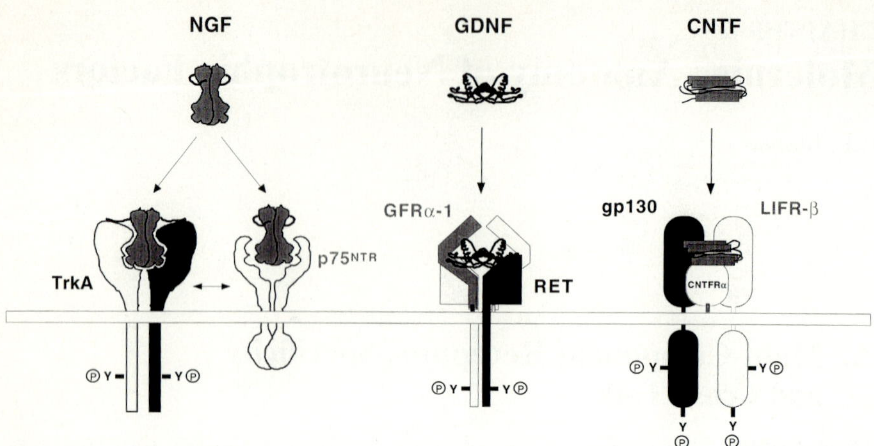

Fig. 1. Multi-component receptor systems of neurotrophic factors. NGF binds separately to p75^{NTR} and TrkA. Interactions between ligand-bound TrkA and p75^{NTR} complexes have been proposed. GDNF binds to a GFRα-1-RET receptor complex in which the GPI-linked α-component (GFRα-1) is essential for ligand binding. CNTF interacts with a tripartite receptor complex formed by a ligand binding α-component (CNTFRα) and two signal-transducing β-components (LIFR-β and gp130). Binding of neurotrophic factors to their receptors leads to receptor tyrosine phosphorylation by either intrinsic (TrkA and RET) or associated cytoplasmic (gp130 and LIFR-β) tyrosine kinase activities

can bind to and elicit biological actions through each of these two receptors independently.

Most neurotrophic factors belong to families of structurally and functionally related molecules. This raises the issue of the specificity of the interaction of structurally similar but distinct ligands with their corresponding receptors. This specificity problem has been solved in different ways during the expansion of the different families of neurotrophic factors (Fig. 2). "Alpha" receptor

Fig. 2. Specificity and cross talk in families of neurotrophic factors and receptors: Ligand–receptor interactions in the neurotrophin (*top*), GDNF (*center*) and neurokine (*bottom*) families is shown. In the neurotrophins, specificity is determined by ligand binding to different members of the Trk receptor tyrosine-kinase family. Cross talk is also apparent in these interactions as more than one neurotrophin may bind to the same Trk receptor, and more than one Trk may bind to the same neurotrophin. Although all members of the neurotrophin family interact with p75^{NTR}, this receptor is also capable of detecting differences between the different neurotrophins. In the GDNF ligand family, GDNF and NTN use the same signaling receptor subunit, *RET*. Differential binding to members of the GFRα receptor family has been proposed as a mechanism of specificity (Buj-Bello et al. 1997; Klein et al. 1997); however, substantial cross talk also exists between GDNF, NTN and GFRα receptors (Baloh et al. 1997; Sanicola et al. 1997). The binding specificities of persephin (*PSP*), a third member of the GDNF ligand family (J. Mildbrant, personal communication) and GFRα-3, a third member of the GFRα receptor family (Trupp et al. 1998), are unknown

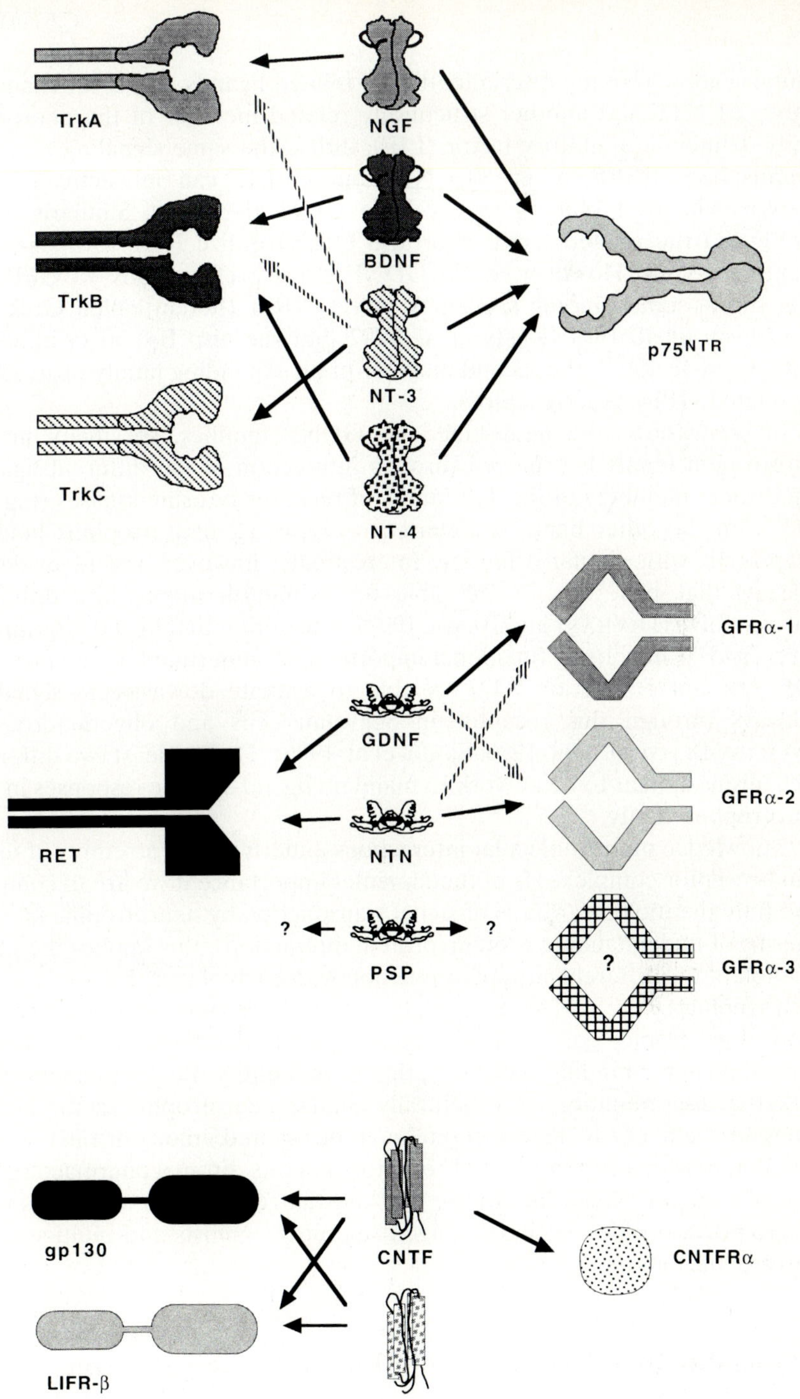
TrkA
NGF
TrkB
BDNF
p75NTR
NT-3
TrkC
NT-4
GFRα-1
GDNF
RET
GFRα-2
NTN
?
?
PSP
?
GFRα-3
gp130
CNTF
CNTFRα
LIFR-β
LIF

subunits can help in the discrimination of related ligands. Thus, for example, although CNTF and another structurally related member of the neurokine family, leukemia inhibitory factor (LIF), utilize the same signaling receptor subunits, i.e., LIFR-β and gp130, CNTF, but not LIF, can only activate these receptors via prior binding to CNTFRα (IP et al. 1993a). Similarly, both GDNF and the related factor neurturin (NTN) utilize RET as a signaling receptor subunit. However, while GDNF binds preferentially to GFRα-1, NTN shows some binding specificity for NTNR-α (herein called GFRα-2) (BUJ-BELLO et al. 1997; KLEIN et al. 1997, but see also BALOH et al. 1997; SANICOLA et al. 1997), the second member of an expanding family of structurally related GPI-linked receptors.

In contrast to the neurokine and GDNF families, specificity in the neurotrophin family is achieved through interaction of the different ligands with distinct members of the Trk family of receptor tyrosine kinases (Fig. 2). $p75^{NTR}$, on the other hand, is a shared receptor, all neurotrophins bind to this protein with similar affinities. Interestingly, however, recent evidence indicates that $p75^{NTR}$ is in fact able to distinguish among the different neurotrophins (DECHANT and BARDE 1997). The notion that ligand discrimination by $p75^{NTR}$ may be of functional importance is underlined by the fact that NGF, but not BDNF or NT-3, is able to activate downstream signaling pathways through this receptor in Schwann cells and oligodendrocytes (CASACCIA-BONNEFIL et al. 1996; FRADE et al. 1996). Thus, at least two different mechanisms appear to be at work to maintain ligand-specific responses in the neurotrophin family.

Knowledge of the molecular interactions underlying the assembly of these ligand-receptor complexes is of fundamental importance if we are to comprehend fully the molecular basis of signal transduction by neurotrophic factors. In terms of understanding protein–protein interactions, this implies the identification of the different sites of interaction with each of its receptors, for any given trophic factor molecule, as well as of the individual chemical groups involved in receptor contact. It also means elucidating the molecular mechanisms of receptor-binding specificity, that is, to identify the determinants that allow the discrimination of structurally similar neurotrophic factor homologues and, conversely, the functional epitopes shared among distinct factors that interact with a common set of receptor subunits. From a pharmacological point of view, we would like to use this knowledge to obtain molecules with novel binding profiles, such as antagonists, super agonists and multi-specific neurotrophic factors.

B. Insights into Neurotrophic-Factor Function from Structural Analyses

A three-dimensional structure, as determined by X-ray crystallographic or nuclear magnetic resonance methods, provides information on the structural environment of each residue in the protein, whether buried or surface accessible, hydrogen bonded or making van der Waal contacts, and identifies which residues are close together spatially. Such information can be helpful in predicting the location of functional sites on the protein surface, features that may guide subsequent mutagenesis experiments.

The structure of NGF revealed a novel tertiary fold dominated by two central pairs of anti-parallel β-strands that define the elongated shape of the molecule (McDonald et al. 1991) (Fig. 3). These β-strands are connected by a number of highly flexible hairpin loops, in which most of the sequence variability among the different neurotrophins is located. The three disulphide bridges of the molecule are clustered, with two disulphide bridges and their connecting residues forming a ring structure through which the third disulphide bridge passes to form a "cystine knot" motif (McDonald and Hendrickson 1993). In the NGF dimer, the two protomers are arranged in a head-to-head conformation and are stabilized by a large hydrophobic interface. All neurotrophins adopt a similar fold and dimer arrangement, as

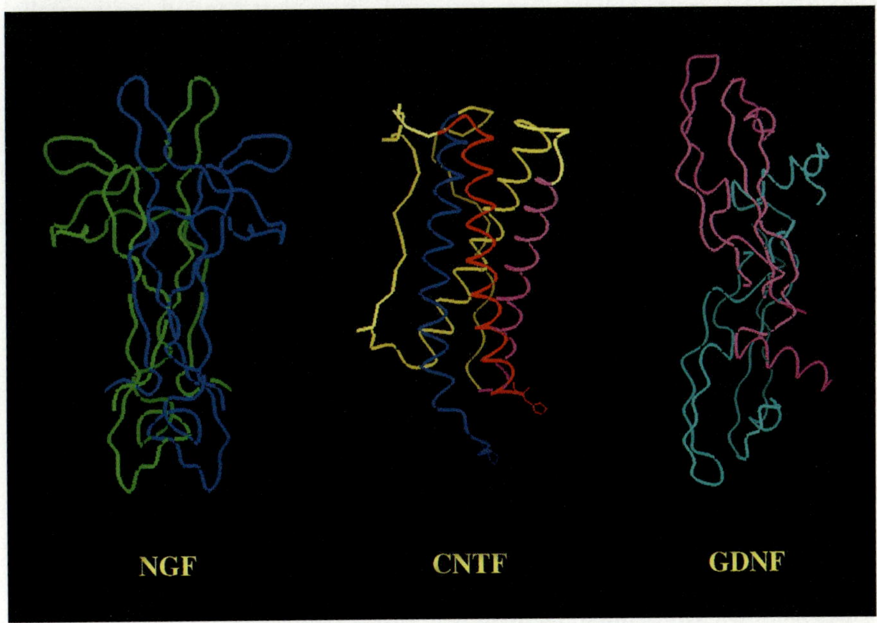

Fig. 3. Three-dimensional structures of NGF, CNTF and GDNF. The Ca chains of NGF (*left*), CNTF (*center*) and GDNF (*right*) are shown. The two NGF protomers are colored blue and green, and are viewed perpendicular to a vertical-symmetry axis. In CNTF, helices A, B, C and D are colored red, yellow, magenta and blue, respectively. The two long loops are colored yellow. The two GDNF protomers are colored magenta and cyan, and are viewed perpendicular to a horizontal symmetry axis. Images were generated with MacImdad

demonstrated by the crystal structure of a BDNF/NT-3 heterodimer (Robinson et al. 1995).

The crystal structure of GDNF reflects, as expected, its structural similarities to transforming growth factor-β (TGF-β), predicted from the conserved pattern of cystine residues in the primary sequences of these two factors (Lin et al. 1993). Noteworthy, TGF-β was the second protein, after NGF, shown to have a cystine-knot motif (Daopin et al. 1992; Schlunegger and Grüter 1992), a feature conserved in the GDNF crystal structure. Like TGF-β, the GDNF structure is characterized by two long "fingers" formed by pairs of antiparallel β-strands connected by loops, and a helical region at the opposite end of the molecule (Eigenbrot and Gerber 1997) (Fig. 3). In contrast to NGF, the two protomers in the GDNF dimer are arranged in a "hand shake"-like, head-to-tail orientation. The amino-acid sequences of the loops in the fingers of GDNF and NTN show high variability. Interestingly, in both the neurotrophins and the GDNF ligand family, variable hairpin loops are spatially close together, indicating possible determinants of receptor binding specificity.

The three-dimensional structure of CNTF revealed a four-helix bundle motif similar to that of LIF and other cytokines (McDonald et al. 1995) (Fig. 3). The four helices are arranged in a left-handed anti-parallel manner and are connected by two long cross-over loops and a shorter loop. The structure of CNTF unexpectedly showed it to be dimeric under the conditions used for crystallization. Solution studies confirmed that CNTF is dimeric at concentrations above 40 μM. However, the high potency and low extracellular concentrations of CNTF suggest that the monomeric form is physiologically relevant. Several features of the CNTF and LIF structures, including pronounced kinks that interrupt the regular main chain hydrogen bonding patterns in two of the helices, appear to be unique to the neurokine family. Remarkably, CNTF and LIF share very little or no sequence identity, despite having very similar structures (Robinson et al. 1994).

C. Electrostatic Forces and the Interaction of Neurotrophic Factors with Their Receptors

Examination of the surface properties of a molecule can help in identifying functionally important regions that may provide binding surfaces to interact with receptors. These might be flexible loops, crevices, hydrophobic patches or charged clusters. The latter contribute electrostatic forces that guide ligands to receptors to bind or collide in a productive fashion. Electrostatic interactions are generally long range and are predicted to affect the association rate of binding. Use of long-range electrostatic forces is likely to be important for recruiting the limiting amounts of neurotrophic factors available in vivo and localizing them at the cell membrane.

The charge distribution in the solvent-accessible surface of NGF reveals a positive electrostatic patch on each protomer, formed primarily by three lysine residues at positions 32, 34 and 95, respectively, from two of the hairpin loops (McDonald et al. 1991) (Fig. 4). Replacement of these lysine residues into alanine by site-directed mutagenesis severely compromises the binding of the mutants to p75^{NTR}, indicating that these positive charges are an important functional epitope for the interaction of NGF with this receptor (Ibáñez et al. 1992). Interestingly, the third and fourth domains of p75^{NTR}, which are important for binding to NGF, contain a number of glutamic and aspartic acid residues that could be important in defining electrostatic interactions with positively charged residues in NGF (Baldwin et al. 1992). Despite the near complete loss of binding to p75^{NTR}, NGF derivatives with mutations that abolish the positive electrostatic patch retain the ability to bind and activate TrkA receptors as well as retaining their biological activity (Ibáñez et al. 1992). Thus, although these positively charged residues are also likely to be buried in the NGF–TrkA complex, these data indicate that they are not directly involved in NGF binding to TrkA.

Despite all neurotrophins being capable of interacting with p75^{NTR}, the lysine residues involved in the binding of NGF to p75^{NTR} are not conserved in other members of the family. However, modeling of BDNF, NT-3 and NT-4, confirms the preservation of a positively charged surface in this region in all the neurotrophins (Rydén et al. 1995), suggesting a similar manner of engaging p75^{NTR}, but with differences in the precise positioning of the charged

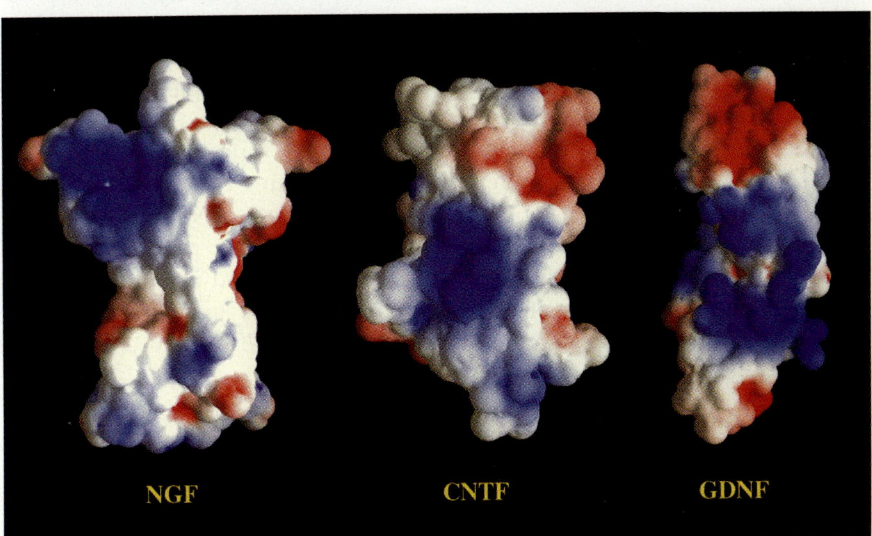

Fig. 4. Electrostatic potential on the surfaces of NGF, CNTF and GDNF. Negative potential is shown in red, positive in blue, and neutral in white. Images were generated with the program GRASP (Nicholls et al. 1991)

surface. In BDNF, the positively charged patch is formed by three consecutive lysine residues (positions 95, 96 and 97) located in one of the hairpin loops known as variable region V (IBÁÑEZ et al. 1991). No positively charged residues are found in loop region I of BDNF, where the critical lysine residues Lys-32 and Lys-34 are found in NGF. In NT-3, arginine and histidine residues are found in place of lysine at these positions and, in NT-4, these two residues are arginines. These differences in the location and spatial arrangement of positive charges may account for the differences in the kinetics of binding to $p75^{NTR}$ seen among the different neurotrophins (RODRIGUEZ-TÉBAR et al. 1992). The functional importance of these positively charged residues in the binding of BDNF, NT-3 and NT-4 to $p75^{NTR}$ has been confirmed by site-directed mutagenesis. Neurotrophins with alanine replacements at these positions are greatly impaired in their ability to bind to $p75^{NTR}$, while retaining substantial binding abilities to their respective cognate Trk receptors (RYDÉN et al. 1995).

A second region of interaction with $p75^{NTR}$ in NGF is formed by another pair of positively charged residues (Lys-74 and His-75) located in a highly conserved and exposed, hydrophilic loop region (bottom loop in the view of NGF shown in Fig. 3). Mutation of these residues into alanine, alone or in combination, reduces NGF binding to $p75^{NTR}$, but not to TrkA (RYDÉN and IBÁÑEZ 1997). Lys-73 in NT-3 (homologous to Lys-74 in NGF) has also been shown to form part of the binding epitope of this neurotrophin to $p75^{NTR}$ (URFER et al. 1994), suggesting a similar role for this region in all neurotrophins. Two other positively charged residues from the NT-3 C-terminus (Arg-114 and Lys-115) are in close proximity to Lys-73 from the other NT-3 protomer, and substitution of these positions into alanine reduces the binding of NT-3 to $p75^{NTR}$ by two orders of magnitude (URFER et al. 1994). Thus, in NT-3, the second binding determinant to $p75^{NTR}$ appears to also be formed by a continuous patch of positive electrostatic potential.

The fact that the two binding epitopes to $p75^{NTR}$ are located at the two opposite ends of the neurotrophin molecule indicates that the interactions between the neurotrophins and $p75^{NTR}$ may be more extensive than previously thought. Again, none of the substitutions made at these positions in NGF or NT-3 affect the ability of these neurotrophins to bind and activate their respective receptors TrkA and TrkC, reinforcing the notion that distinct sites mediate the interaction of neurotrophins with $p75^{NTR}$ and cognate Trk receptors.

A similar analysis of the electrostatic surface of CNTF shows a cluster of three Arg residues at positions 25, 28 and 177 that are highly conserved among CNTF sequences from different species but not in other neurokines. These residues are solvent accessible and form a prominent patch of positive electrostatic potential on the surface of CNTF (MCDONALD et al. 1995) (Fig. 4). The positioning of these residues in the first and fourth helices are analogous to those from the high-affinity site of growth hormone (GH), which also has a four-helix bundle structure. Site-directed mutagenesis analyses have established the importance of these positively charged positions for the interaction of CNTF with the CNTFRα receptor. Replacement of either arginine 25 or 28 into alanine disrupts functional interactions with CNTFRα, but does not affect low-affinity interactions with gp130 or LIFR-β (PANAYOTATOS et al. 1995). Substitution of arginine 177 had a much lower, but still significant, effect. In addition to these three arginines, other residues identified as being part of the binding epitope to CNTFRα, including Gln-63, Trp-64 and Gln-64, also clustered in the same region. Interestingly, substitution of glutamine 63 for arginine, which adds a fourth positive charge to this cluster, creates a protein with greatly enhanced potency and affinity for CNTFRα (PANAYOTATOS et al. 1995). Thus, not only do these observations underline the importance of electrostatic interactions for receptor binding, but they also point to a plausible strategy for the design of ligands with enhanced binding affinities and super-agonists.

In GDNF, the negatively, positively and uncharged regions are well segregated (Fig. 4). A continuous band of net positive charge forms along one side of the dimer, including positively charged residues Lys-81, Lys-84, Arg-88, Arg-90 and Arg-91 from the exposed surface of the α-helix, residues from the N-terminal region of the first finger (Lys-37 and Arg-39) and Lys-129 and Arg-130 from the second protomer.

Another feature emerging from the analysis of the charge distribution in the solvent-accessible surface of GDNF are two symmetric clusters of negatively charged residues one at each end of the elongated GDNF dimer (Fig. 4). This region of negative electrostatic potential is formed by residues Asp-52, Glu-58, Glu-61 and Glu-62 from the loop region of the first finger, and Asp-115 and Asp-116 from the loop in the second finger (EIGENBROT and GERBER 1997). The picture that emerges from these analyses shows GDNF as an elongated, “cigar-shaped” molecule with a central band of positive electrostatic potential flanked by regions of negative potential at the two ends of the protein (Fig. 4).

At the time of writing this manuscript, no information is yet available from mutagenesis analyses of GDNF. However, based on what we have learned so far, from studies on NGF, CNTF and other growth factors and cytokines, it is safe to speculate on the functional importance of the charged regions in GDNF. The available evidence supports a stoichiometry of $(GFR\alpha\text{-}1)_2\,(RET)_2$ GDNF for the ligand–receptor complex (JING et al. 1996). Although cross-linking studies indicate that GDNF contacts RET in this complex, GDNF does not bind this receptor in the absence of GFRα-1, indicating a limited, low-energy interaction. The negatively charged loop regions in the fingers could be sites of contact to GFRα receptors, as these show high sequence variability between GDNF and NTN. Thus, in one possible scenario of complex assembly, two GFRα-1 molecules could clamp GDNF at the two ends of the molecule through contacts with negatively charged residues in the loops, thereby generating a composite surface formed by residues from GFRα-1 and

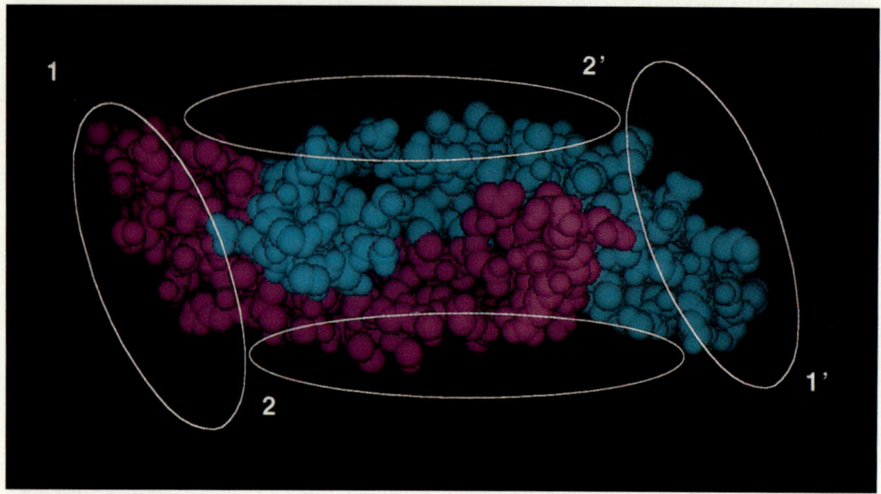

Fig. 5. Hypothetical receptor binding surfaces in GDNF. A filled model of the GDNF dimer, viewed along the two-fold symmetry axis (from the right-hand side of the views shown in Figs. 3 and 4) The cell membrane is hypothesized to be parallel to the plane of the image. Symmetrically related putative binding surfaces of GFRα-1 and RET receptors are denoted, respectively, by *1* and *1'*, and *2* and *2'*. The image was generated with MacImdad

the positively charged central region of GDNF, available for interaction with RET (Fig. 5). A definitive demonstration of the importance of the charged regions in GDNF awaits the results of ongoing site-directed mutagenesis studies.

D. Site-Directed Mutagenesis and Structure–Activity Relationships

Although analysis of the surface properties of a ligand gives information regarding the possible sites of interaction with receptors, the functional importance of individual residues needs to be assessed directly by site-directed mutagenesis. Moreover, predictions based on three-dimensional structures of ligand–receptor complexes (not yet available for neurotrophic factors) need also to be confirmed by direct functional studies.

Alanine-scanning mutagenesis, the systematic replacement of amino-acid residues into alanine, is a widely used technique for obtaining a preliminary profile of the functionally important regions of a polypeptide. Alanine is best suited to the scanning approach, since it can accommodate to most elements of the secondary structure of proteins to conveniently combine small size with minimal structural distortion. Loss of function after alanine replacement is indicative of the functional importance of the mutated position as long as the structural integrity of the mutant polypeptide can be demonstrated.

Homologue-scanning mutagenesis is another strategy that consists of the replacement of single residues, parts, or whole variable regions with homologous sequences from another family member with a different receptor specificity, although it is only applicable to families of proteins. This approach allows the identification of those variable residues that are absolutely critical for receptor binding. The use of residues from a homologous protein minimizes the occurrence of undesired structural changes. Mutant molecules may be analyzed for either loss or gain of function, as swaps of variable regions among homologous proteins may result in the recruitment of additional receptor specificities. Interestingly, numerous studies have shown that using homologue-scanning mutagenesis, gain of function is more readily obtained than loss of function. This strategy has the additional advantage that parallel assays for loss and gain of function mutually control for possible structural side-effects of the mutations.

Alanine- and homologue-scanning mutagenesis of variable regions of the neurotrophins have served to establish their importance for receptor binding and specificity (reviewed in IBÁÑEZ 1995). In NGF, determinants of binding to the TrkA receptor are distributed along the two-fold symmetry axis of the molecule, following the interface between the two protomers. Interestingly, the *N*-terminus of NGF, which does not have enough electron density to be visualized in the crystal structure, is an important binding determinant as truncation (KAHLE et al. 1992), deletion (DRINKWATER et al. 1993), point mutation (SHIH et al. 1994) or replacement with BDNF sequences (IBÁÑEZ et al. 1993) results in decreased binding to TrkA. Other residues contributing to TrkA binding in NGF include Ile-31, several variable residues in the loop between positions 41 and 49, His-84 from the central β-strand bundle, as well as Gln-96, Ala-97 and Ala-98 from loop region V (IBÁÑEZ et al. 1993; ILAG et al. 1994; KULLANDER and EBENDAL 1994; KULLANDER et al. 1997). Several of these residues can transfer TrkA-binding activity to other members of the neurotrophin family. However, mutations at the majority of these positions result in little change in activity when made individually, suggesting that they contribute synergistically to receptor binding.

The *N*-terminus of NGF is so far unique in its importance for NGF binding to TrkA, as mutation or deletion of *N*-terminal sequences in BDNF or NT-3 do not appear to affect biological activity or receptor binding in these neurotrophins. In BDNF, amino-acid residues in variable-loop regions and non-conserved residues in the central β-strand bundle are important for TrkB binding, as shown in studies using NGF/BDNF chimeric molecules (IBÁÑEZ et al. 1991; SUTER et al. 1992; IBÁÑEZ et al. 1993). In NT-3, the binding site to TrkC is dominated by Arg-103, a conserved residue in the central β-strand bundle at the interface of both protomers (URFER et al. 1994). Specificity is achieved by recruiting variable residues from a loop region (ILAG et al. 1994) and the central β-strand bundle (URFER et al. 1997) to the binding surface. Thus, it appears that all neurotrophins make use of residues clustered along the dimer interface from the central β-strand bundle and loop regions for

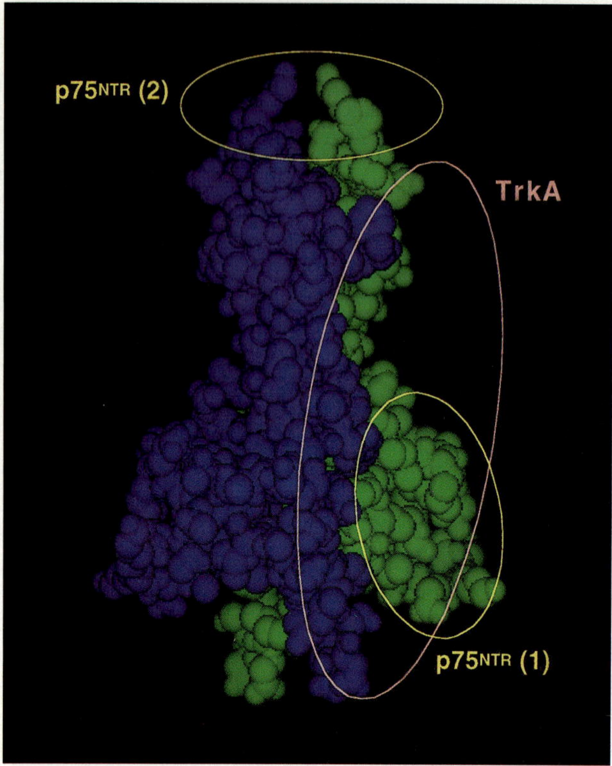

Fig. 6. Receptor-binding surfaces in NGF. A filled model of the NGF dimer ("upside down" compared to the views shown in Figs. 3 and 4) The cell membrane is hypothesized to be at the bottom, perpendicular to the plane of the image. The binding surface of TrkA, and the two sites of interaction with p75^{NTR} are indicated. Analogous surfaces in other members of the neurotrophin family are also predicted to be used for receptor binding. The image was generated with MacImdad

contact with Trk receptors (Fig. 6). However, there are variations among the neurotrophins in the specific residues utilized and in the contribution of the *N*-terminus.

In addition to the binding determinants of CNTFRα mentioned above, site-directed mutagenesis studies on CNTF have also identified candidate regions for interaction with gp130 and LIFR-β. The results from these analyses show that distinct surfaces in the CNTF molecule interact with CNTFR-α, gp130 and LIFR-β, consistent with the notion of a tripartite multi-component receptor complex (Fig. 7). A region important for CNTF binding to gp130 is centered around Asp-30 from the first helix (helix A) (PANAYOTATOS et al. 1995). Mutation of Asp-30 into Gln greatly diminishes CNTF biological activity, without affecting binding to CNTFRα. Mutation of a nearby residue,

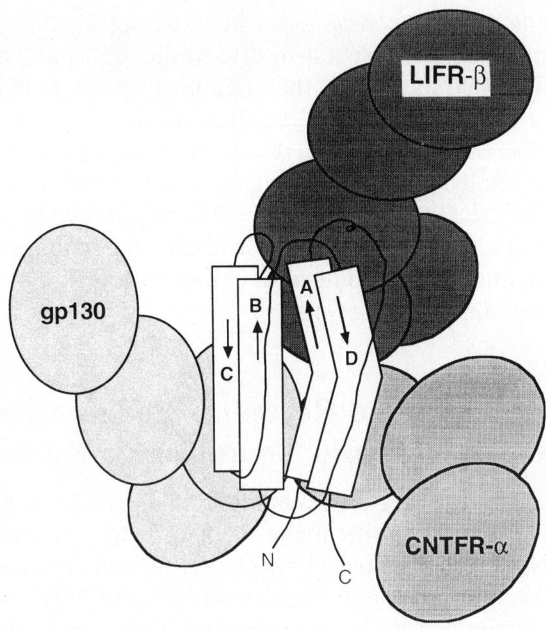

Fig. 7. Model of the tripartite CNTF receptor, viewed above the cell membrane (adapted from McDonald et al. 1995). The shaded ellipsoids represent the extracellular domains of the receptors CNTFRα, LIFR-β and gp130. Helices A, B, C and D in CNTF are denoted by *cylinders* and are labeled

Lys-26, into alanine also reduces biological activity (Panayotatos et al. 1995). Remarkably, the CNTF crystal structure shows that the side chains of these two residues in helix A are solvent accessible, interact via a salt bridge, and are positioned away from the face of helix A that contributes to CNTFRα receptor binding.

Interestingly, super positions of the Ca atoms of human CNTF and human GH show that the Ca atom of Lys-26 is superimposable on the Ca atom of GH Arg-19, which is one of the residues in the second receptor-binding epitope of GH (De Vos et al. 1992). Moreover, alignment of the sequences of CNTF and interleukin-6 (IL-6) shows that residues Asp-30 and Lys-26 of human CNTF correspond to residues Tyr-31 and Gly-35 of human IL-6, which have been reported to affect binding of IL-6 to gp130 (Savino et al. 1994). These observations indicate that Asp-30 and Lys-26 define, on the surface of CNTF, a partial epitope for binding to gp130 (Panayotatos et al. 1995).

In CNTF, the locations of the first two epitopes in the crystal structure show that the loops between the second and third helix (BC loop), the third and fourth (CD loop) and the beginning of the fourth helix (D helix) lie in an area that would be uniformly accessible to a third receptor component such as LIFR-β. An analogous site has been proposed on LIF for interaction of this cytokine with the LIFR-β component (Robinson et al. 1994). Site-directed mutagenesis studies appear to confirm this prediction as individual mutation of Phe-152 or Lys-155, located at the beginning of the D helix, specifically inhibited CNTF interaction with LIFR-β without affecting binding to CNTFRα or gp130 (Di Marco et al. 1996). Simultaneous alanine substitution of both residues totally abolished biological activity. Thus, residues in the so called D1 motif at the *N*-terminus of helix D form a binding epitope of CNTF to LIFR-β. Together, the results from site-directed mutagenesis delineate three discrete and non-overlapping surfaces for interaction of CNTF with its tripartite receptor complex (Fig. 7).

E. Ligands with Altered Receptor-Binding Specificity Offer New Insights into Neurotrophic Factor Function

Taking advantage of its TrkA-only binding profile, a NGF mutant deficient in the ability to bind to $p75^{NTR}$, with alanine replacements at positions 32, 34 and 35 (termed triNGF), has been used to probe for possible roles of $p75^{NTR}$ in the survival responses of primary embryonic neurons to NGF (Rydén et al. 1997). The mutant was found to be less potent than wild-type NGF at low ligand concentrations, similar to or below the high-affinity dissociation binding constant. The reduced responsiveness to the mutant NGF was increasingly evident at later developmental stages; late embryonic neurons did not respond to concentrations of triNGF that were saturating at earlier developmental stages. Likewise, although no difference could be seen between wild-type and mutant NGF on the survival responses of the embryonic rat superior cervical ganglion (SCG) sympathetic neurons, the mutant was much less potent than native NGF on postnatal sympathetic neurons. These results indicate that NGF binding to $p75^{NTR}$ enhances the responsiveness to the ligand, particularly, when this is present at limiting concentrations. In addition, during development, $p75^{NTR}$ appears to modulate responsiveness to NGF, so that binding to $p75^{NTR}$ becomes increasingly important for a biological response at later stages.

NT-3 appears to be unique among the neurotrophins in its ability to bind to all members of the Trk receptor family. Although TrkC is the preferred NT-3 receptor, low-affinity interactions also occur with TrkA and TrkB (Cordon-Cardo et al. 1991; Soppet et al. 1991; Squinto et al. 1991; Ip et al. 1993b). Interestingly, NT-3 utilizes a different binding site for binding to TrkA and TrkB which overlaps with residues involved in binding to $p75^{NTR}$, namely Arg-31 and His-33 (Rydén and Ibáñez 1996). Mutations in these positively charged residues that abolish binding to $p75^{NTR}$ also impair binding to and activation of TrkA and TrkB by NT-3. Binding to TrkC is however unaffected by these mutations. The physiological significance of the interactions of NT-3 with TrkA and TrkB is unclear, but it has been proposed that binding of NT-3 to these two Trk receptors may be an archaic trait maintained during neurotrophin evolution due to the complete overlap of this binding site with residues critical for binding of NT-3 to p75^{NTR} (Rydén and Ibáñez 1996).

Because neurotrophins are being developed as therapeutic agents for nerve injury and neurodegenerative diseases, it is important to consider the potential effects of NT-3 on neurons expressing TrkA and TrkB in addition to those that express TrkC. Since the double mutation of Arg-31 and His-33 into alanine generates a monospecific NT-3 that exhibits normal activities towards TrkC but it is unable to bind or to activate TrkA and TrkB, this mutant may be of greater advantage than native NT-3 when a therapeutic treatment needs to be specifically targeted to TrkC-expressing neurons.

In addition to ligands with a more restricted receptor binding specificity, neurotrophins with a broader spectrum of activities have also been engineered. Taking advantage of the extended binding surface to Trk receptors, as well as distinctive features of the binding determinants of individual neurotrophins, site-directed mutagenesis has been used to engineer multifunctional molecules combining portions of the binding sites of several neurotrophins. Using an NT-3 skeleton, molecules combining NGF, BDNF and NT-3 specific activities into a single polypeptide have been constructed (Ibáñez et al. 1993; Urfer et al. 1994). Neurotrophin molecules with multiple specificities offer an alternative approach to combination therapy and may be particularly useful for the treatment of peripheral sensory neuropathies in which the survival of neurons with different neurotrophic requirements is compromised. In this regard, some of the in vivo activities of multi-specific neurotrophins characterized so far are promising, including axonal retrograde transport to neurons of different sizes in rat dorsal root ganglia (Ilag et al. 1995) and accelerated regeneration of sensory and motor axons after crush or transection of the rat sciatic nerve (Funakoshi et al. 1998).

Provided a high-throughput assay for screening is available, random mutagenesis, followed by selection using phage display, is a very powerful method for the identification of high-affinity binding variants of a ligand (super agonists). This approach has been applied to select for high-affinity CNTFRα binders after random mutagenesis of the fourth helix (helix D) in CNTF (Saggio et al. 1995). This resulted in the preferred replacement of Gln-167, either alone or in combination with neighboring mutations on the hydrophilic side of the C-terminal portion of the D helix (Saggio et al. 1995). The epitope to CNTFRα, defined by this analysis, is adjacent to the positively charged surface defined by arginine residues 25, 28 and 177 and, together, they define the binding site to this receptor in CNTF.

An increase in binding affinity of up to 20-fold was observed in some of the variants recovered which correlated with enhanced biological effects mediated by binding to CNTFRα, including survival of chicken ciliary neurons (Saggio et al. 1995). Taking advantage of this increased affinity and, with the knowledge of residues important for the interaction of CNTF with the LIFR-β signaling receptor, the same authors combined these two mutations to generate a very potent competitive antagonist of CNTF (Di Marco et al. 1996).

This double CNTF mutant showed enhanced binding to CNTFRα, but did not display any biological activity as it was incapable of interacting with LIFR-β. Moreover, the mutant inhibited the activity of wild-type CNTF and the CNTF super agonist in several cell lines (Di Marco et al. 1996). Because the pleiotropic activities of CNTF and related neurokines may be due, in part, to the sharing and cross-activation of receptor subunits, specific CNTF agonists and antagonists constitute new tools with which to explore the therapeutic potential of this molecule.

F. Conclusions

Understanding of structure–function relationships in families of neurotrophic factors has not only furthered our knowledge of important aspects of the biology of these proteins, but it has also provided molecules with novel activity profiles, thereby expanding the repertoire of tools with which to explore the therapeutic applications of neurotrophic factors.

Acknowledgements. Work at the author's laboratory is supported by grants from the Swedish Medical Research Council, the Swedish Cancer Society and the European Commission.

References

Baldwin AN, Bitler CM, Welcher AA, Shooter EM (1992) Studies on the structure and binding properties of the cysteine-rich domain of rat low affinity nerve growth factor receptor (p75NGFR). J Biol Chem 267:8352–8359

Baloh RH, Tansey MG, Golden JP, Creedon DJ, Heuckeroth RO, Keck CL, Zimonjic DB, Popescu NC, Johnson EM, Milbrandt J (1997) Trnr2, a novel receptor that mediates neurturin and GDNF signaling through RET. Neuron 18:793–802

Barbacid M (1994) The Trk family of neurotrophin receptors. J Neurobiol 25:1386–1403

Buj-Bello A, Adu J, Pinon L, Horton A, Thompson J, Rosenthal A, Chinchetru M, Buchman VL, Davies AM (1997) Neurturin responsiveness requires a GPI-linked receptor and the RET receptor tyrosine kinase. Nature 387:721–724

Casaccia-Bonnefil P, Carter BD, Dobrowsky RT, Chao MV (1996) Death of oligodendrocytes mediated by the interaction of nerve growth factor with its receptor p75. Nature 383:716–719

Chao MV (1994) The p75 neurotrophin receptor. J Neurobiol 25:1373–1385

Cordon-Cardo C, Tapley P, Jing S, Nanduri V, O'Rourke E, Lambelle F, Kovary K, Klein R, Jones K, Reichardt L and Barbacid M (1991) The Trk tyrosine kinase mediates the mitogenic properties of nerve growth factor and neurotrophin-3. Cell 66:173–183

Daopin S, Piez K, Ogawa Y, Davies D (1992) Crystal structure of transforming growth factor-β2: an unusual fold for the superfamily. Science 257:369–373

Davis S, Aldrich TH, Ip NY, Stahl N, Scherer S, Farruggella T, Distefano PS, Curtis R, Panayotatos N, Gascan H, Chevalier S, Yancopoulos GD (1993a) Released form of CNTF receptor-alpha component as a soluble mediator of CNTF responses. Science 259:1736–1739

Davis S, Aldrich TH, Stahl N, Pan L, Taga T, Kishimoto T, Ip NY, Yancopoulos GD (1993b) LIFR beta and gp130 as heterodimerizing signal transducers of the tripartite CNTF receptor. Science 260:1805–1808

De Vos A, Ultsch M, Kossiakoff A (1992) Human growth hormone and extracellular domain of its receptor: crystal structure of the complex. Science 255:306–312

Dechant G, Barde Y-A (1997) Signaling through the neurotrophin receptor $p75^{NTR}$. Curr Opin Neurobiol 7:413–418

Di Marco A, Gloaguen I, Graziani R, Paonessa G, Saggio I, Hudson KR, Laufer R (1996) Identification of ciliary neurotrophic factor (cntf) residues essential for leukemia inhibitory factor receptor binding and generation of cntf receptor antagonists. Proc Natl Acad Sci USA 93:9247–9252

Drinkwater CC, Barker PA, Shooter EM (1993) The carboxyl terminus of nerve growth factor is required for biological activity. J Biol Chem 268:23202–23207

Eigenbrot C, Gerber N (1997) X-ray structure of glial cell-derived neurotrophic factor at 1.9 angstrom resolution and implications for receptor binding. Nat Struct Biol 4:435–438

Frade JM, Rodriguez-Tébar A, Barde YA (1996) Induction of cell death by endogenous nerve growth factor through its p75 receptor. Nature 383:166–168

Funakoshi H, Risling M, Carlstedt T, Lendahl U, Timmusk T, Metsis M, Yamamoto Y, Ibáñez CF (1998) Targeted expression of a multifunctional chimeric neurotrophin in the lesioned sciatic nerve accelerates regeneration of sensory and motor axons. Proc Natl Acad Sci USA 95:5269–5274

Ibáñez CF (1995) Neurotrophic factors: from structure-function relationships to designing efficient therapeutics. Trends Biotechnol 13:217–227

Ibáñez CF, Ebendal T, Persson H (1991) Chimeric molecules with multiple neurotrophic activities reveal structural elements determining the specificities of NGF and BDNF. EMBO J 10:2105–2110

Ibáñez CF, Ebendal T, Barbany G, Murray-Rust J, Blundell TL, Persson H (1992) Disruption of the low affinity receptor-binding site in NGF allows neuronal survival and differentiation by binding to the Trk gene product. Cell 69:329–341

Ibáñez CF, Ilag LL, Murray-Rust J, Persson H (1993) An extended surface of binding to Trk tyrosine kinase receptors in NGF and BDNF allows the engineering of a multifunctional pan-neurotrophin. EMBO J 12:2281–2293

Ilag LL, Lönnerberg P, Persson H, Ibáñez CF (1994) Role of variable β-hairpin loop in determining biological specificities in neurotrophin family. J Biol Chem 269:19941–19946

Ilag LL, Curtis R, Glass D, Funakoshi H, Tobkes N, Ryan T, Acheson A, Lindsay R, Persson H, Yancopoulos GD, DiStefano P, Ibáñez CF (1995) Pan-neurotrophin 1: A genetically engineered neurotrophic factor displaying multiple specificities in peripheral neurons in vitro and in vivo. Proc Natl Acad Sci USA 92:607–611

Ip NY, Nye SH, Boulton TG, Davis S, Taga T, Li YP, Birren SJ, Yasukawa K, Kishimoto T, Anderson DJ, Stahl N, Yancopoulos GD (1992) CNTF and LIF act on neuronal cells via shared signaling pathways that involve the IL-6 signal transducing receptor component gp130. Cell 69:1121–1132

Ip NY, McClain J, Barrezueta NX, Aldrich TH, Pan L, Li Y, Wiegand SJ, Friedman B, Davis S and Yancopoulos GD (1993a) The alpha component of the CNTF receptor is required for signaling and defines potential CNTF targets in the adult and during development. Neuron 10:89–102

Ip NY, Stitt TN, Tapley P, Klein R, Glass DJ, Fandl J, Greene LA, Barbacid M, Yancopoulos GD (1993b) Similarities and differences in the way neurotrophins interact with the Trk receptors in neuronal and nonneuronal cells. Neuron 10:137–149

Jing SQ, Wen DZ, Yu YB, Holst PL, Luo Y, Fang M, Tamir R, Antonio L, Hu Z, Cupples R, Louis JC, Hu S, Altrock BW, Fox GM (1996) GDNF-induced activation of the RET protein tyrosine kinase is mediated by GDNFR-alpha, a novel receptor for GDNF. Cell 85:1113–1124

Kahle P, Burton LE, Schmelzer CH, Hertel C (1992) The amino terminus of nerve growth factor is involved in the interaction with the receptor tyrosine kinase p140^{trkA}. J Biol Chem 267:22707–22710

Klein RD, Sherman D, Ho WH, Stone D, Bennett GL, Moffat B, Vandlen R, Simmons L, Gu QM, Hongo JA, Devaux B, Poulsen K, Armanini M, Nozaki C, Asai N, Goddard A, Phillips H, Henderson CE, Takahashi M, Rosenthal A (1997) A GPI-linked protein that interacts with RET to form a candidate neurturin receptor. Nature 387:717–721

Kullander K, Ebendal T (1994) Neurotrophin-3 acquires NGF-Like activity after exchange to five NGF amino acid residues: molecular analysis of the sites in NGF mediating the specific interaction with the NGF high affinity receptor. J Neurosci Res 39:195–210

Kullander K, Kaplan D, Ebendal T (1997) Two restricted sites on the surface of the nerve growth factor molecule independently determine specific TrkA receptor binding and activation. J Biol Chem 272:9300–9307

Lin L-FH, Doherty D, Lile J, Bektesh S, Collins F (1993) GDNF: a glial cell line-derived neurotrophic factor for midbrain dopaminergic neurons. Science 260: 1130–1132

McDonald NQ, Hendrickson WA (1993) A structural superfamily of growth factors containing a cysteine knot motif. Cell 73:421–424

McDonald N, Lapatto R, Murray-Rust J, Gunning J, Wlodawer A, Blundell T (1991) New protein fold revealed by a 2.3-Å resolution crystal structure of nerve growth factor. Nature 354:411–414

McDonald NQ, Panayotatos N, Hendrickson WA (1995) Crystal structure of dimeric human ciliary neurotrophic factor determined by MAD phasing. EMBO J 14:2689–2699

Nicholls A, Sharp KA, Honig B (1991) Protein folding and association: insights from the interfacial and thermodynamic properties of hydrocarbons. Proteins 11:281–296

Panayotatos N, Radziejewska E, Acheson A, Somogyi R, Thadani A, Hendrickson WA, Mcdonald NQ (1995) Localization of functional receptor epitopes on the structure of ciliary neurotrophic factor indicates a conserved, function-related epitope topography among helical cytokines. J Biol Chem 270:14007–14014

Robinson RC, Grey LM, Staunton D, Vankelecom H, Vernallis AB, Moreau JF, Stuart DI, Heath JK, Jones EY (1994) The crystal structure and biological function of leukemia inhibitory factor: implications for receptor binding. Cell 77:1101–1116

Robinson RC, Radziejewski C, Stuart DI, Jones EY (1995) Structure of the brain-derived neurotrophic factor/neurotrophin 3 heterodimer. Biochemistry 34:4139–4146

Rodriguez-Tébar A, Dechant G, Gotz R, Barde YA (1992) Binding of neurotrophin-3 to its neuronal receptors and interactions with nerve growth factor and brain-derived neurotrophic factor. EMBO J 11:917–922

Rydén M, Ibáñez CF (1996) Binding of neurotrophin-3 to P75^{LNGFR}, TrkA and TrkB mediated by a single functional epitope distinct from that recognized by TrkC. J Biol Chem 271:5623–5637

Rydén M, Ibáñez CF (1997) A second determinant of binding to the p75 neurotrophin receptor revealed by alanine-scanning mutagenesis of a conserved loop in NGF. J Biol Chem 272:33085–33091

Rydén M, Murray-Rust J, Glass D, Ilag LL, Trupp M, Yancopoulos GD, McDonald NQ, Ibáñez CF (1995) Functional analysis of mutant neurotrophins deficient in low-affinity binding reveals a role for p75^{LNGFR} in NT-4 signalling. EMBO J 14:1979–1990

Rydén M, Hempstead B, Ibáñez CF (1997) Differential modulation of neuron survival during development by nerve growth factor binding to the p75 neurotrophin receptor. J Biol Chem 272:16322–16328

Saggio I, Gloaguen I, Laufer R (1995) Functional phage display of ciliary neurotrophic factor. Gene 152:35–39

Sanicola M, Hession C, Worley D, Carmillo P, Ehrenfels C, Walus L, Robinson S, Jaworski G, Wei H, Tizard R, Whitty A, Pepinsky RB, Cate RL (1997) Glial cell line-derived neurotrophic factor-dependent RET activation can be mediated by two different cell-surface accessory proteins. Proc Natl Acad USA 94:6238–6243

Savino R, Lahm A, Salvati AL, Ciapponi L, Sporeno E, Altamura S, Paonessa G, Toniatti C, Ciliberto G (1994) Generation of interleukin-6 receptor antagonists by molecular-modeling guided mutagenesis of residues important for gp130 activation. EMBO J 13:1357–1367

Schlunegger M, Grüter M (1992) An unusual feature revealed by the crystal structure at 2.2 Å resolution of human transforming growth factor-β2. Nature 358:430–434

Shih A, Laramee GR, Schmelzer CH, Burton LE, Winslow JW (1994) Mutagenesis identifies amino-terminal residues of nerve growth factor necessary for Trk receptor binding and biological activity. J Biol Chem 269:27679–27686

Soppet D, Escandon E, Maragos J, Middlemas D, Reid S, Blair J, Burton L, Stanton B, Kaplan D, Hunter T, Nikolics K, Parada L (1991) The neurotrophic factors brain-derived neurotrophic factor and neurotrophin-3 are ligands for the TrkB tyrosina kinase receptor. Cell 65:895–903

Squinto S, Stitt T, Aldrich T, Davis S, Bianco S, Radziejewski C, Glass D, Masiakowski P, Furth M, Valenzuela D, DiStefano P, Yancopoulos G (1991) TrkB encodes a functional receptor for brain-derived neurotrophic factor and neurotrophin-3 but not nerve growth factor. Cell 65:885–893

Suter U, Angst C, Tien CL, Drinkwater CC, Lindsay RM, Shooter EM (1992) NGF/BDNF chimeric proteins – Analysis of neurotrophin specificity by homologue-scanning mutagenesis. J Neurosci 12:306–318

Treanor J, Goodman L, Desauvage F, Stone DM, Poulsen KT, Beck CD, Gray C, Armanini MP, Pollock RA, Hefti F, Phillips HS, Goddard A, Moore MW, Buj-Bello A, Davies AM, Asai N, Takahashi M, Vandlen R, Henderson CE, Rosenthal A (1996) Characterization of a multi-component receptor for GDNF. Nature 382:80–83

Trupp M, Arenas E, Fainzilber M, Nilsson A-S, Sieber BA, Grigoriou M, Kilkenny C, Salazar-Grueso E, Pachnis V, Arumäe U, Sariola H, Saarma M, Ibáñez CF (1996) Functional receptor for glial cell line-derived neurotrophic factor encoded by the c-RET proto-oncogene product. Nature 381:785–789

Trupp M, Belluardo N, Funakoshi H, Ibáñez CF (1997a) Complementary and overlapping roles of GDNF, RET and GDNF receptor-alpha indicates multiple mechanisms of trophic actions in the adult rat CNS. J Neurosci 17:3554–3567

Trupp M, Raynoschek C, Ibáñez CF (1998) Multiple GPI-anchored receptors control GDNF-dependent and independent activation of the c-Ret receptor tyrosine kinase. Mol Cell Neurosci 11:47–63

Urfer R, Tsoulfas P, Soppet D, Escandón E, Parada L, Presta L (1994) The binding epitopes of neurotrophin-3 to its receptors TrkC and gp75 and the design of a multifunctional human neurotrophin. EMBO J 13:5896–5909

Urfer R, Tsoulfas P, Oconnell L, Presta LG (1997) Specificity determinants in neurotrophin-3 and design of nerve growth factor-based TrkC agonists by changing central beta-strand bundle residues to their neurotrophin-3 analogs. Biochemistry 36:4775–4781

CHAPTER 3

Neurotrophin Treatment of Peripheral Sensory Neuropathies

C.A. RASK and E. ESCANDON

Abbreviations

ANS	autonomic nervous system
bFGF	basic fibroblast growth factor
BDNF	brain derived neurotrophic factor
CGRP	calcitonin gene-related peptide
CNS	central nervous system
CNTF	ciliary neurotrophic factor
CMAP	compound muscle action potential
CDT	cooling detection threshold
DCCT	Diabetes Control and Complications Trial Research Group
DM	diabetes mellitus
DRG	dorsal root ganglia
GDNF	glial-derived neurotrophic factor
HB DB	heart beat to deep breathing
HIV	human immunodeficiency virus
LIF	leukemia inhibitory factor
MTD	maximum tolerated dose
MNCV	motor nerve conduction velocity
MNDL	motor nerve distal latency
NC	nerve conduction
NGF	nerve growth factor
NIS	neuropathy impairment score
NIS-LL	neuropathy impairment score for the lower limbs
NSP	neuropathy symptom profile
NSC	neuropathy symptoms and change
NPY	neuropeptide Y
NTN	neurturin
NT-3	neurotrophin 3
NT-4/5	neurotrophin 4/5
PNS	peripheral nervous system
PD	pharmacodynamic
rhNGF	recombinant human nerve growth factor
RDNS	Rochester Diabetic Neuropathy Study
SNAP	sensory nerve action potential

STZ	streptozotocin
SC	subcutaneous
SCG	superior cervical ganglion
TGF	transforming growth factor
VIP	vasoactive intestinal peptide
VDT	vibratory detection threshold

A. Introduction

Peripheral sensory neuropathies result from many known etiologies, including diabetes and other metabolic disorders; toxicity from chemotherapeutic agents, such as taxol, cisplatin and vincristine; mechanical compression; ischemia; HIV and other viral infections; hereditary causes; and inflammatory and immune diseases. The etiology of some peripheral neuropathies remains obscure, despite thorough evaluations of the known causes; these are classified as idiopathic neuropathies. Diabetic polyneuropathy comprises the largest group of peripheral sensory neuropathies world-wide and, thus, is the targeted population in many ongoing clinical trials, including NGF. However, as will be illustrated below, neurotrophins, such as NGF, have the potential to be effective therapies for various types of peripheral sensory neuropathies, regardless of etiology.

Peripheral sensory neuropathies are among the first neurological diseases for which therapeutic trials of neurotrophins are currently being conducted. The PNS is much simpler in structure and organization than the CNS. There are relatively few major populations of neurons in the PNS compared with the CNS and it is, thus, easier to identify subpopulations both anatomically and functionally. The simpler anatomy and relative accessibility of peripheral neurons to the systemic circulation make the PNS less difficult than the CNS for the study of neurotrophin treatment of neurological diseases in humans.

B. Organization of the Peripheral Nervous System

I. Sensory Neurons

Somatic sensory neurons exist as pseudo-unipolar neurons with their cell bodies in the DRG, and processes going both to the periphery and to the spinal cord via the dorsal nerve root. These neurons are derived embryologically from the neural crest, an important distinction from some of the cranial sensory nerves of the CNS, since embryonic origin appears to be one important factor in determining responsiveness of neurons to a particular neurotrophic factor. For example, NGF, the first neurotrophic factor discovered, is trophic for some neural crest-derived sensory neurons, but not for those derived from the placode.

Table 1. DRG neurons by fiber type

Fiber type	Size	Sensation(s) mediated
Aα	13–20 μm myelinated	Limb proprioception
Aβ	6–12 μm myelinated	Limb proprioception, pressure, vibration
Aδ	1–5 μm myelinated	Mechanical sharp pain
C	0.2–1.5 μm unmyelinated	Thermal pain, mechanical pain

Sensory ganglion cells are a hetereogeneous group of cells. They vary morphologically in cell-body size, fiber type, sensory-receptor subtype, and they also vary physiologically in neuropeptide content and signaling properties. Table 1 summarizes the general morphological differences among neurons of the DRG, but one must keep in mind that there is also considerable overlap in the function of differently sized groups. In general, large sensory-fiber neurons are attached to muscle spindles and Golgi tendon organs in muscle and, thus, mediate proprioception primarily. Medium-sized fiber neurons subserve mechanoreceptors and, thus, mediate touch, pressure, and vibratory sensations primarily. These receptors are located chiefly in joints and deep cutaneous layers of the skin. Small-fiber sensory neurons may either be myelinated or unmyelinated; they mediate pain and temperature sensation. The terminals for small-fiber sensory neurons are located primarily in the superficial cutaneous layers of the skin (Mense 1990; Mu et al. 1993; Eide et al. 1993; Apfel et al. 1997).

Most studies agree that there is an approximate positive correlation between soma size and fiber type, but the variation is so great that it is difficult to determine the diameter of a particular axon on the basis of its cell-body size. In general, however, larger cell bodies are associated with larger axonal diameters. This correlation, though rough, has enabled investigators to correlate specific neurotrophin receptors with functional subpopulations of neurons in the sensory ganglia, the DRG. TrkA, the high affinity receptor for NGF, is expressed predominantly on small-diameter sensory neurons, some of which are nociceptors. TrkB, the high affinity receptor for BDNF and NT-4/5, is expressed on medium-sized sensory neurons which are generally mechanoreceptors. TrkC, the high affinity receptor for NT-3, is expressed on the large-size sensory neurons which mediate proprioception. In support of these functional associations are studies which have localized neurotrophin mRNA expression in the appropriate target tissues; NGF mRNA in the superficial epidermis, BDNF mRNA in deeper dermal layers and NT-3 mRNA in muscle fibers (Mense 1990; Mu et al. 1993; Eide et al. 1993; Apfel et al. 1997).

II. Sympathetic Neurons

The sympathetic neurons of the ANS are comprised of preganglionic and postganglionic neurons. The preganglionic neuronal cell bodies reside in the intermediolateral gray matter of the thoracolumbar spinal cord. Axons emerge through the ventral root and go through the white rami communicants to the paravertebral sympathetic ganglia. The cell bodies of the postganglionic neurons are located in the paravertebral ganglia, from which they send processes through the gray rami communicants to their target tissues. Some preganglionic fibers pass through the paravertebral ganglia and synapse on neurons of the prevertebral ganglia.

Levi-Montalcini demonstrated in 1951 that administration of NGF to embryonic sympathetic ganglia resulted in massive cellular hypertrophy, fiber outgrowth and increased cell survival in culture (LEVI-MONTALCINI and HAMBURGER 1951). It was subsequently shown that neurotransmitter synthesis was also increased. A number of experiments have shown that nearly all postganglionic sympathetic neurons are NGF-responsive. BDNF, NT-3 and NT-4/5 do not have significant survival-promoting activity on sympathetic neurons. Neurotrophic factors outside the neurotrophin family that are trophic for sympathetic ganglia include ciliary neurotrophic factor (CNTF), basic fibroblast growth factor, (bFGF), the insulin-like growth factor family and leukemia inhibitory factor (LIF) (RECIO-PINTO et al. 1986; ECKENSTEIN et al. 1990; EIDE et al. 1993; KOTZBAUER et al. 1994; APFEL et al. 1997).

More recently, a new family of neuronal trophic factors has been characterized. They comprise a family of TGFβ-related neurotrophic proteins, including GDNF and NTN. They promote the survival of a variety of neuronal populations, including sensory and sympathetic cells (LIN et al. 1993; HENDERSON et al. 1994; BUJ-BELLO et al. 1995; TRUPP et al. 1995; KOTZBAUER et al. 1996).

III. Parasympathetic Neurons

The cell bodies of the parasympathetic division of the ANS are located in the brainstem and in the sacral portion of the spinal cord. Like the sympathetic nervous system, the parasympathetic division of the ANS is comprised of preganglionic and postganglionic neurons, but the parasympathetic ganglia differ in that they are closely associated with their target organs. Much less is known about the effects of neurotrophins on parasympathetic neurons than is known about neurotrophin effects on sympathetic neurons. One of the best studied parasympathetic ganglia is the ciliary ganglion. However, only CNTF, which was discovered in ciliary target tissue extract, has been demonstrated to promote the survival of neurons in the ciliary ganglion. None of the other neurotrophins has demonstrated well-characterized, consistent effects on parasympathetic neurons (BARBIN et al. 1984; APFEL et al. 1997).

C. Role of NGF in PNS Development

The assembly and formation of the PNS are complex and regulated processes involving the interaction of multiple cellular components and biochemical signals. NGF was discovered when mouse sarcoma cells (which were found later to secrete NGF) were transplanted into chick embryos, and it was observed that the transplants induced a dramatic increase in the size of spinal sensory and sympathetic ganglia and innervation of the transplants (BUEKER 1948; LEVI-MONTALCINI and HAMBURGER, 1951, 1953; LEVI-MONTALCINI et al. 1954). Most of the information about the structure and biological function of NGF has been derived from studies using the NGF protein isolated from the mouse submaxillary gland (PURVES and LICHTMAN 1985; THOENEN et al. 1987). Mouse-derived NGF and human NGF are identical in 92% of their primary sequence residues (KORSCHING et al. 1986). NGF protein sequences from several other species are remarkably similar to mouse and human NGF (ULLRICH et al. 1983).

In addition to neuronal survival, a variety of responses in sensory and sympathetic neurons are induced by NGF administered in vitro and in vivo. These effects include chemotaxis (CAMPENOT 1982; LEVI-MONTALCINI 1983; ZETTLER et al. 1991; HOYLE et al. 1993), peripheral axonal branching (DIAMOND et al. 1992), dendritic and terminal arborization (SNIDER 1988; HOYLE et al. 1993), regulation of neurotransmitter production, including catecholamine synthesis and regulation of neuropeptide levels (THOENEN et al. 1971; KESSLER and BLACK 1980a,b, 1981; LINDSAY and HARMAR 1989), establishment of functional synapsis (DIAMOND and COUGHLIN 1987; HOYLE et al. 1993), long-term control of metabolic functions, including cellular size (BRADSHAW 1978; THOENEN and BARDE 1980; LEVI-MONTALCINI 1987; RUSH et al. 1995), and local regulation of nerve terminal growth (CAMPENOT 1994).

A physiological role for NGF during development of the PNS was clearly demonstrated by the dramatic induction of sensory and sympathetic neuronal degeneration when embryonic or newborn animals were exposed to neutralizing antibodies against NGF (LEVI-MONTALCINI 1972; GOEDERT et al. 1978). Recently, using specific antibodies that do not cross-react with any other known member of the NGF family of growth factors, RUIT et al. (1992) demonstrated that approximately 70% of developing sensory DRG neurons are dependent on NGF for survival. These results were recently confirmed by transgenic gene-target disruption (knockout) studies in which the NGF gene was specifically disrupted. These homozygous mice showed extensive sensory and sympathetic neuronal cell loss (CROWLEY et al. 1994; MCMAHON and PRIESTLEY 1995). In concordance with previous anti-NGF antibody studies, the neuronal loss in the DRG is selective, involving mostly small peptidergic, nociceptive, and thermal receptive neurons. By 10 days after birth, the NGF knockout mice have lost all their sympathetic ganglia.

D. Role of NGF in the Adult PNS

Anti-NGF antibody studies, similar to those described above, were performed using adult rodents. These experiments demonstrated that sympathetic, but not sensory neurons continue to be strictly dependent on NGF for survival throughout adulthood (Bjerre et al. 1975; Gorin and Johnson 1980; Ruit et al. 1990). However, a potential physiological role for target-derived endogenous NGF in adult sensory neurons was indicated by Stockel et al. (1975), who demonstrated that adult sensory neurons retrogradely transport NGF from the periphery to the cell body. It was later found that adult sensory neurons retain specific responsiveness to endogenous NGF (Goedert et al. 1981; Verge et al. 1995).

DRG cells from adult animals chronically deprived of target-derived NGF due to auto-antibodies against this trophic factor display mild atrophy (Rich et al. 1984), reduction of axonal caliber (Gold et al. 1991) and a substantial decrease in the levels of the neuropeptide substance P (Schwartz et al. 1982). These studies demonstrated that normal adult DRG sensory neurons require endogenous NGF for maintenance of their normal morphological homeostasis and biochemical functioning (Johnson et al. 1986; Vantini 1992; Longo et al. 1993). This lifelong responsiveness of sensory and sympathetic neurons to NGF is directly relevant to clinical pharmacological intervention. In addition, because these neurons require NGF for regulation of their normal properties, decreased production of NGF and/or an impaired retrograde axonal transport of this trophic factor may underlie or modulate some of the clinical manifestations of specific peripheral neuropathies.

E. NGF Receptors

All of the direct biological actions of NGF require binding to specific cell-surface membrane receptors expressed by the responsive tissues. There are two receptor classes for NGF with different affinities and functions (Sutter et al. 1979; Raffioni et al. 1993; Dechant et al. 1994). The gene encoding the human low-affinity NGF receptor was isolated by gene transfer and molecular cloning. This gene codes for a glycoprotein of approximately 75 kDa, referred to as p75. It contains an extracellular ligand-binding region, a membrane-spanning domain and a short intracellular sequence that lacks a consensus tyrosine kinase (Chao et al. 1986; Johnson et al. 1986; Radeke et al. 1987; Escandon and Chao 1989; Large et al. 1989). p75 also acts as a low-affinity receptor for all the members of the neurotrophin family (Rodriguez-Tebar et al. 1990, 1992; Escandon et al. 1993, 1994).

The high-affinity NGF receptor has a molecular mass of 140 kDa and is encoded by the proto-oncogene *trk*. It is a tyrosine kinase signal-transducing receptor and is referred to as trkA (Kaplan et al. 1991; Longo et al. 1993; Barbacid 1994; Kaplan and Stephens 1994). Transgenic knockout deletions of NGF and trkA result in very similar phenotypes, characterized by a dramatic depletion of nociceptive sensory and most of the sympathetic neurons (Crowley et al. 1994; Smeyne et al. 1994; Snider 1994). There is evidence that the low-affinity p75 NGF receptor is required for some of the normal activities of the functional high-affinity trkA receptor (BERG et al. 1991; LEE et al. 1992, 1994; DAVIES et al. 1993; BARKER and SHOOTER 1994; SALTIEL and DECKER 1994; SNIDER 1994). p75 may also play an active role in modulating NGF binding and responsiveness (HEMPSTEAD et al. 1991; SALTIEL and DECKER 1994).

I. Expression in Normal Nerves

Both p75 and trkA NGF receptors are expressed in most adult sympathetic and many primary sensory DRG neurons (RICHARDSON et al. 1986; VERGE et al. 1989; MCMAHON et al. 1994; AVERILL et al. 1995; KASHIBA et al. 1995; SHELTON et al. 1995; WETMORE and OLSON 1995; WRIGHT and SNIDER 1995). In agreement with the hypothesis of a target-derived trophic supply, the levels of NGF in the target organs correlate with the density (KORSHING and THEONEN 1983; HEUMANN et al. 1984; SHELTON and REICHARDT 1984) and properties (HEUMANN et al. 1987; ENGLISH et al. 1994) of the innervating fibers.

II. Expression in Injured Nerves

Following sciatic nerve transection, there is a rapid increase in NGF and NGF receptors, mediated by Schwann cells distal to the transected region (TANIUCHI et al. 1986; HEUMANN et al. 1987; VERGE et al. 1992; YAMAMOTO 1992). Once re-innervation takes place and contact of the regenerating axons with Schwann cells is re-established, expression of NGF and p75 disappears from these cells (TANIUCHI et al. 1988). SOBUE et al. (1988) have also reported an increase in the expression of NGF receptors in sural nerve biopsies from patients suffering from axonal neuropathies.

III. Alterations in NGF and NGF-Receptor Expression in Human Diabetic Neuropathy

In a recent study in humans, ANAND et al. (1996) compared alterations in sensory and autonomic function in subjects with diabetic neuropathy and measured NGF and neuropeptide levels in the affected skin. They found that NGF levels are significantly reduced in diabetic skin when compared with matched controls. The depletion of endogenous NGF correlates significantly with decreased skin axon reflex vasodilation and with lower levels of the sensory neuropeptide substance P. The authors suggested that NGF deprivation may affect small sensory-fiber function in early diabetic neuropathy. FARADJI and SOTELO (1990) have also described reduced levels of NGF in the serum of patients with diabetic neuropathy. HRUSKA et al. (1993) showed increased levels of a truncated form of the NGF low-affinity receptor in plasma and urine of patients with diabetic neuropathy. They also demonstrated an increase in p75 expression in Schwann cells.

F. The Role of Neurotrophins in the Pathogenesis of Peripheral Sensory Neuropathies

I. Pharmacology of Neurotrophins in Chemotherapeutic-Induced (Toxic) Peripheral Sensory Neuropathies

In addition to its putative beneficial effects during nerve regeneration following axonal trauma, there is also evidence that NGF may reverse or ameliorate the peripheral neuropathies experimentally induced in mice by several chemotherapeutic agents, including taxol and cisplatin (Johnson et al. 1978; Apfel et al. 1991, 1992). All of these cytostatic drugs, including vincristine, affect sensory neurons, and each one produces a characteristic neuropathy. The studies with cisplatin (Roelofs et al. 1984; Mollman 1990; Apfel et al. 1991, 1992) measured proprioception (rotating dowel balance), tail NC velocity and sensory ganglion levels of the peptide transmitter CGRP. The studies with taxol (Lipton et al. 1989) evaluated the threshold to thermally induced pain (tail flick), amplitude of the compound action potential for the caudal nerve, and levels of substance P in the DRG.

In both the cisplatin and taxol studies, NGF significantly prevented the development of neuropathies induced by these chemotherapeutic agents. The NGF-treated animals exhibited peripheral nerve-function evaluations matching those of control animals (Roelofs et al. 1984; Bleecker 1985; Wiernik et al. 1987; Lipton et al. 1989; Mollman 1990; APFEL et al. 1991, 1992). Additional evidence in vitro has shown a neuroprotective effect of NGF in adult DRG and sympathetic SCG explants, cultured in the presence of taxol, cisplatin or vincristine (Hayakawa et al. 1994; Konings et al. 1994; Malgrange 1994). In cancer patients, the manifestation of a sensory neuropathy is often a dose-limiting factor in the clinical use of these antiblastic agents. Thus, the clinical administration of rhNGF, in combination with cancer chemotherapy drugs, may potentially minimize the peripheral nerve degeneration caused by the chemotherapeutic agents and allow the administration of higher chemotherapy doses.

In an animal model of cisplatin-induced neuropathy, Gao et al. (1995) have shown that NT-3 prevents the pathological changes in nerve conduction velocity associated with large-DRG, trkC-positive sensory neuron loss.

II. Pharmacology of NGF in Experimental Diabetic Neuropathy

Many of the peripheral sensory and sympathetic cells that are predominately affected in human diabetic neuropathy are precisely those neurons continually dependent on the trophic effects of NGF for maintenance and functioning in experimental animal models. The hypothesis that NGF-related alterations underlie some of the manifestations present in diabetic polyneuropathy has been the subject of intense investigation reviewed by Brewster et al. (1994); McMahon and Priestley (1995); Schmidt (1993); and Vantini (1992).

A physiological connection between these events was explored by JAKOBSEN et al. (1981) using STZ-treated rodents as an animal model for diabetes-induced neuropathy (SCHMIDT et al. 1981). Since then, several laboratories have successfully identified NGF and NGF-related alterations that seem functionally tied to the diabetic and neuropathic manifestations. These changes include reduced axonal retrograde transport of NGF (JAKOBSEN et al. 1981; SCHMIDT et al. 1983, 1985, 1986; SCHMIDT and YIP 1985; SCHMIDT 1993; HELLWEG et al. 1994) and reduced levels of endogenous NGF in the sciatic nerve and the SCG (HELLWEG et al. 1990), a condition that is alleviated by insulin treatment or transplantation of pancreatic islet tissue to restore glucose control (HELLWEG et al. 1991). Using the same experimental model, additional studies have reported decreased levels of NGF protein (FERNYHOUGH et al. 1995) and mRNA (FERNYHOUGH et al. 1994; ORDONEZ et al. 1994) in several tissues, including skeletal muscle and skin. Reductions of NGF levels in foot skin, but not in muscle, are reversed by insulin treatment (BREWSTER et al. 1994) and worsened with the increased duration of the diabetes (FERNYHOUGH et al. 1993).

1. Therapeutic Effects of NGF in Experimental Diabetic Neuropathy

The most compelling evidence in support of the potential clinical application of NGF for the treatment of diabetic neuropathies comes from the analysis of the therapeutic effects of NGF in experimentally STZ-induced diabetic neuropathy in rodents. APFEL et al. (1994) were the first to demonstrate that administration of NGF can reverse some of the STZ-induced neuropathic changes. For example, NGF treatment prevents the increase in tail-flick threshold (hypoalgesia) and the decreases in substance P and CGRP. DIEMEL et al. (1994) showed that NGF administration prevents the alterations in substance P and CGRP in the sciatic nerve and normalizes the mRNA levels of *g*-preprotachykinin and CGRP in DRG cells in rats. Similar results were obtained by SANGO et al. (1994) who showed that NGF reverses the depletion of substance P and CGRP in sensory neurons in diabetic mice. In a different animal model of peripheral neuropathy using transgenic diabetic mice, Elias and colleagues (unpublished observations) demonstrated that NGF administration successfully restores C-fiber function.

III. Summary

While the actual role that endogenous NGF plays in the development and progression of diabetic-induced and chemotherapeutic-induced (toxic) and other peripheral sensory neuropathies is unknown, cumulative pre-clinical experimental evidence clearly demonstrates that some of the damaging consequences of diabetes and chemotherapeutic agents in the PNS can be effectively reversed or alleviated by NGF. The potential pharmacological use for rhNGF in the treatment of diabetic neuropathies in humans, involving sensory and sympathetic neuronal components, is currently being studied. In addition, the potential pharmacological use for rhNGF in the treatment of HIV-associated peripheral sensory neuropathy is also under study in the clinic.

G. Clinical Peripheral Sensory Neuropathies: Diabetic Polyneuropathy

Sensory and autonomic neuropathies are the most common form of neuropathy in diabetic patients (EWING and CLARKE 1987). Diabetic neuropathy is most frequently manifested in humans as an insidious, distal, symmetrical polyneuropathy that affects sensory and autonomic function and may also affect motor nerves. The signs and symptoms include pain and paresthesias in the limbs, loss of deep tendon reflexes, weakness and sensory loss, sensory ataxia and autonomic dysfunction. The manifestations of autonomic dysfunction include cardiac arrhythmias, orthostatic hypotension, erectile dysfunction (impotence), gastroparesis, and bladder and bowel dysfunction.

Long-term complications of diabetic neuropathy include non-healing foot ulcers, limb amputations and, possibly, death due to cardiac autonomic neuropathy. Cellular atrophy is frequently present in the DRG, sympathetic ganglia, and the ventral horn of the spinal cord. Structural changes in the peripheral nerves include axonal degeneration, reduction in axonal caliber and demyelination of fibers proximal to the axonal degeneration (SUGIMURA and DYCK 1981; SAID et al. 1983; BREWSTER et al. 1994; THOMAS 1994; MCMAHON and PRIESTLY 1995). Typically, the fiber degeneration affects the more distal nerve trunks with the longest axons. In a sural-nerve morphometric study of diabetic peripheral neuropathy, LLEWELYN et al. (1991) demonstrated the presence of axonal regeneration only in the earlier stages of neuropathy. Axonal sprouting is also seen in diabetic nerves.

I. Epidemiology of Diabetic Neuropathy

DM affects between 2% and 5% of the general population of countries in the developed world. According to the latest estimates, announced in November 1994 in Japan at the World Congress of the International Diabetes Federation, there are now approximately 110 million patients with diabetes worldwide. The figures have more than tripled over the past decade – 1987 estimates put the prevalence at just 30 million cases – the prevalence is forecasted to exceed 175 million in the year 2000 and approach 240 million by 2010 (Fig. 1).

Estimates of the prevalence of diabetic neuropathy vary widely and reflect differences in definitions and methods of patient assessment and selection. The overall prevalence of clinically defined neuropathy has been estimated at

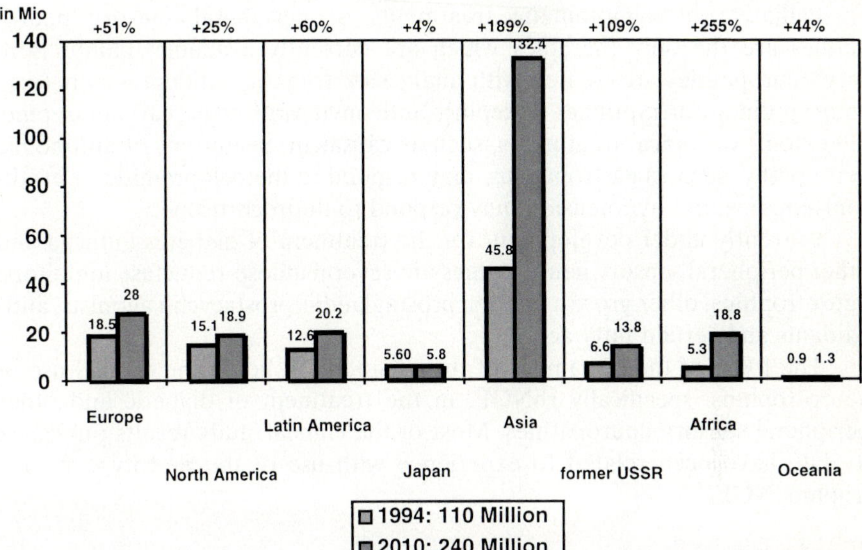

Fig. 1. Regional estimates and projections of diabetes 1994 (*light shading*)–2010 (*dark shading*). The numbers above the bars indicate regional estimates of the prevalence of diabetes mellitus in millions of people. The numbers in the bottom box indicate the total world estimates of the prevalence of diabetes mellitus in millions of people

approximately 30% of patients with DM in the UK and Germany. The RDNS found much higher prevalence rates for diabetic polyneuropathy in a representative group of diabetic residents of Rochester (US) in 1986: 66% of Type I and 59% of Type II patients had some form of neuropathy, although only 20% experienced symptoms when evaluated.

It is generally accepted that neuropathy is the most common and only diabetic complication that is currently untreatable: the probability of a diabetic patient developing secondary complications, including neuropathy, retinopathy and/or nephropathy is dependent on the duration of their disease and the severity of their hyperglycemia. Thus, given the increasing prevalence of DM, the prevalence of diabetic neuropathy will continue to increase over the ensuing decades.

II. Current Treatment of Peripheral Sensory Neuropathies

Although rigorous glycemic control can prevent neuropathic pain in diabetic neuropathy even after symptoms appear and has been shown to decrease the occurrence of clinically detectable neuropathy by 60% (DCCT, 1993), this approach may not work in severe neuropathies and may be limited to patients with Type I DM.

Palliative or symptomatic treatments of peripheral sensory neuropathies are the only therapies which are currently available: painful sensory neuropathies are treated with analgesics, tricyclic antidepressants (e.g., amitryptiline, nortryptiline, doxepin), anticonvulsants (e.g., carbamazepine, phenytoin) or topical treatments, such as capsaicin. Symptoms of autonomic neuropathy, such as gastroparesis, may respond to metoclopramide or erythromycin; postural hypotension may respond to fludrocortisone.

Currently under development for the treatment of diabetes-induced and other peripheral sensory neuropathies are several aldose-reductase inhibitors, neurotrophins, other growth factors, prostaglandin/prostacyclin agonists, antioxidants and certain fatty acids.

The focus of the remainder of this chapter will be on the clinical use of neurotrophins, specifically rhNGF, in the treatment of diabetic and other peripheral sensory neuropathies. Most of the clinical-study results published to date have been related to experience with use of the prototype neurotrophin, NGF.

H. Trial Design Considerations for the Study of Peripheral Sensory Neuropathies

I. Selection of Study Endpoints

In the past, clinical studies conducted to assess the efficacy of agents for the treatment of peripheral sensory neuropathies have relied on electrophysiology, namely attributes of nerve conduction, and also on sural-nerve morphology, assessed pre-and post-treatment. However, determination of what constitutes a clinically meaningful improvement for the patient with regard to changes in attributes of nerve conduction and sural-nerve morphology has been the subject of considerable discussion and debate for years. Dyck and O'Brien (1989) suggested that, in controlled clinical trials, a mean change of two points on the neurological disability score (subsequently renamed the NIS) is clinically detectable and meaningful. Based on their previously published data on the RDNS Cohort study, this would correspond to a change of motor-nerve conduction velocity of the average ulnar, median and peroneal nerves of 2.9 m/s. The corresponding changes in nerve amplitude would be 1.2 (ulnar and median) and 0.7 mV.

However, although abnormalities of nerve conduction are known to be associated with severity of neuropathic symptoms and neurological impairments, direct translation of such specific increments of improvements in nerve conduction attributes, as described above, to a meaningful clinical benefit noticeable to the patient and his/her physician has not been fully established or widely accepted. Thus, there have been continuing efforts to establish study endpoints or criteria which would better reflect the overall status of patients' neuropathy.

In 1992, Dyck et al. suggested that the percentile approach, based on normal limits for various neuropathic tests, considering physical variables influencing neuropathic endpoints (the test itself, the anatomical site being tested, and the patient's age, sex, height, weight and level of physical fitness) might be adopted by laboratories interested in clinical electromyography and the sensory and autonomic nervous system. Such a percentile approach would enable clinicians to better determine estimates of normality for a given patient and for groups of patients participating in controlled clinical trials. Such a percentile approach might be used in controlled clinical trials to determine the response to treatment.

In 1995, the Peripheral Nerve Society, comprising international experts in the subject, published a consensus report on diabetic polyneuropathy in controlled clinical trials. In this report, the society acknowledged the need to establish a meaningful level of prevention, stabilization or improvement of diabetic polyneuropathy that indicates efficacy and which could be used in prospective, double-blind, controlled clinical trials comparing new therapies with placebo. The difference between the effects of the new drug being studied and placebo must be statistically significant and of sufficient magnitude to be considered clinically useful (Peripheral Nerve Society 1995). Neuropathic symptoms, neurological impairments present on examination, nerve conduction studies, quantitative sensory testing, quantitative autonomic testing and morphometric assessment of the sural nerve (number and size of nerve fibers, pathological abnormalities of teased fibers and frequency of regenerating sprouts) are all useful in characterizing and quantifying the severity of neuropathy. Since the results of one evaluation tend to correlate with the results of the other evaluations, any of these assessments and measurement of a change in the rate of complications due to the neuropathy might be used as endpoints in clinical trials assessing the efficacy of a new treatments for peripheral sensory neuropathies.

The Peripheral Nerve Society consensus report concludes that "perhaps the most convincing evidence that a pharmaceutical product is efficacious is if it prevents, stabilizes or improves global neuropathic deficit (impairment) to a defined degree." (Peripheral Nerve Society 1995) They suggest that such a degree of change is twice (for the two sides of the body) the least degree of neurological abnormality a physician can recognize among change in sensation, activity of tendon reflexes (both graded as normal, decreased or absent), or muscle weakness (graded as normal, 25% weak, 50% weak, 75% weak or paralyzed). This degree of change would correspond to a change of two points on the NIS (Dyck et al. 1987).

Subsequent to this consensus report, Dyck et al. (1997b) have shown that the NIS-LL plus seven tests , a composite score which is calculated as shown in Table 2, provides a more comprehensive assessment of neuropathic

Table 2. Method of calculating the NIS-LL +7 tests score

- Sum individual scores of the NIS for the lower limbs, NIS-LL
- In NIS-LL, substitute transformed points for percentile abnormality[a] of VDT for each great toe (obtained with CASE IV) for the clinical vibration sensation point score of great toes
- Add transformed points for percentile abnormality[a] of HB DB[b] (one time only)
- Summate transformed points for percentile abnormality[a] of the five attributes of – NC lower limb (peroneal nerve [CMAP[c], MNCV[d], MNDL[e]], tibal nerve [MNDL[e]] and sural nerve [SNAP[f]]), divided by the number of attributes with obtainable values[g], multiply by five (the number of attributes) and add this number to the global score

[a] <95th = 0; >95th–99th = 1; >99th–99.9th = 2; >99.9th = 3 (or >5th = 0 to <0.1th = 3, whichever end of the distribution is abnormal).
[b] Heart beat to deep breathing.
[c] Compound muscle action potential.
[d] Motor nerve conduction velocity.
[e] Motor nerve distal latency.
[f] Sensory nerve action potential.
[g] MNCV and MNDL cannot be estimated when CMAP is 0.

impairment and that it avoids an overestimated frequency of diabetic polyneuropathy when the more usually used minimal criteria for diagnosis of diabetic polyneuropathy was used (any one or two abnormalities from among multiple evaluations). In addition, the NIS-LL+ 7 tests was much better at showing a magnitude of monotone worsening in the RDNS Cohort, which could perhaps be used to assess the response to treatment compared with placebo in clinical trials over time, than any one single measure of diabetic polyneuropathy. Using the composite score of NIS-LL+7 tests to assess overall neuropathic impairments, the average diabetic patient in the RDNS cohort worsened by 0.34 points per year, whereas patients who had diabetic polyneuropathy worsened by 0.85 points per year.

If a new therapeutic agent for treatment is able to prevent worsening of diabetic polyneuropathy, but not cause improvement of the neuropathy, a controlled clinical trial would need to be conducted on a sufficient number of patients for 3 years to detect a meaningful change of two points on the NIS, the degree of change the Peripheral Nerve Society consensus group considered to be clinically meaningful (Peripheral Nerve Society 1995). Further study of this composite score in other cohorts of neuropathic patients will be required to determine its widespread applicability and usefulness as an endpoint in controlled clinical studies (Table 2).

II. Study Endpoints for Evaluation of Efficacy of rhNGF

As summarized in the previous section, rhNGF has been demonstrated in numerous experiments to promote the survival, differentiation and maintenance of small-fiber sensory and sympathetic neurons in the PNS. NGF is expressed in the skin and other target tissues of its responsive neuronal populations. There, it binds to its high-affinity receptor, trkA, on nerve terminals and is retrogradely transported back to the neuronal perikaryon, where it exerts its trophic effects.

Clinical studies of the effects of rhNGF must, therefore, include endpoints which measure small-fiber sensory and/or sympathetic functions. In addition, studies should be designed to determine whether rhNGF treatment conveys a meaningful clinical benefit to patients. Study endpoints which would meet these criteria include: (1) measures of neurological impairment, specifically evaluations of pain, temperature and touch pressure sensations on clinical neurological examination; (2) quantitative sensory evaluations of cooling detection threshold and heat pain; (3) neuropathic symptom assessments; and (4) quantitative autonomic evaluations. Attributes of nerve conduction should be used for selection and staging of patients for inclusion in the studies in addition to the four groups of tests listed and should be evaluated at the end of treatment to determine whether NGF has other indirect or more widespread effects in the PNS following chronic administration.

I. Clinical Studies of Nerve Growth Factor

I. Safety, Pharmacokinetics and Pharmacodynamic Effects of rhNGF

Phase-I clinical studies of rhNGF conducted in healthy volunteers and patients with neuropathy (Rask et al. 1995), and a Phase-II clinical study of rhNGF conducted in patients with diabetic polyneuropathy have provided a preliminary safety and efficacy profile for rhNGF. The MTD in both healthy volunteers and patients with various types of neuropathy has been determined to be less than 1.0 μg/kg. Doses of 1.0 μg/kg or greater produce generalized myalgias often accompanied by visceral pain (Petty et al. 1994; Apfel et al. 1995, 1997; Apfel et al. unpublished observations).

At the time of writing this publication, eight documented instances of unintentional overdoses, occurring in seven patients, had been reported in the Phase-II study of diabetic neuropathy (Apfel et al. 1998). Several additional unintentional overdoses have been reported in an ongoing study in HIV-associated neuropathy (personal communication). These incidents were all due to patients forgetting to dilute the concentrated solution as they had been instructed to do. The errors in dilution resulted in administration of approximately 70 μg/kg or approximately 700 times the dose currently being studied in the U.S. Phase-III study. These unintentional overdoses resulted in symptoms of generalized myalgias accompanied by visceral pain in all patients. The symptoms lasted for 24–96 h before resolving completely. No abnormalities were detectable on physical examination (other than mild tenderness to muscle palpation), laboratory testing or monitoring of vital signs and cardiac function. There were no further symptoms upon subsequent rechallenge with the appropriate dose of rhNGF in those five of the seven subjects who continued to participate in the diabetic polyneuropathy study.

The most frequent adverse event associated with administration of rhNGF is local injection site hyperalgesia/allodynia, which is generally described as a mild to moderate discomfort to palpation at the site of the injection. Generally, this begins 1.5–4h following the injection and lasts for variable periods of time. This symptom has not usually required specific treatment; if required, non-steroidal anti-inflammatory agents have generally been effective in ameliorating the discomfort (APFEL et al. unpublished observations).

A study was conducted in healthy volunteers to evaluate the pharmacokinetic profile of those doses of rhNGF used in the Phase-II safety and efficacy study of rhNGF for the treatment of diabetic polyneuropathy and the treatment of HIV-associated neuropathy. The results revealed rhNGF to have a plasma concentration–time under the concentration curve half-life ($T_{1/2}$) of approximately 6–8h following administration of a single dose.

PD effects of intradermal injection of very small doses (1 or 3μg) of rhNGF were studied by DYCK et al. (1997a). They included injection-site hyperalgesia/pressure allodynia and lowered heat-pain threshold at the site of the injection, which was not measurable on the contralateral limb following administration of 1 or 3μg of rhNGF, with the symptoms and signs beginning as early as 3h following a single intradermal dose and lasting for up to 21 days (Table 3).

II. Preliminary Evidence of Efficacy of rhNGF in the Treatment of Peripheral Sensory Neuropathies

The first phase-II study of the safety and efficacy of rhNGF for the treatment of diabetic polyneuropathy was recently completed (APFEL et al. 1998). Fifteen U.S. study sites recruited 250 subjects aged 18–60 years with stage-II neuropathy, as defined by DYCK (1988). Subjects received SC injections of placebo, rhNGF 0.1 or rhNGF 0.3μg/kg three times per week for 6 months.

The following measures were considered as independent endpoints for efficacy: the quantitative neurological examination of the lower limbs (NIS-LL), quantitative measures of sensory function (CDT, VDT and intermediate level of heat pain [HP = 5.0]), and the symptom questionnaires (NSP, NSC, and the global symptom assessment). In addition, in order to better evaluate a subject's overall neuropathy, three different groups of measures of neuropathy were prospectively identified for multiple endpoint analyses prior to unblinding the study. The first group was thought to be most objective and included: NIS-LL, CDT, VDT, HP = 5.0. The second group added subjective measures of neuropathy: NIS-LL, CDT, VDT, HP = 5.0, NSP and the global

Table 3. Studies of recombinant human nerve growth factor in humans

Subjects	Study type	No. of rhNGF	Subjects Placebo	Gender M/F	Dose Regimen[a,b]	Comments
Healthy	Single-dose/placebo-controlled/dose-escalation/double-blind/randomized	32	13	33/12	1.0, 0.3, 0.1, 0.03 μg/kg rhNGF or placebo IV and SC	1 μg/kg produced myalgias, myalgias, visceral pain; injection-site hyperalgesia nondose-related (S.C. 75%) MTD determined to be <1 μg/kg
Healthy	Single-dose/randomized/open-label	12	0	5/7	0.3 or 0.1 μg/kg rhNGF SC	No myalgias, injection-site hyperalgesia in approx. 50% of subjects PK: $T_{1/2}$: approx. 8 h, linear kinetics
Healthy	Single-dose/open-label	16	16	13/3	1.0 or 3.0 μg rhNGF ID and placebo	No myalgias, injection-site hyperalgesia in 15/16 (94%) subjects. Physician-sponsored, localized PD effects starting at 3 h, lasting up to 21 days
Neuropathy	Multiple-dose/open-label	41	0	21/20	1.0, 0.3, 0.1, or 0.03 μg/kg rhNGF SC: 1 day every other week, 1 day per week, or 3 days per week	1 μg/kg produced myalgias, visceral pain; injection-site hyperalgesia nondose-related (S.C. 75%) MTD confirmed in patients
Diabetic neuropathy	Multiple-dose/randomized/double-blind/placebo-controlled/parallel-group	168	82	163/87	0.3 or 0.1 μg/kg rhNGF SC: 3 days per week	See section I, II pages 68–70

symptom assessment. The third group included measures considered most sensitive to small-fiber sensory function: NIS-LL, CDT, HP = 5.0.

This phase-II study was powered to detect large differences between the treatment groups. Any differences that reached a statistical difference of $p \leq .20$ were pre-specified prior to unblinding to be evidence of rhNGF's biological activity and preliminary evidence of efficacy. The results of the study indicated that subjects receiving both doses of rhNGF demonstrated a strong trend ($p = 0.17$) toward improvement in their quantitative neurological examination (NIS-LL) following 6 months of treatment compared with the placebo group. The small-fiber components of the examination were primarily responsible for the improvements in the measurement (pinprick sensation, $p = 0.01$; light touch, $p = 0.19$), whereas motor strength, reflexes, vibration and joint position sense (all large-fiber functions) were not significantly changed compared with placebo. A post-hoc responder analysis performed on the NIS-LL (carried out at the request of FDA) revealed that there was a 30% decrease in the proportion of patients in the rhNGF treatment group who worsened over the 6-month study period compared with placebo.

The neuropathy symptoms questionnaires showed no significant differences among the treatment groups, with the exception of the NSC Score, which demonstrated a trend toward improvement in the severity of symptoms in the rhNGF treatment groups ($p = 0.19$). The global symptom assessment, one question which queries the patients whether their neuropathic symptoms have changed from pre-treatment to post-treatment, revealed a strong beneficial effect of rhNGF treatment on the patients' overall perception of their neuropathic symptoms ($p = 0.001$).

The prospective multiple-endpoint analyses (O'Brien 1984) indicated rhNGF to be highly efficacious. The measures thought to be most objective, namely NIS-LL, CDT, VDT and HP = 5.0, indicated that rhNGF administration resulted in an overall improvement compared with placebo ($p = 0.032$). When more subjective values were added to the analysis (NIS-LL, CDT, VDT, HP = 5.0, NSP and the global symptom assessment), the improvement over placebo in the rhNGF treatment groups increased substantially ($p = 0.008$). When only small-fiber function tests were analyzed (NIS-LL, CDT, HP = 5.0), a highly significant beneficial effect of rhNGF administration was demonstrated ($p = 0.005$).

A trial of rhNGF in the treatment of HIV-associated neuropathy will soon be completed, in 1998. In addition to measuring the effects of rhNGF administration on the study endpoints used in the phase-II diabetic polyneuropathy study, this study evaluates the effects of rhNGF administration on neuropathic pain, using the Gracely pain scale (Max et al. 1992) as a study endpoint. This study includes a pilot evaluation of the use of skin biopsy as a morphological endpoint for measuring response to neurotrophin treatment. The effects of rhNGF on viral burden will also be examined (personal communications).

J. Interpretation of Clinical-Trial Results

Neurotrophins, including the prototype NGF, have been demonstrated in vivo to restore peripheral nerve function. However, the precise mechanism(s) by which NGF and other neurotrophins, such as NT-3, may restore nerve function is (are) unclear. Prior studies have demonstrated deficits in production and retrograde axonal transport of NGF released from sensory and sympathetic target tissues in diabetic models (JAKOBSEN et al. 1981; SCHMIDT et al. 1986; KASAYAMA and OKA 1989; FERNYHOUGH et al. 1994; HELLWEG et al. 1990, 1994; ORDONEZ et al. 1994; ANAND et al. 1996).

Systemic administration of rhNGF may bypass the need for retrograde axonal transport and allow the protein to reach sensory ganglion cells directly. This would enhance resistance of responsive neurons to injury and promote reparative mechanisms. NGF promotes the survival and morphological differentiation of sympathetic neurons and subpopulations of developing sensory neurons and stimulates neuropeptide expression (KESSLER and BLACK 1980b; MACLEAN et al. 1989). It also increases overall protein synthesis, sensory nerve-fiber sprouting, and free-radical scavenging (TIERCY and SHOOTER 1986; JACKSON et al. 1990; DIAMOND et al. 1992) among its other physiological effects on mature neurons.

Some of the benefits of rhNGF, reported in the clinical studies completed to date, including improved thermal sensation, increased normal pain perception, reduction in neuropathic pain and dysesthesias, could be related to increased neuropeptide expression rather than nerve regeneration. Some patients reported subjective improvements within the first 2 months of the rhNGF treatment period, earlier than nerve regeneration or sprouting could be anticipated. On the other hand, some of the observed improvements were still measurably improved for 1 month post-treatment, suggesting a relatively persistent – possibly structural – effect. Since animal and clinical studies suggest that neuropeptide depletion may be an important feature of diabetic neuropathy (DIEMEL et al. 1994; ANAND et al. 1996), either mechanism would be clinically significant.

K. Conclusions

rhNGF appears to be safe as well as potentially efficacious for treating symptomatic diabetes-induced peripheral sensory neuropathy. In the diabetic patients studied to date, rhNGF appears to promote improved sensory perception and reduce the severity of neuropathic symptoms. Larger and longer clinical trials of this neurotrophic agent will ultimately determine its efficacy in the treatment of peripheral sensory neuropathies.

References

Anand P, Terenghi G, Warner G, Kopelman P, Williams-Chestnut RE, Sinicropi DV (1996) The role of endogenous nerve growth factor in human diabetic neuropathy. Nat Med 2:703–707

Angeletti PU, Levi-Montalcini R (1970) Sympathetic nerve cell destruction in newborn mammals by 6-hydroxydopamine. Proc Natl Acad Sci U S A 65:114–121

Angeletti PU, Levi-Montalcini R, Caramia F (1971) Ultrastructural changes in sympathetic neurons of newborn and adult mice treated with nerve growth factor. J Ultrastruct Res 36:24–36

Apfel SC, Lipton RB, Arezzo JC, Kessler JA (1991) Nerve growth factor prevents toxic neuropathy in mice. Ann Neurol 29:87–90

Apfel SC, Arezzo JC, Lipson L, Kessler JA (1992) Nerve growth factor prevents experimental cisplatin neuropathy. Ann Neurol 31:76–80

Apfel SC, Arezzo JC, Brownlee M, Federoff H, Kessler JA (1994) Nerve growth factor administration protects against experimental diabetic sensory neuropathy. Brain Res 634:7–12

Apfel SC, Adornato BT, Cornblath D, Kessler JA, Petty B, Chaudhry V, Schwartz S, Rask CA (1995) Clinical trial of recombinant human nerve growth factor (rhNGF) in peripheral neuropathy. Neurology 45[Suppl 4]:A278–A279

Apfel SC, Kessler JA, Adornato BT, Litchy WJ, Sanders C, Rask CA and The NGF Study Group (1998) Recombinant Human Nerve Growth Factor in the Treatment of Diabetic Polyneuropathy. Neurology 50 (Sept. 1998, in Press)

Apfel SC, Kozer S, Van De Water TR (1997) Treatment of peripheral nervous system disorders. In: Apfel SC (ed) Clinical applications of neurotrophic factors. Lippincott-Raven, Philadelphia, pp 63–81

Averill S, McMahon SB, Clary DO, Reichardt LF, Priestley JV (1995) Immunocytochemical localization of trkA receptors in chemically identified subgroups of adult rat sensory neurons. Eur J Neurosci 7:1484–1494

Barbacid M (1994) The Trk family of neurotrophin receptors. J Neurobiol 25:1386–1403

Barbin G, Manthorpe M, Varon S (1984) Purification of the chick eye ciliary neurotrophic factor. J Neurochem 43:1468–1478

Barker PA, Shooter EM (1994) Disruption of NGF binding to the low affinity neurotrophin receptor p75LNTR reduces NGF binding to TrkA on PC12 cells. Neuron 13:203–215

Berg MM, Sternberg DW, Hempstead BL, Chao MV (1991) The low-affinity p75 nerve growth factor (NGF) receptor mediates NGF-induced tyrosine phosphorylation. Proc Natl Acad Sci USA 88:7106–7110

Bjerre B, Bjorklund A, Mobley W, Rosengren E (1975) Short- and long-term effects of nerve growth factor on the sympathetic nervous system in the adult mouse. Brain Res 94(2):263–277

Bleecker ML (1985) Quantifying sensory loss in peripheral neuropathies. Neurobehav Toxicol Teratol 7:305–308

Bradshaw RA (1978) Nerve growth factor. Annu Rev Biochem 47:191–216

Brewster WJ, Fernyhough P, Diemel LT, Mohiuddin L, Tomlinson DR (1994) Diabetic neuropathy, nerve growth factor and other neurotrophic factors. Trends Neurosci 17:321–325

Bueker ED (1948) Implantation of tumors in the hind limb field of the embryonic chick and the developmental response of the lumbosacral nervous system. Anat Rec 102:369–89

Buj-Bello A, Buchman VL, Horton A, Rosenthal A, Davies AM (1995) GDNF is an age-specific survival factor for sensory and autonomic neurons. Neuron 15(4):821–828

Campenot RB (1982) Development of sympathetic neurons in compartmentalized cultures. II. Local control of neurite growth by nerve growth factor. Dev Biol 93:1–12

Campenot RB (1994) NGF and the local control of nerve terminal growth. J Neurobiol 25:599–611

Chao MV, Bothwell MA, Ross AH, Koprowski H, Lanahan AA, Buck CR, Sehgal A (1986) Gene transfer and molecular cloning of the human NGF receptor. Science 232(4749):518–521

Crowley C, Spencer SD, Nishimura MC, Chen KS, Pitts-Meek S, Armanini MP, Ling LH, McMahon SB, Shelton DL, Levinson AD (1994) Mice lacking nerve growth factor display perinatal loss of sensory and sympathetic neurons yet develop basal forebrain cholinergic neurons. Cell 76:1001–1011

Davies AM, Lee KF, Jaenisch R (1993) p75-deficient trigeminal sensory neurons have an altered response to NGF but not to other neurotrophins. Neuron 11:565–574

Dechant G, Rodriguez-Tebar A, Barde YA (1994) Neurotrophin receptors. Prog Neurobiol 42:347–352

Diabetes Control and Complications Trial Research Group (DCCT) (1993) The effect of intensive treatment of diabetes on the development and progression of long-term complications in insulin-dependent diabetes mellitus. N Engl J Med 329:977–986

Diamond J, Coughlin M, Macintyre L, Holmes M, Visheau B (1987) Evidence that endogenous beta nerve growth factor is responsible for the collateral sprouting, but not the regeneration, of nociceptive axons in adult rats. Proc Natl Acad Sci USA 84:6596–6600

Diamond J, Holmes M, Coughlin M (1992) Endogenous NGF and nerve impulses regulate the collateral sprouting of sensory axons in the skin of the adult rat. J Neurosci 12:1454–1466

Diemel LT, Brewster WJ, Fernyhough P, Tomlinson DR (1994) Expression of neuropeptides in experimental diabetes; effects of treatment with nerve growth factor or brain-derived neurotrophic factor. Mol Brain Res 21(1–2):171–175

Dyck PJ (1988) Detection, characterization, and staging of polyneoropathy: assessed in diabetics. Muscle Nerve 11:21–32

Dyck PJ, O'Brien PC (1989) Meaningful degrees of prevention or improvement of nerve conduction in controlled clinical trials of diabetic neuropathy. Diabetes Care 12:649–652

Dyck PJ, Thomas PK, Asbury AK et al. (1987) Diabetic neuropathy. WB Saunders, Philadelphia

Dyck PJ, Karnes JL, O'Brien PC, Litchy WJ, Low PA, Melton LJ (1992) The Rochester diabetic neuropathy study: reassessment of tests and criteria for diagnosis and staged severity. Neurology 42:1164–1170

Dyck PJ, Peroutka S, Rask CA, Burton E, Baker MK, Lehman DA, Gillen LPN, Hokanson BA, O'Brien, PC (1997a) Intradermal recombinant human nerve growth factor induces pressure allodynia and lowered heat-pain threshold in humans. Neurology 48:501–505

Dyck PJ, Davies JL, Litchy WJ, O'Brien PC (1997b) Longitudinal assessment of diabetic polyneuropathy using a composite score in the Rochester diabetic neuropathy study cohort. Neurology 49:229–239

Eckenstein FP, Esch F, Holbert T, Blacher RW, Nishi R (1990) Purification and characterization of a trophic factor for embryonic peripheral neurons: comparison with fibroblast growth factors. Neuron 4:623–631

Eide FF, Lowenstein DH, Reichart LF (1993) Neurotrophins and their receptors-current concepts and implications for neurologic disease. Exp Neurol 121:200–214

English KB, Harper S, Stayner N, Wang ZM, Davies AM (1994) Localization of nerve growth factor (NGF) and low-affinity NGF receptors in touch domes and quantification of NGF mRNA in keratinocytes of adult rats. J Comp Neurol 344:470–480

Escandon E, Chao MV (1989) Developmental expression of the chicken nerve growth factor receptor gene during brain morphogenesis. Brain Res Dev 47:187–196

Escandon E, Burton LE, Szonyi E, Nikolics K (1993) Characterization of neurotrophin receptors by affinity crosslinking. J Neurosci Res 34(6):601–613

Escandon E, Soppet D, Rosenthal A, Mendoza-Ramirez JL, Szonyi E, Burton LE, Henderson CE, Parada LF, Nikolics K (1994) Regulation of neurotrophin receptor expression during embryonic and postnatal development. J Neurosci 14:2054–2068

Ewing DJ, Clarke BF (1987) Diabetic autonomic neuropathy: a clinical viewpoint. In: Diabetic neuropathy. W.B. Saunders, Philadelphia, p 66

Faradji V, Sotelo J (1990) Low serum levels of nerve growth factor in diabetic neuropathy. Acta Neurol Scand 81:402–406

Fernyhough P, Brewster WJ, Diemel LT, Tomlinson DR (1993) Nerve growth factor mRNA in diabetic rat sciatic nerve: effects of neurotrophic factor treatment. Br J Pharmacol 110:1P–186P

Fernyhough P, Diemel LT, Brewster WJ, Tomlinson DR (1994) Deficits in sciatic nerve neuropeptide content coincide with a reduction in target tissue nerve growth factor messenger RNA in streptozotocin-diabetic rats: effects of insulin treatment. Neuroscience 62:337–344

Fernyhough P, Diemel LT, Brewster WJ, Tomlinson DR (1995) Altered neurotrophin mRNA levels in peripheral nerve and skeletal muscle of experimentally diabetic rats. J Neurochem 64:1231–1237

Gao WQ, Dybdal N, Shinsky N, Murname A, Schmelzer C, Siegel M, Keller G, Hefti F, Phillips H, Winslow JW (1995) Neurotrophin-3 reverses experimental cisplatin-induced peripheral sensory neuropathy. Ann Neurol 38:30–37

Goedert M, Otten U, Thoenen H (1978) Biochemical effects of antibodies against nerve growth factor on developing and differentiated sympathetic ganglia. Brain Res 148:264–268

Goedert M, Stoeckel K, Otten U (1981) Biological importance of the retrograde axonal transport of nerve growth factor in sensory neurons. Proc Natl Acad Sci USA 78:5895–5898

Gold BG, Mobley WC, Matheson SF. (1991) Regulation of axonal caliber, neurofilament content, and nuclear localization in mature sensory neurons by nerve growth factor. J Neurosci 11:943–955

Gorin PD, Johnson EM Jr (1980) Effects of long-term nerve growth factor deprivation on the nervous system of the adult rat: an experimental autoimmune approach. Brain Res 198:27–42

Hayakawa K, Sobue G, Itoh T, Mitsuma T (1994) Nerve growth factor prevents neurotoxic effects of cisplatin, vincristine and taxol, on adult rat sympathetic ganglion explants in vitro. Life Sci 55(7):519–525

Hellweg R, Hartung HD (1990) Endogenous levels of nerve growth factor (NGF) are altered in experimental diabetes mellitus: a possible role for NGF in the pathogenesis of diabetic neuropathy. J Neurosci Res 26:258–267

Hellweg R, Wohrle M, Hartung HD, Stracke H, Hock C, Federlin K (1991) Diabetes mellitus-associated decrease in nerve growth factor levels is reversed by allogenic pancreatic islet transplantation. Neurosci Lett 125:1–4

Hellweg R, Raivich G, Hartung HD, Hock C, Kreutzberg GW (1994) Axonal transport of endogenous nerve growth factor (NGF) and NGF receptor in experimental diabetic neuropathy. Exp Neurol 130:24–30

Hempstead BL, Martin-Zanca D, Kaplan DR, Parada LF, Chao MV (1991) High-affinity NGF binding requires coexpression of the trk proto-oncogene and the low-affinity NGF receptor. Nature 350:678–683

Henderson CE, Phillips HS, Pollack RA, Davies AM, Lemeulle C, Armanini M, Simmons L, Moffet B, Vandlen RA, Simpson LC (1994) GDNF: a potent survival factor for motoneurons present in peripheral nerve and muscle. Science 266(5187):1062–1064

Heumann R, Korsching S, Scott J, Thoenen H (1984) Relationship between levels of nerve growth factor (NGF) and its messenger RNA in sympathetic ganglia and peripheral target tissues. EMBO J 3:3183–3189

Heumann R, Korsching S, Bandtlow C, Thoenen H (1987) Changes of nerve growth factor synthesis in nonneuronal cells in response to sciatic nerve transection. J Cell Biol 104:1623–1631

referHoyle GW, Mercer EH, Palmiter RD, Brinster RL (1993) Expression of NGF in sympathetic neurons leads to excessive axon outgrowth from ganglia but decreased terminal innervation within tissues. Neuron 10:1019–1034

Hruska RE, Chertack MM, Kravis D (1993) Elevation of nerve growth factor receptor-truncated in the urine of patients with diabetic neuropathy. Ann NY Acad Sci 679:349–351

Jackson GR, Apffel L, Werrbach-Perez K, Perez-Polo JR (1990) Role of nerve growth factor in oxidant-antioxidant balance and neuronal injury. I. Stimulation of hydrogen peroxidase resistance. J Neurosci Res 25:360–368

Jakobsen J, Brimijoin S, Skau K, Sidenius P, Wells D (1981) Retrograde axonal transport of transmitter enzymes, fucose-labeled protein, and nerve growth factor in streptozotocin-diabetic rats. Diabetes 30:797–803

Johnson EM Jr, Andres RY, Bradshaw RA (1978) Characterization of the retrograde transport of nerve growth factor (NGF) using high specific activity [^{125}I] NGF. Brain Res 150:319–331

Johnson EM Jr, Rich KM, Yip HR (1986) The role of NGF in sensory neurons in vivo. Trends Neurosci 9:33–37

Kaplan DR, Stephens RM (1994) Neurotrophin signal transduction by the Trk receptor. J Neurobiol 25:1404–1417

Kaplan DR, Hempstead BL, Martin-Zanca D, Chao MV, Parada LF (1991) The trk proto-oncogene product: a signal transducing receptor for nerve growth factor. Science 252:554–558

Kasayama S, Oka T (1989) Impaired production of nerve growth factor in submandibular gland of diabetic mice. Am J Physiol 257:E400–E404

Kashiba H, Noguchi K, Ueda Y, Senba E (1995) Coexpression of trk family members and low-affinity neurotrophin receptors in rat dorsal root ganglion neurons. Brain Res Mol Brain Res 30:158–164

Kessler JA, Black IB (1980a) Nerve growth factor stimulates the development of substance P in sensory ganglia. Proc Natl Acad Sci USA 77:113–122

Kessler JA, Black IB (1980b) The effects of nerve growth factor (NGF) and antiserum to NGF on the development of embryonic sympathetic neurons in vivo. Brain Res 189:157–168

Kessler JA, Black IB (1981) Similarities in development of substance P and somatostatin in peripheral sensory neurons: effects of capsaicin and nerve growth factor. Proc Natl Acad Sci USA 78:4644–4647

Konings PN, Makkink WK, van Delft AM, Ruigt GS (1994) Reversal by NGF of cytostatic drug-induced reduction of neurite outgrowth in rat dorsal root ganglia in vitro. Brain Res 640(1–2):195–204

Korsching S, Thoenen H (1983) Nerve growth factor in sympathetic ganglia and corresponding target organs of the rat: correlation with density of sympathetic innervation. Proc Natl Acad Sci USA 80:3513–3516

Korsching S, Heumann R, Thoenen H, Hefti F (1986) Cholinergic denervation of the rat hippocampus by fimbrial transection leads to a transient accumulation of nerve growth factor (NGF) without change in mRNANGF content. Neurosci Lett 66:175–180

Kotzbauer PT, Lampe PA, Estus S, Milbrandt J, Johnson Jr EM (1994) Postnatal development of survival responsiveness in rat sympathetic neurons to leukemia inhibitory factor and ciliary neurotrophic factor. Neuron 12:763–773

Kotzbauer PT, Lampe PA, Heuckeroth RO, Golden JP, Creedon DJ, Johnson EM Jr., Milbrandt J (1996) Neurturin, a relative of glial-derived-cell-line-derived neurotrophic factor. Nature 384(6608):467–470

Large TH, Weskamp G, Helder JC, Radeke MJ, Misko TP, Shooter EM, Reichardt LF (1989) Structure and developmental expression of the nerve growth factor receptor in the chicken central nervous system. Neuron 2:1123–1134

Lee KF, Li E, Huber LJ, Landis SC, Sharpe AH, Chao MV, Jaenisch R (1992) Targeted mutation of the gene encoding the low affinity NGF receptor p75 leads to deficits in the peripheral sensory nervous system. Cell 69:737–749

Lee KF, Bachman K, Landis S, Jaenisch R (1994) Dependence on p75 for innervation of some sympathetic targets. Science 263(5152):1447–1449

Levi-Montalcini R (1972) The morphological effects of immunosymphathectomy. In: Steiner G, Schonbaum E (eds) Immunosymphathectomy. Elsevier, Amsterdam, pp 55–78

Levi-Montalcini R (1983) The nerve growth factor-target cells interaction: a model system for the study of directed axonal growth and regeneration. In: Huner B, Perez-Polo JR, Hashim GA, Stella AM (eds) Nervous system regeneration. Proceedings of an International Symposium, Satellite Meetings of International Society for Neurochemistry. 1981 Sept. Catania, Italy. Alan R. Liss, New York

Levi-Montalcini R (1987) The nerve growth factor 35 years later. Science 237:1154–1162

Levi-Montalcini R, Hamburger V (1951) Selective growth stimulating effects of mouse sarcoma on the sensory and sympathetic nervous system of the chick embryo. J Exp Zool 116:321–362

Levi-Montalcini R, Hamburger V (1953) A diffusible agent of mouse sarcoma, producing hyperplasia of sympathetic ganglia and hyperneurotization of viscera in the chick embryo. J Exp Zool 123:233–288

Levi-Montalcini R, Meyer H, Hamburger V (1954) In vitro experiments on the effects of mouse sarcomas 180 and 37 on the spinal and sympathetic ganglia of the chick embryo. Cancer Res 14:49–57

Lin LF, Doherty DH, Lile JD, Bektesh S, Collins F (1993) GDNF: a glial cell line – derived neurotrophic factor for midbrain dopaminergic neurons Science 260(5111):1130–1132

Lindsay RM, Harmar AJ (1989) Nerve growth factor regulates expression of neuropeptide genes in adult sensory neurons. Nature 337:362–364

Lipton RB, Apfel SC, Dutcher JP, Rosenberg R, Kaplan J, Berger A, Einzig AI, Wiernik P, Schaumburg HH (1989) Taxol produces a predominantly sensory neuropathy. Neurology 39:368–373

Llewelyn JG, Gilbey SG, Thomas PK, King RH, Muddle JR, Watkins PJ (1991) Sural nerve morphometry in diabetic autonomic and painful sensory neuropathy. A clinic pathological study. Brain 114(Pt 2):867–892

Longo FM, Holtzman DM, Grimes ML, Mobley WC (1993) Nerve growth factor: actions in the peripheral and central nervous system. In: Loughlin SE, Fallon JH (eds) Neurotrophic factors. Academic Press, Orlando, pp 209–256

MacLean DB, Bennett B, Morris M, Wheeler FB (1989) Differential regulation of calcitonin gene related peptide in substance P in cultured neonatal rat vagal sensory neurons. Brain Res 478:349–355

Malgrange B, Delree P, Rigo JM, Baron H, Moonen G (1994) Image analysis of neuritic regeneration by adult rat dorsal root ganglion neurons in culture: quantification of the neurotoxicity of anticancer agents and of its prevention by nerve growth factor or basic fibroblast growth factor but not brain-derived neurotrophic factor or neurotrophin-3. J Neurosci Methods 53:111–122

Max MB, Lunch SA, Muir J, Shoaf SE, Smoller B, Dubner R (1992) Effects of desipramine, amitriptyline, and fluoxetine on pain in diabetic neuropathy. N Engl J Med 326:1250–1256

McMahon SB, Priestley JV (1995) Peripheral neuropathies and neurotrophic factors: animal models and clinical perspectives. Curr Opin Neurobiol 5:616–624

McMahon SB, Armanini MP, Ling LH, Phillips HS (1994) Expression and coexpression of Trk receptors in subpopulations of adult primary sensory neurons projecting to identified peripheral targets. Neuron 12:1161–1171

Mense S (1990) Structure function relationships in identified afferent neurones. Anat Embryol 181:1–17

Mollman JE (1990) Cisplatin neurotoxicity (editorial). N Engl J Med 322:126–127

Mu X, Silos-Santiago I, Carroll SL, Snider WD (1993) Neurotrophin receptor genes are expressed in distinct patterns in developing dorsal root ganglia. J Neurosci 13:4029–4041

O'Brien PC (1984) Procedures for comparing samples with multiple endpoints. Biometrics 40:1079–1087

Ordonez G, Fernandez A, Perez A, Sotelo J (1994) Low contents of nerve growth factor in serum and submaxillary gland of diabetic mice. A possible etiological element of diabetic neuropathy. J Neurol Sci 121:163–166

Peripheral Nerve Society (1995) Diabetic polyneuropathy in controlled clinical trials: consensus report of the peripheral nerve society. Ann Neurol 38:478–482

Petty BG, Cornblath DR, Adornato BT, Chaudhry V, Flexner C, Wachsman M, Sinicropi D, Burton LE, Peroutka SJ (1994) The effect of systemically administered recombinant human nerve growth factor in healthy human subjects. Ann Neurol 36:244–246

Purves D, Lichtman JW (1985) Trophic effects of targets on neurons. Principles of neural development. Sinauer, Boston, pp 155–178

Radeke MJ, Misko TP, Hsu C, Herzenberg LA, Shooter EM (1987) Gene transfer and molecular cloning of the rat nerve growth factor receptor. Nature 325:593–597

Raffioni S, Bradshaw RA, Buxser SE (1993) The receptors for nerve growth factor and other neurotrophins. Annu Rev Biochem 62:823–850

Rask CA, Apfel SC, Adornato BT, Cornblath D, Kessler J, Petty B, Chaudhry V, Schwartz S, Dyck P, Burton LE (1995) An overview of the clinical experience with systemic administration of nerve growth factor in treating peripheral nervous system disorders. Ann Neurol 38:317

Recio-Pinto E, Reichler MM, Ishii DN (1986) Effects of insulin, insulin like growth factor-II, and nerve growth factor on neurite formation and survival in cultured sympathetic and sensory neurons. J Neurosci 6:1211–1219

Rich KM, Yip HK, Osborne PA, Schmidt RE, Johnson EM Jr (1984) Role of nerve growth factor in the adult dorsal root ganglia neuron and its response to injury. J Comp Neurol 230:110–118

Richardson PM, Issa VM, Riopelle RJ (1986) Distribution of neuronal receptors for nerve growth factor in the rat. J Neurosci 6:2312–2321

Rodriguez-Tebar A, Dechant G, Barde YA (1990) Binding of brain-derived neurotrophic factor to the nerve growth factor receptor. Neuron 4:487–492

Rodriguez-Tebar A, Dechant G, Gotz R, Barde YA (1992) Binding of neurotrophin-3 to its neuronal receptors and interactions with nerve growth factor and brain-derived neurotrophic factor. EMBO J 11:917–922

Roelofs RI, Hrushesky W, Rogin J, Rosenberg L (1984) Peripheral sensory neuropathy and cisplatin chemotherapy. Neurology 34:934–938

Ruit KG, Elliott JL (1992) Selective dependence of mammalian dorsal root ganglion neurons on nerve growth factor during embryonic development. Neuron 8:573–587

Ruit KG, Osborne PA, Schmidt RE (1990) Nerve growth factor regulates sympathetic ganglion cell morphology and survival in the adult mouse. J Neurosci 10:2412–2419

Rush RA, Mayo R, Zettler C (1995) The regulation of nerve growth factor synthesis and delivery to peripheral neurons. Pharmacol Ther 65:93–123

Said G, Slama G, Selva J (1983) Progressive centripetal degeneration of axons in small fibre diabetic polyneuropathy. Brain 106(Pt 4):791–807

Saltiel AR, Decker SJ (1994) Cellular mechanisms of signal transduction for neurotrophins. Bioessays 16:405–411

Sango K, Verdes JM, Hikawa N, Horie H, Tanaka S, Inoue S, Sotelo JR, Takenaka T (1994) Nerve growth factor (NGF) restores depletions of calcitonin gene-related peptide and substance P in sensory neurons from diabetic mice in vitro. J Neurol Sci 126:1–5

Schmidt RE (1993) The role of nerve growth factor in the pathogenesis and therapy of diabetic neuropathy. Diabet Med 10 [Suppl 2]:10S–13S

Schmidt RE, Nelson JS, Johnson EM Jr (1981) Experimental diabetic autonomic neuropathy. Am J Pathol 103:210–225

Schmidt RE, Modert CW, Yip HK, Johnson EM Jr (1983) Retrograde axonal transport of intravenously administered ^{125}I-nerve growth factor in rats with streptozotocin-induced diabetes. Diabetes 32:654–663

Schmidt RE, Yip HK (1985) Retrograde axonal transport in rat ileal mesenteric nerves. Characterization using intravenously administered ^{125}I-nerve growth factor and effect of chemical sympathectomy. Diabetes 34:1222–1229

Schmidt RE, Plurad SB, Saffitz JE, Grabau GG, Yip HK (1985) Retrograde axonal transport of ^{125}I-nerve growth factor in rat ileal mesenteric nerves. Effect of streptozocin diabetes. Diabetes 34:1230–1240

Schmidt RE, Grabau GG, Yip HK (1986) Retrograde axonal transport of [^{125}I] nerve growth factor in ileal mesenteric nerves in vitro: effect of streptozotocin diabetes. Brain Res 378:325–336

Schwartz JP, Pearson J, Johnson EM (1982) Effect of exposure to anti-NGF on sensory neurons of adult rats and guinea pigs. Brain Res 244:378–381

Shelton DL, Reichardt LF (1984) Expression of the beta-nerve growth factor gene correlates with the density of sympathetic innervation in effector organs. Proc Natl Acad Sci USA 81:7951–7955

Shelton DL, Sutherland J, Gripp J, Camerato T, Armanini MP, Phillips HS, Carroll K, Spencer SD, Levinson AD (1995) Human trks: molecular cloning, tissue distribution, and expression of extracellular domain immunoadhesins. J Neurosci 15(1 Pt 2):477–491

Smeyne RJ, Klein R, Schnapp A, Long LK, Bryant S, Lewin A, Lira SA, Barbacid M (1994) Severe sensory and sympathetic neuropathies in mice carrying a disrupted Trk/NGF receptor gene. Nature 368:246–249

Snider WD (1988) Nerve growth factor enhances dendritic arborization of sympathetic ganglion cells in developing mammals. J Neurosci 8:2628–2634

Snider WD (1994) Functions of the neurotrophins during nervous system development: what the knockouts are teaching us. Cell 77:627–638

Sobue G, Yasuda T, Mitsuma T, Ross AH, Pleasure D (1988) Expression of nerve growth factor receptor in human peripheral neuropathies. Ann Neurol 24:64–72

Stockel K, Schwab M, Thoenen H (1975) Comparison between the retrograde axonal transport of nerve growth factor and tetanus toxin in motor, sensory and adrenergic neurons. Brain Res 99:1–16

Sugimura K, Dyck PJ (1981) Sural nerve myelin thickness and axis cylinder caliber in human diabetes. Neurology 31:1087–1091

Sutter A, Riopelle RJ, Harris-Warrick RM, Shooter EM (1979) Nerve growth factor receptors. Characterization of two distinct classes of binding sites on chick embryo sensory ganglia cells. J Biol Chem 254:5972–5982

Taniuchi M, Schweitzer JB, Johnson EM Jr (1986) Nerve growth factor receptor molecules in rat brain. Proc Natl Acad Sci USA 83:1950–1954

Taniuchi M, Clark HB, Schweitzer JB, Johnson EM Jr (1988) Expression of nerve growth factor receptors by Schwann cells of axotomized peripheral nerves: ultrastructural location, suppression by axonal contact, and binding properties. J Neurosci 8:664–681

Thoenen H, Barde YA (1980) Physiology of nerve growth factor. Physiol Rev 60:1284–1335

Thoenen H, Angeletti PU, Levi-Montalcini R, Kettler R (1971) Selective induction by nerve growth factor of tyrosine hydroxylase and dopamine-hydroxylase in the rat superior cervical ganglia. Proc Natl Acad Sci USA 68:1598–1602

Thoenen H, Bandtlow C, Heumann R (1987) The physiological function of nerve growth factor in the central nervous system: comparison with the periphery. Rev Physiol Biochem Pharmacol 109:145–178

Thomas PK (1994) Growth factors and diabetic neuropathy. Diabet Med 11:732–739

Tiercy JM, Shooter EM (1986) Early changes in the synthesis of nuclear and cytoplasmic proteins are induced by nerve growth factor in differentiating rat PC12 cells. J Cell Biol 103:2367–2378

Trupp M, Ryden, Jornvall H, Funakoshi H, Timmusk T, Arenas E, Ibanez CF (1995) Peripheral expression and biological activities of GDNF, a new neurotrophic factor for avian and mammalian peripheral neurons. J Cell Biol 130(1):137–148

Ullrich A, Gray A, Berman C, Dull TJ (1983) Human beta–nerve growth factor gene sequence highly homologous to that of mouse. Nature 303:821–825

Vantini G (1992) The pharmacological potential of neurotrophins: a perspective. Psychoneuroendocrinology 17:401–410

Verge VM, Richardson PM, Benoit R, Riopelle RJ (1989) Histochemical characterization of sensory neurons with high-affinity receptors for nerve growth factor. J Neurocytol 18:583–591

Verge VM, Richardson PM, Wiesenfeld-Hallin Z, Hokfelt T (1995) Differential influence of nerve growth factor on neuropeptide expression in vivo: a novel role in peptide suppression in adult sensory neurons. J Neurosci 15(3 Pt 1):2081–2096

Verge VMK, Merlioo JP, Grondin J, Emfors P, Perrson H, Riopelle RJ, Hokfelt T, Richardson PM (1992) Colocalization of NGF binding sites, trk RNA, and low affinity NGF mRNA in primary sensory neurons: response to injury and infusion of NGF. J Neurosci 12:4011–4022

Wetmore C, Olson L (1995) Neuronal and nonneuronal expression of neurotrophins and their receptors in sensory and sympathetic ganglia suggest new intercellular trophic interactions. J Comp Neurol 353:143–159

Wiernik PH, Schwartz EL, Einzig A, Strauman JJ, Lipton RB, Dutcher JP (1987) Phase I trial of taxol given as a 24-hour infusion every 21 days: responses observed in metastatic melanoma. J Clin Oncol 5(8):1232–1239

Wright DE, Snider WD (1995) Neurotrophin receptor mRNA expression defines distinct populations of neurons in rat dorsal root ganglia. J Comp Neurol 351:329–338

Yamamoto M, Kondo H, Iseki S (1992) Nerve growth factor receptor NGFR-like immunoreactivity in the perineurial cell in normal and sectioned peripheral nerves of rats. Anat Rec 233:301–308

Zettler C, Head RJ, Rush RA (1991) Chronic nerve growth factor treatment of normotensive rats. Brain Res 538:251–262

CHAPTER 4

Neurotrophic Factors and Amyotrophic Lateral Sclerosis

M. Sendtner

A. Introduction

I. Developmental Cell Death of Motoneurons

In higher vertebrates, motoneurons are generated in excess during embryonic development, and a significant proportion of the newly generated cells that have already, at that time, made functional contact with their target field, the skeletal muscle, are eliminated. In 6-day-old chick embryos, the lumbar part of the spinal cord contains about 20000 motoneurons, of which about 8000 are lost until embryonic day 12 (see Oppenheim 1991 for review). This loss of motoneurons has been named "physiological cell death" in contrast to "pathological cell death" which is characteristic of various forms of motoneuron disease. Such diseases lead to paresis of the musculature and finally result in death, in most cases, as a consequence of respiratory failure (see Smith 1992, for review). As the cellular mechanisms underlying the various forms of human motoneuron disease (MND) are still incompletely understood, the embryonic form of motoneuron loss serves as an important model for these diseases.

Experiments performed to understand the mechanisms of developmental cell death of motoneurons have played an essential role in establishing the concept that target tissues influence the development of innervating neurons. Experiments in the first half of this century showed that the removal of leg or wing buds in early chick embryos leads to virtually complete loss of corresponding motoneurons (Hamburger 1934, 1958). Conversely, the implantation of an additional limb anlage results in an increase of the number of motoneurons projecting into the enlarged target area (Hollyday and Hamburger 1975).

These experiments were the first steps in the discovery of the nerve growth factor (NGF). However, the replacement of target tissue by sarcoma tissue (Levi-Montalcini et al. 1954) did not lead to an increased number of motoneurons, but only to enhanced cell numbers of sympathetic neurons in the paravertebral ganglia and subpopulations of sensory neurons. A series of experiments has shown that NGF is produced in the target of these neurons and is retrogradely transported in the axons to the cell bodies, after binding to specific receptors (see Thoenen and Barde 1980, for review). These findings with NGF have guided research in the field of neurotrophic factors for motoneurons. Throughout the past decades, researchers have concentrated on discovering factors with analogous function for motoneurons.

Despite this strong evidence that one or more neurotrophic factors exist in skeletal muscle and regulate motoneuron survival during development (reviewed by THOENEN et al. 1993), molecules with survival-promoting effects on embryonic motoneurons were only identified in the last 10 years. This list now includes molecules of several gene families and is still incomplete. None of the factors identified so far seems to be the physiological neurotrophic factor from skeletal muscle that regulates survival of developing motoneurons.

Important steps which helped to identify such molecules were improved cell culture methods for isolated motoneurons. For example, the survival effects of semi-purified CNTF were missed in earlier experiments applying mixed spinal cord cultures (LONGO et al. 1982). They were only discovered when techniques for enrichment and appropriate survival (not only of minor subpopulations of isolated motoneurons) were developed (O'BRIEN and FISCHBACH 1986; ARAKAWA et al. 1990; CAMU and HENDERSON 1992). Nevertheless, despite the discovery of many factors with survival-promoting activities on motoneurons, it is still unclear which of these molecules regulates motoneuron survival during the period of developmental cell death, and what the specific functions of these factors are for motoneurons during postnatal development. Therefore, all attempts to apply these factors as drug candidates for the treatment of human motoneuron disease have to be considered as preliminary and serve as part of the puzzle which has to be solved in understanding both the molecular mechanisms leading to motoneuron disease and the specific function of neurotrophic factors for survival, and the function of motoneurons during postnatal development.

II. Pathological Cell Death of Motoneurons and Human Motoneuron Disease

Amyotrophic lateral sclerosis (ALS) is a neurodegenerative disorder which mainly affects motoneurons in the spinal cord and brain stem, as well as neurons in the motor cortex (CHOU 1992). More than 90% of all cases appear sporadic; approximately 5%–10% of cases are inherited. The molecular mechanisms of this disease are still far from being understood. Therefore, great efforts have been made in the last 10 years to identify the gene defects responsible for the inherited forms (Table 1). Both autosomal recessive and dominant forms of familial ALS are distinguished. Mutations have been identified in the gene for superoxide dismutase-1 (SOD-1) on chromosome 21q33 in about 20% of the cases of autosomal dominant ALS (ROSEN et al. 1993). Other cases of autosomal dominant forms of motoneuron disease (spastic paraplegia), characterized by degeneration of the neurons in the motor cortex, have been linked to chromosome 2p (HENTATI et al. 1994a), 14q and 15q.

Cases of autosomal recessive ALS are linked to chromosome 2q33-q35 (HENTATI et al. 1994b); autosomal recessive familial spastic paraplegia links to

Table 1. Inherited forms of motoneuron disease

Disease	Defect	Locus	Reference
Lower motoneuron disease			
Spinal muscular atrophy	SMN, NAIP	5q13	Roy et al., 1995, Lefebvre et al. 1995
X-linked spinal muscular atrophy	Androgen receptor	Xq11	LaSpada et al. 1991
Upper and lower motoneuron disease (ALS)			
Autosomal dominant ALS	SOD-1	21q33	Rosen et al. 1993
Autosomal recessive ALS	?	2q33-q35	Hentati et al. 1994b
Juvenile-onset ALS with Parkinsonism and frontotemporal dementia	?	17	Wilhelmsen et al. 1994
Upper motoneuron disease			
Autosomal-dominant familial spastic paraplegia	?	2p	Hentati et al. 1994a
	?	14q	Hazan et al. 1993
	?	15q	Fink et al. 1995
Autosomal-recessive familial spastic paraplegia	?	8q	Hentati et al. 1994c

chromosome 8 (Hentati et al. 1994c). Spinal muscular atrophy, which is the most common form of motoneuron disease in childhood, is linked to chromosome 5q13, and two candidate genes (survival motor neuron gene *SMN* and neural apoptosis inhibitory gene *NAIP*) have been identified in this region (Lefebvre et al. 1995; Roy et al. 1995).

Another form of spinal muscular atrophy (SMA) has been linked to the X-chromosome. It is the only form of motoneuron disease, known so far, that is caused by a trinucleotide (CAG) expansion located in the gene for androgen receptors (La Spada et al. 1991). Affected men develop muscle paralysis, which is (in contrast to ALS) usually symmetrical and slowly progressive. In many cases, brain-stem motoneurons are affected, which leads to difficulties in swallowing and articulation. Heterozygous female carriers of this gene alteration appear healthy. Histological analysis in autopsy cases has shown that sensory neurons in dorsal root ganglia (DRG) are also reduced in number (Sobue et al. 1989).

The androgen receptor belongs to a family of steroid, thyroid-hormone receptors. The CAG expansion is localized within the first exon of the androgen-receptor gene. Usually, about 10–30 CAG triplets are found within this gene in healthy individuals; patients with X-linked SMA have 20–60 CAG triplets. This leads to an expanded polyglutamine domain within the androgen receptor protein. However, the hormone-binding domain of the protein is not affected (BROOKS and FISCHBECK 1995). Also, the ability of the mutated protein to bind DNA is preserved. Therefore, it is assumed that the alteration leads to changes in transcriptional activity.

Interestingly, loss of androgen receptor function does not lead to motoneuron disease. Other mutations of this gene, abolishing its biological activity, are known to cause testicular feminization. Affected individuals are male by XY karyotype (genotype), but are phenotypically female. The symptoms of this disease are caused by unresponsiveness of various organs to androgens. Such patients are not affected by motoneuron disease. Therefore, gene-therapeutic approaches to transfer a "normal" androgen-receptor gene to patients with X-linked SMA do not appear promising. In contrast, approaches such as treatment with "anti-androgens" (BROOKS and FISCHBECK 1995) or interference with the mechanisms which are the down-stream effectors of cell death in motoneurons are discussed as strategies that should be tested in the future.

In addition to these well-characterized familial forms of motoneuron disease, a variety of additional loci have been identified by linkage studies (summarized by SIDDIQUE et al. 1996), indicating that even the familial forms of motoneuron disease, which are less frequent than sporadic ALS, represent a heterogeneous group. This variety of gene defects underlying familial motoneuron disease indicates that motoneuron disease, and in particular ALS, are heterogeneous disorders that can be caused by a variety of cellular mechanisms leading to the same phenotype, namely the degeneration of motoneurons. Patients with sporadic ALS have been screened for defects in SOD-1, SMN and NAIP genes (JONES et al. 1993; JACKSON et al. 1996). Mutations in these genes have been identified only in very few cases, and it is not clear whether they play a crucial role for the pathogenesis of the disease. Thus, it has to be assumed that additional mechanisms exist that are responsible for the development of motoneuron disease in the majority of sporadic ALS cases.

III. Why Should Neurotrophic Factors Interfere with the Pathogenic Mechanisms in Sporadic ALS?

Only very little is known about the mechanisms that contribute to the degeneration of motoneurons in sporadic ALS. The clinical appearance of the disease is quite heterogeneous (SMITH 1992). In addition, multiple gene defects, found in familial forms of motoneuron disease (SIDDIQUE et al. 1996), point to the existence of various genetic and epigenetic mechanisms which could be responsible for the disease. Variances exist, in particular with respect to the onset of disease, the disease progression and the involvement of different subpopulations of motoneurons. Most ALS patients are older than 50 years when the first symptoms occur, but younger patients have also been reported. The interval from first symptoms to complete failure of the respiratory musculature or other important body functions can vary between a few months and more than 30 years. In addition, the involvement of upper motoneurons varies from case to case. Subgroups of the disease can be distinguished by the predominant involvement of bulbar versus spinal motoneurons. This distinction has been relevant for the treatment effect of an anti-glutamatergic drug, Riluzole (BENSIMON et al. 1994).

This heterogeneity of ALS makes it very difficult to predict which treatment strategy might be successful. All clinical studies using drug candidates that should interfere with presumptive disease mechanisms have shown that some patients show positive treatment effects (if any), whereas the majority of treated patients do not differ from untreated controls. The absence of molecular markers that could help to define subgroups of ALS patients and the restriction to measure the outcome of treatment studies only by clinical signs, such as muscle strength, respiratory parameters or survival time, limit the conclusions which can be drawn from previous clinical tests. For example, drug candidates or mechanisms which lead to significantly improved survival of motoneuron cell bodies, without any positive effects on the degeneration of axons (SAGOT et al. 1995a), would not be recognized by the trial designs currently applied. This might be relevant, in particular for trials with neurotrophic factors. For example, treatment with glial-derived neurotrophic factor (GDNF) significantly rescues motoneuron cell bodies, but not the peripheral axons in an animal model, the *pmn* mouse, and, thus, does not lead to increased muscle strength or prolonged survival time of the animals (SAGOT et al. 1996). The same effect can be seen in *pmn* or wobbler mice in which the anti-apoptotic gene *bcl-2* is overexpressed (AIT IKHLEF et al. 1995; SAGOT et al. 1995a). Therefore, such positive effects would be missed in clinical trials with ALS patients.

Recent data have shown that overexpression of *bcl-2* can delay the onset of disease in mice transgenic for a mutated form of SOD-1, but not the duration of the disease (KOSTIC et al. 1997). Such data are, at the moment, without relevance for the treatment of sporadic cases of ALS caused by the same disease mechanism, as the disease is only recognized after the first symptoms have occurred.

Histological analysis at autopsy has shown that the extent of motoneuron loss in ALS is very variable (CHOU 1992). This has been discussed as a consequence of the fact that the disease can start in any group of motoneurons (cortical, bulbar or spinal motoneurons) and progresses to other groups of motoneurons without any recognizable regularity. Interestingly, the motoneurons in the third, fourth and fifth brain-stem motor nuclei are spared in most cases, and α-motoneurons in the spinal cord are usually much more affected than γ-motoneurons which innervate the muscle spindles.

Occasionally, no loss of motoneurons is observed by autopsy in patients who have been clinically diagnosed as ALS (CHOU 1992), suggesting that loss of motoneuron function and motoneuron cell death do not appear synchronously, but successively. This is important for the design of therapeutic approaches. Degeneration of the motor endplates, which are the most distal structures of the motoneurons, leads to muscle denervation, which guides the clinical appearance of this disease. However, time intervals of several years can exist between this event and cell death of the corresponding motoneuron cell body. During this time, compensatory effects, by sprouting of neighboring motoneurons which are still functional, are usually observed. The time interval between loss of motoneuron function and the ultimate death of the cells makes the use of neurotrophic factors very attractive: a variety of experiments has shown that these factors can:

1. induce regrowth of axons which have lost contact with their target cell
2. induce sprouting and, thus, at least partial re-innervation of denervated muscle fibers
3. increase transmitter synthesis and
4. help to maintain the motoneurons which are still functional when initial disease symptoms are seen.

The latter of these points is still controversial. Indeed, it is not known, so far, whether the cell death of motoneurons in sporadic ALS is apoptotic or necrotic. The histomorphological analysis indicates that the shrinkage of the cells, the changes in chromatin structure, the absence of inflammatory cells and the apparently random distribution of dying cells (HIRANO and IWATA 1979) in the tissue argue in favor of apoptotic cell death. As most neurotrophic factors have been shown to prevent apoptotic neuronal cell death under a variety of experimental conditions both in vivo and in vitro, it is very likely that they should also interfere with at least some of the cellular mechanisms responsible for human ALS. Of course, such effects are only expected at stages when many motoneurons are still alive, and not at late stages of the disease when most motoneurons have already been lost.

IV. Ciliary Neurotrophic Factor (CNTF) and Related Molecules

CNTF has originally been identified as a survival-promoting activity for cultured embryonic-chick ciliary neurons, present in high quantities in chick-eye extracts (ADLER et al. 1979; BARBIN et al. 1984). When this protein was purified from chick-eye extracts, it became apparent that extracts of adult rat sciatic nerves contained a protein with very similar biochemical and biological properties (MANTHORPE et al. 1986). This activity was purified to homogeneity, and the corresponding gene was cloned (LIN et al. 1989; STÖCKLI et al. 1989). CNTF lacks a hydrophobic signal peptide and is not released from transfected cell lines. Moreover, it is not expressed during embryonic development at a time when physiological cell death of motoneurons occurs.

1. The CNTF Receptor Complex: Actions of Leukemia Inhibitory Factor, Oncostatin M and Cardiotrophin-1 Are Mediated Through Shared Receptor Subunits

CNTF acts on responsive neurons via a receptor complex involving at least 3 subunits (STAHL and YANCOPOULOS 1994). The low affinity receptor CNTFRα exists both in membrane bound form and as a soluble binding protein in body fluids (DAVIS et al. 1993). The cell membrane-bound CNTFRα is linked via a glycosyl phosphatidylinositol (GPI) anchor to the outer layer of the cell membrane and lacks a transmembrane domain. The expression of this receptor component is relatively high in the nervous system and in skeletal muscle. Low amounts of CNTFRα mRNA have also been found in liver cells (WONG et al. 1995).

The high affinity receptor for CNTF involves two additional components: gp130, which has originally been identified as the signal-transducing component of the IL-6 receptor, and LIFRβ. This latter component can bind Leukemia inhibitory factor (LIF) with low affinity (GEARING et al. 1991). Involvement of gp130 and LIFRβ in the receptor complexes for CNTF, LIF, oncostatin-M (OSM) and cardiotrophin-1 (CT-1) (GEARING and BRUCE 1992; PENNICA et al. 1995) explains the overlapping activities of these factors in supporting motoneuron survival and function.

Mice have been produced in which the receptor components CNTFRα, LIFRβ and gp130 have been eliminated (DECHIARA et al. 1995; LI et al. 1995; YOSHIDA et al. 1996). In all cases, the introduced gene defects are lethal which contrasts with mice in which the genes for the ligands of these receptors were eliminated (MASU et al. 1993; SENDTNER et al. 1996). Therefore, although CNTF, LIF, OSM and CT-1 share little homology at the amino-acid sequence level, they show a remarkable overlap in cellular functions, which is apparently the basis for compensatory activities in case of deficiency of these ligands. This, however, should not distract from the fact that the individual ligands have specific physiological functions which might differ significantly from each other.

2. The Function of Endogenous CNTF and Related Factors for Motoneurons

Originally, it was assumed that CNTF is a target-derived neurotrophic factor for ciliary neurons and for responsive motoneurons (MANTHORPE et al. 1980). The high quantities of this protein in peripheral nerves was interpreted as a consequence of retrograde transport of CNTF from skeletal muscle and skin to responsive sensory, sympathetic and motor neurons (WILLIAMS et al. 1984). Indeed, several studies reported the presence of CNTF mRNA in embryonic and adult rat skeletal muscle (IP et al. 1993). In the meantime, it became apparent that this was not the case. CNTF is produced in myelinating Schwann cells (FRIEDMAN et al. 1992; SENDTNER et al. 1992c), and the presence of small quantities of CNTF mRNA in skeletal muscle can be explained by the presence of CNTF in the Schwann cells of innervating nerves within the target tissue (reviewed in SENDTNER et al. 1994a).

CNTF lacks a classic hydrophobic leader sequence and, thus, is not released from synthesizing cells by the constitutive secretory pathway. Immunohistochemistry with specific antibodies indicates that the protein is located in the cytosol of myelinated Schwann cells (FRIEDMAN et al. 1992; SENDTNER et al. 1992c). It is still unclear how the protein is released from these cells. After nerve lesion in adult rodents, CNTF immunoreactivity can be identified in association with myelin breakdown products at extracellular locations (SENDTNER et al. 1992c). The amounts of CNTF present at the nerve lesion site are several orders of magnitude higher than, for example, levels of NGF, despite the fact that CNTF mRNA expression is downregulated and NGF mRNA is upregulated after nerve lesion. Therefore, it was suggested that endogenous CNTF might serve as a lesion factor.

Mice with homozygous targeted disruption of the CNTF gene (MASU et al. 1993) appear normal at birth, which supports the concept that endogenous CNTF is not necessary for the development of motoneurons. The number of motoneurons was unchanged in comparison with controls until 4 weeks after birth, when endogenous CNTF production has reached the high levels that are present in adult animals. However, after this period, a significant loss of about 20% of motoneurons could be observed. This means that CNTF is necessary for the postnatal maintenance of motoneurons, at least in a subpopulation of these cells. Therefore, it has to be assumed that the protein might be released from the Schwann cells in order to elicit this effect. Apparently, there is an overlap in the functions of endogenous CNTF and LIF for lesioned motoneurons. LIF expression in peripheral nerves is very low, but increases dramatically after nerve lesion (CURTIS et al. 1994). Interestingly, this upregulation of LIF expression is not seen in *pmn* mice, which represent an animal model of human motoneuron disease, and it would be interesting to know whether this mechanism could play a pathogenic role for the disease (SENDTNER et al. 1997b).

Mice lacking endogenous LIF do not show any defects in motoneurons. However, mice which lack both CNTF and LIF show increased motoneuron loss compared with CNTF knockout mice, and functional deficits in muscle strength are more severe (SENDTNER et al. 1996). Nothing is known about the role of endogenous OSM for motoneurons. CT-1, which resembles CNTF in the lack of a hydrophobic leader sequence, is highly produced in skeletal muscle and, thus, could control distinct functions of motoneurons compared with those influenced by CNTF (PENNICA et al. 1996).

3. Pharmacological Effects of CNTF on Lesioned Motoneurons

In newborn rodents, transection of peripheral nerves leads to cell death of corresponding motoneurons within few days (SCHMALBRUCH 1984). This high vulnerability decreases during the 4 weeks after birth. The molecular mechanisms regulating this change are still not understood. Both the presence of higher levels of endogenous neurotrophic factors in adult versus newborn peripheral nerves as well as decreased dependence on exogenous support have been suggested as possible reasons for this change in lesion-induced cell death during postnatal development (SNIDER and THANEDAR 1989; YAN et al. 1993).

The local application of CNTF to the proximal nerve stump of lesioned facial nerves (SENDTNER et al. 1990) can reduce the amount of cell death of the corresponding motoneuron cell bodies significantly. This experiment showed that CNTF is a survival factor for postnatal motoneurons and that it also acts in vivo after local application to lesioned motoneurons. In adult rodents, retrograde transport of CNTF has been shown to be increased after peripheral nerve lesion (CURTIS et al. 1993). However, several studies have been reported in which recombinant human CNTF (rhCNTF) did not enhance survival of motoneurons after ventral root avulsion (KOLIATSOS et al. 1994b); this led to complete removal of the peripheral nerve from the spinal cord and, thus, to deprivation of endogenous survival factors provided by Schwann cells.

The reason for this discrepancy is not clear. On the one hand, rapid degradation of the protein at the application site could be responsible, but also the low specific activity of rh- in comparison with rat CNTF (PANAYOTATOS et al. 1993; SENDTNER et al. 1994b). When CNTF or BDNF were applied to lesioned motoneurons in newborn rodents, survival effects were only observed during the first week, but not at 3 or 5 weeks after lesion (VEJSADA et al. 1995; ERIKSSON et al. 1994). Under such circumstances, the endogenous continuous production and release by means of recombinant adenoviruses have been shown to be very effective (GRAVEL et al. 1997), and it remains to be demonstrated whether the mode of CNTF delivery could influence the results of such nerve avulsion studies in adult rodents.

Evidence that CNTF can influence the survival of adult motoneurons comes from murine animal models of motoneuron disease. In particular, the *pmn* mouse mutant showed significant survival of motoneurons after CNTF treatment (SENDTNER et al. 1992b; SAGOT et al. 1995b), despite the fact that endogenous CNTF was present in high quantities and in biologically active form in the cytoplasm of peripheral nerve Schwann cells in these mice. Apparently, the CNTF was not available to the degenerating Schwann cells. However, peripheral nerve lesion in *pmn* mice led to increased survival of lesioned motoneurons (SENDTNER et al. 1997b). This survival effect was absent in *pmn* mice lacking endogenous CNTF, indicating that endogenous CNTF can preserve lesioned motoneurons in the adult and interfere with the disease mechanisms in *pmn* mice.

4. Effects of CNTF and Other Neurotrophic Factors in Murine Animal Models for Motoneuron Disease

CNTF has been successfully used for experimental therapy in murine animal models for motoneuron disease (Fig. 1). Systemic administration of CNTF to

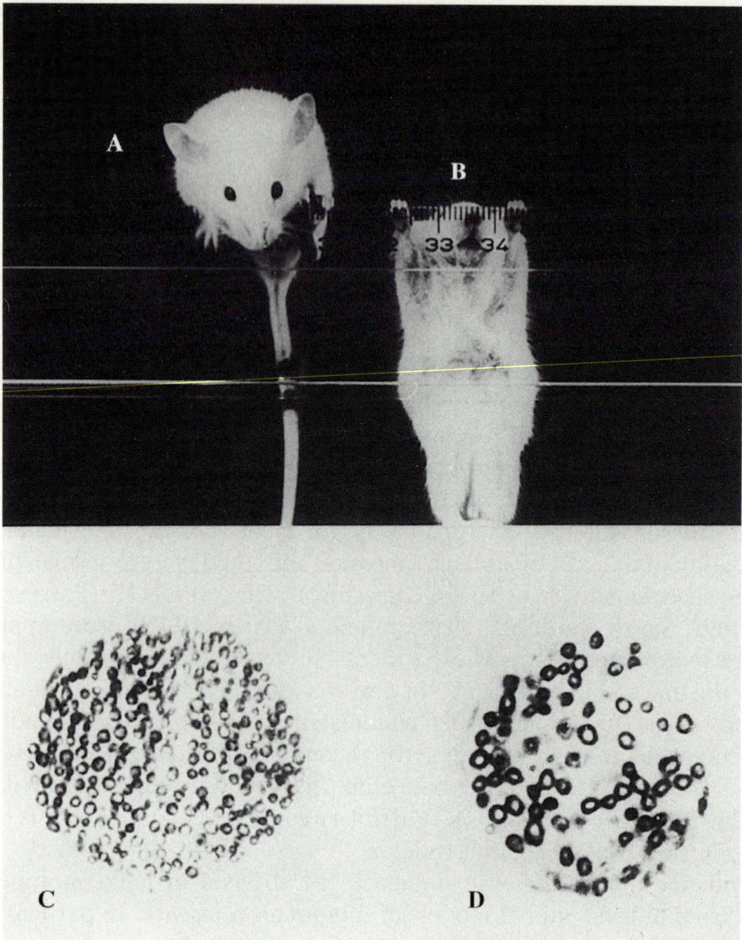

Fig. 1. Effect of CNTF treatment in *pmn* mice. Two homozygous *pmn* mice were (**A**) treated either with CNTF-secreting D3 cells or (**B**) with untransfected control cells (SENDTNER et al. 1992b). The cells were injected intraperitoneally after first symptoms could be detected in these mice at postnatal day 20. The mice shown are 36 days old. The CNTF-treated mice survived longer and showed improved motor performance. Morphology of the phrenic nerve of a CNTF-treated (**C**) and untreated (**D**) *pmn* mouse. In CNTF-treated *pmn* mice, more myelinated axons could be detected in the phrenic nerve, suggesting that the CNTF treatment did not only maintain motoneuron cell bodies, but led to axonal preservation and regeneration

pmn (SENDTNER et al. 1992b; SAGOT et al. 1995b), wobbler (MITSUMOTO et al. 1994a) and *mnd* (HELGREN et al. 1992) mice showed significant effects on the course of the disease, although the mechanisms how CNTF achieves this effect might be different. The underlying gene defects in these mouse mutants have not been identified so far. However, chromosomal-linkage data and experiments searching for mutations in candidate genes indicate that they are unrelated and that these mice are not defective of genes coding for these neurotrophic factors or their receptors.

In the case of the *mnd* and wobbler mice, large inclusion bodies were observed in motoneurons that appeared during the course of the disease. Whereas the content of these inclusion bodies has not been identified in wobbler mice (DUCHEN et al. 1968; BLONDET et al. 1995), the *mnd* mouse has been described as an animal model of neural ceroid lipofuscinosis (corresponding to Batten's disease in humans) (BRONSON et al. 1993); this mouse mutant, therefore, should be classified in a context other than motoneuron disease. Nevertheless, significant effects of CNTF have been observed in this mouse mutant (HELGREN et al. 1992). Whether CNTF signaling interferes with the mechanisms leading to this storage disease, is still unclear. These data indicate that the application of CNTF, and most probably of other neurotrophic factors as well, could interfere with disease mechanisms which primarily have nothing to do with programmed cell death. Similar beneficial effects have also been observed in wobbler mice with CNTF, BDNF and IGF-I (MITSUMOTO et al. 1994a,b; HANTAI et al. 1995; IKEDA et al. 1995), and the data obtained in this mouse mutant have been the basis of previous clinical studies using these factors in ALS patients.

The *pmn* mouse differs from wobbler and *mnd* mice by the lack of large vacuolar inclusion bodies and a more rapid course of the disease (SCHMALBRUCH et al. 1991). First symptoms are detectable during the third postnatal week, and all homozygous animals die by postnatal weeks 5–7 by respiratory failure due to paralysis of the diaphragm and other muscles necessary for respiratory activity. The disease starts at the muscle endplates, and the dying back process leads to degeneration of axons and motoneuron cell bodies in a successive manner. Thus, the disease process resembles that of human sporadic ALS (CHOU 1992). At postnatal week 5, about 40% of the motoneurons in the facial nucleus are lost.

We tried to treat these mice with daily subcutaneous injections of 10mg CNTF/kg body weight. This treatment did not alter the course of the disease. However, the implantation of CNTF-secreting cell lines either into the peritoneal cavity (SENDTNER et al. 1992b) or under the skin (SAGOT et al. 1995b) could significantly reduce loss of motoneurons and prolong the survival of these mice. We have concluded from these findings that CNTF and possibly other factors need to be continuously available to motoneurons in order to exert a protective effect and to prevent their degeneration in the course of motoneuron disorders.

Interestingly, the amounts of CNTF that could be detected in the circulation after the implantation of CNTF-releasing cell lines were much lower than the amounts of endogenous CNTF present in peripheral nerves of *pmn* mice. Only after nerve lesion, could the endogenous CNTF act on the degenerating motoneurons (SENDTNER et al. 1997). Thus, it can be concluded that pharmacological application of CNTF rescues motoneurons even in situations when endogenous CNTF is present. This applies to both *pmn* mice and most ALS patients (Anand et al. 1995).

5. Pharmacological Effects of Systemically Applied CNTF

When radiolabelled CNTF is injected intravenously in adult rats, it is removed very rapidly from the circulation (Dittrich et al. 1994). The initial half-life is in the range of a few minutes. Originally, it was assumed that the expression of CNTFRα in skeletal muscle and the nervous system leads to local binding of CNTF in these tissues (Ip et al. 1993), and thus, concentrates CNTF at the muscle endplate where it could be taken up by innervating motoneurons and retrogradely transported in their axons to the cell bodies. However, no accumulation of CNTF could be observed in skeletal muscle after intravenous injection. On the contrary, about 50% of the injected factor binds to liver cells within less than 1 h. This is probably due to the association of CNTF with soluble CNTFRα in the circulation. This complex can then bind to cells expressing gp130 and LIFRβ, including liver cells, cells in the immune system and many others.

Two clinical trials in which rhCNTF was injected subcutaneously to ALS patients showed the factor to have no efficacy (THE ALS CNTF TREATMENT STUDY GROUP 1995a, 1995b, 1996; Miller et al. 1996). On the contrary, severe side-effects were observed, including fever and cachexia. Those could be explained by the induction of acute-phase responses in liver cells (Dittrich et al. 1994), which are induced through functional CNTF receptors that form after binding of the CNTF/CNTFRα complex to LIF receptors on the surface of liver cells. As low levels of CNTFRα are also expressed in liver cells, they could also contribute in mediating these side-effects. In addition, severe cough was observed in most of the CNTF-treated ALS patients (Brooks et al. 1993). This could be caused by activation of alveolar macrophages after binding of the CNTF/CNTFRα complex to gp130 and LIFRβ.

Initial data obtained from a phase I/II trial with CNTF in ALS patients gave a more optimistic view than the recent results (Brooks et al. 1993). Indeed, the progression of the disease as measured by muscle strength and respiratory parameters, in particular peak inspiratory force and forced vital capacity, seem to be slowed down. However, the difference after a 20-week treatment period was not significant. It cannot be excluded that the negative side-effects have covered a potential positive effect of CNTF on motoneuron survival and regeneration. Nevertheless, these data indicated that the mode of delivery (subcutaneous injection at 24-h or 48-h intervals) was not applicable. This parallels findings in *pmn* mouse mutants, which did not respond to daily subcutaneous injections of recombinant CNTF, but only when the factor was continuously released from injected tumor cells or encapsulated cell implants (Sendtner et al. 1992b; Sagot et al. 1995b).

The low levels of CNTF detectable in the circulation of CNTF-treated *pmn* mice (corresponding to about 10ng/ml of biologically active CNTF) did not lead to side-effects such as significant loss of body weight, cough or severe alterations of the immune system. Such side-effects were only observed in rodents when high levels of CNTF were injected (HENDERSON et al. 1994b). This dose effect could be due to the binding kinetics of CNTF to soluble CNTFRα and to the tripartite high-affinity receptor on the cell surface. Indeed, the CNTFRα binds CNTF with only low affinity, and saturation requires about 100-fold higher quantities than saturation of the functional cellular high-affinity receptor (HUBER et al. 1993; WONG et al. 1995). Therefore, it is possible that low concentrations which saturate the cellular high-affinity receptors could lead to cellular effects only in neurons and in those cells expressing functional CNTF receptors, whereas very high concentrations, leading to saturation of soluble CNTFRα, are responsible for the side-effects in the liver and cells of the immune system.

There is experimental evidence that supports this hypothesis. In order to reduce the side-effects caused by systemic injection of recombinant CNTF, a phase-I clinical trial with intrathecal administration of CNTF to ALS patients was carried out (PENN et al. 1997). These patients were treated with increasing doses up to about 200μg/day. Steady-state concentrations of rhCNTF in the lumbar subarachnoidal space ranged between 50 and 1230ng/ml. For comparison, saturation of high-affinity CNTF receptors is reached in the range 100–500pg/ml in responsive isolated neuronal cells (HUBER et al. 1993). At those high levels, intrathecally administrated CNTF caused meningeal irritation, lymphocytic infiltration and other side-effects were observed (PENN et al. 1997). On the other hand, the implantation of encapsulated CNTF-producing BHK (baby hamster kidney) cells into the subarachnoidal space of ALS patients resulted in the release of about 0.5µg of human CNTF per day (AEBISCHER et al. 1996). Steady-state levels in patients' cerebrospinal fluid were in the range of 0.2–6ng/ml. The patients treated with encapsulated cells did not show any side-effects such as those observed after intrathecal administration of high levels of rhCNTF. However, CNTF at a concentration of 0.5–6ng should be sufficient for saturation of high-affinity receptors, provided that no major obstacle exists in the subarachnoidal space for free diffusion of the protein to the high-affinity binding sites on the motoneurons. Therefore, it would be very interesting to learn whether the therapeutic approach, using CNTF-secreting encapsulated cell lines, has an influence, which has not been determined so far, on the progression of the disease in ALS patients (AEBISCHER et al. 1996).

First pharmacokinetic and toxicological trials with LIF have shown that these neurotrophic cytokines show side-effects which are at least as severe as those of CNTF after systemic application. Therefore, systemic injection of LIF apparently does not offer any advantages over CNTF. However, cardiotrophin-1 does not bind to the CNTFRα (PENNICA et al. 1996) and, therefore, pharmacokinetic and toxicological properties are expected to differ from those of CNTF. Nevertheless, nothing is known so far about the effects of cardiotrophin-1 after systemic or intrathecal administration, so that clinical trials cannot be envisaged at present.

V. The Effects of Neurotrophins on Motoneurons

1. Nerve Growth Factor

Nerve growth factor (NGF) is the prototypic target-derived retrogradely transported trophic factor (reviewed by BARDE 1990). Its biological activities are limited to specific populations of peripheral and central neurons. The biological effects of nerve growth factor on responsive neurons are mediated by a low-affinity receptor that is common to all neurotrophins ($p75^{NTR}$) and through a specific high-affinity receptor (trkA) (see EIDE et al. 1993 for review). The p75 receptor is highly expressed in motoneurons during embryonic development, but the expression drops to undetectable levels after birth and, only after nerve lesion or in degenerative diseases, in particular in ALS, is it re-expressed in these cells (KERKHOFF et al. 1991; SEEBURGER et al. 1993). Under no such condition has any expression of trkA been observed in motoneurons.

The high expression of p75 explains why NGF can be taken up and retrogradely transported in embryonic motoneurons of newborn, but not adult, rats (STOECKEL and THOENEN 1975; YAN et al. 1988). Some effects of NGF have been observed in motoneurons, among them hypertrophy of a subpopulation of NGF receptor-positive lumbar motoneurons (KOLIATSOS et al. 1991) or a short-term effect on dendritic outgrowth in cultured embryonic motoneurons (WAYNE and HEATON 1990). In other experimental paradigms, negative trophic effects of NGF on motoneurons were found. For example, in newborn rats, the administration of NGF increases the number of degenerating motoneurons after sciatic nerve (MIYATA et al. 1986) and facial nerve lesions (SENDTNER et al. 1992a). It is very likely that these effects are mediated through the p75 neurotrophin receptor. Binding of NGF to p75 can lead to specific signals within the cells, in particular of NFkB (CARTER et al. 1996), but also of other events.

During embryonic development, endogenous NGF can induce cell death through its p75 receptor (FRADE et al. 1996). This scenario could be particularly relevant to this condition when p75 is re-expressed in motoneurons, such as in patients with ALS (KERKHOFF et al. 1991; SEEBURGER et al. 1993). Therefore, potential endogenous effects of neurotrophins, including NGF on the degenerating motoneurons in ALS patients, are possible.

2. The Effects of Brain-Derived Neurotrophic Factor (BDNF), Neurotrophin-3 (NT-3) and Neurotrophin-4/5 (NT-4/5) on Motoneurons

In contrast to trkA, which is part of the high-affinity NGF receptor, motoneurons express significant levels of full-length trkB. A subpopulation of motoneurons also expresses trkC, which is a specific cellular receptor for NT-3 (HENDERSON et al. 1993; GRIESBECK et al. 1995). The positive effects of BDNF and NT-3 were discovered when these proteins were applied to lesioned motoneurons in newborn rats (SENDTNER et al. 1992; YAN et al. 1992) or to the allantoic membrane of developing chick embryos (OPPENHEIM et al. 1992). Although virtually all of the motoneurons express trkB, only a subpopulation of about 50%–60% of the motoneurons survive after BDNF administration in vivo (SENDTNER et al. 1992a; YAN et al. 1992) or in vitro (HENDERSON et al. 1993; HUGHES et al. 1993). The reason for this apparent discrepancy is not clear. As this effect is observed both in cultured motoneurons from different embryonic stages and in vivo in postnatal motoneurons, it has to be assumed that the responsiveness of motoneurons to BDNF through trkB does not simply increase during embryonic development, but is regulated by other cellular or extracellular signals.

Motoneurons also express trkC, which is a specific receptor for NT-3. This appears relevant, as NT-3 is the most abundantly expressed neurotrophin in skeletal muscle, both during development and in the adult. For comparison, levels of BDNF expression in muscle are very low (GRIESBECK et al. 1995). From trkC and NT-3 knockout mice, there is good evidence that the γ-motoneurons innervating the muscle spindles are dependent on NT-3 for their physiological development (ERNFORS et al. 1995; KUCERA et al. 1995). However, NT-3 also supports survival of facial motoneurons after nerve lesion, a population of motoneurons which does not contain γ-motoneurons (SENDTNER et al. 1992a). Therefore, it has to be assumed that subpopulations of α-motoneurons are also responsive to NT-3, which is paralleled by the high expression of trkC mRNA in spinal and brain-stem motoneurons.

During embryonic development, the spinal motoneurons express NT-3 at relatively high levels (ERNFORS and PERSSON 1991). This finding suggested that NT-3 could function as an autocrine factor during this period. However, gene ablation of NT-3 did not lead to reduced numbers of α-motoneurons. It is likely that the NT-3 produced in motoneurons serves as a neurotrophic or even tropic molecule for proprioceptive neurons that invade the spinal cord through the dorsal horn and make contacts with the ventral motoneurons. In addition, NT-3 from motoneurons could function on upper motoneurons that have been shown to respond to this factor (SCHNELL et al. 1994).

NT-4/5 can also bind to trkB and support motoneurons, most probably through this receptor. Therefore, redundancy of these two ligands in their function on motoneurons has been suggested (HUGHES et al. 1993; KOLIATSOS et al. 1994a; CONOVER et al. 1995; LIU et al. 1995). However, this is not necessarily the case. Recently, splice variants of trkB have been identified with increased specificity for BDNF (STROHMAIER et al. 1996), and it is not clear so far whether such splice variants with increased specificity for each of these ligands are expressed on motoneurons. This could be relevant for consideration of the therapeutic potential of these two ligands for treatment of human ALS.

NT-3 expression is detectable in skeletal muscle both during development and in the adult. After muscle denervation either by nerve transection or by transient blockade of neuronal transmission by injection of tetrodotoxin into the sciatic nerve, NT-4 expression is rapidly downregulated in adult rats (Griesbeck et al. 1995). Electrical stimulation of motor nerves leads to the opposite effect, a significant upregulation of NT-4 expression (Funakoshi et al. 1995). These data suggest that neuronal activity at the neuromuscular endplate has a significant influence on NT-4 expression in skeletal muscle and that NT-4 could be involved in regulating efficacy of neuromuscular transmission, as has been shown in co-cultures of xenopus motoneurons and skeletal muscle after addition of NT-3 or BDNF (Lohoff et al. 1993).

3. Physiological Functions of Neurotrophins for Motoneurons, As Revealed by Gene Targeting

Gene ablation of BDNF leads to death of homozygous animals, usually within 2 days after birth; some mice survive until 4 weeks of age (Ernfors et al. 1995). Histologically, a marked loss of neurons in the vestibular and nodose ganglia is observed as well as a loss of specific subpopulations of myelinated sensory nerve fibers, most probably including the mechanoreceptors, but not BDNF-responsive motoneurons. Similarly, mice lacking NT-4 do not show any reduction in the number of motoneurons (Conover et al. 1995; Liu et al. 1995). The possibility that BNDF and NT-4 compensate for each other in such mice, thus explaining the apparent lack of motoneuron loss, was excluded by the generation of double-knockout mice, which show normal numbers of motoneurons in their spinal cord and in brain-stem nuclei (Conover et al. 1995; Liu et al. 1995). Originally, it was described that mice lacking trkB expression show a 70% reduction of motoneurons at birth (Klein et al. 1993). However, these results could not be reproduced (DeChiara et al. 1995); therefore, trkB-mediated signaling by BDNF or NT-4 apparently does not regulate survival of motoneurons during the critical period of developmental cell death.

4. Pharmacological Potential of Neurotrophins for Treatment of Amyotrophic Lateral Sclerosis

In contrast to CNTF, the systemic application of BDNF or NT-3 is apparently well tolerated in animal models and in patients, as revealed by clinical studies in which these drugs were tested for their efficacy in treating ALS or neuropathies (Lindsay 1996). However, animal studies in which these factors were applied for maintaining survival of motoneurons under various experimental conditions pointed to potential problems which have to be solved for effective use of these factors as drug candidates for motoneuron disease. The pharmacological application of BDNF, NT-4 or NT-3 to cell cultures or lesioned motoneurons in vivo supports less motoneurons than one would expect from the expression of trkB or trkC (Yan et al. 1992; Sendtner et al. 1992a; Henderson et al. 1993; Hughes et al. 1993). Moreover, the local administration of high amounts of BDNF to lesioned motor nerves in newborn rodents has only a transient effect in rescuing the corresponding motoneurons (Eriksson et al. 1994; Vejsada et al. 1994, 1995). In order to test the possibility that rapid degradation of the factor was due to this effect, either gel pieces soaked with the factor were replaced after 1 week or high levels of BDNF were injected systemically in order to make the factor available for longer time periods to the lesioned motoneurons. None of the attempts was successful.

Levels of endogenous BDNF mRNA are extremely low in skeletal muscle, and are only upregulated after lesion of the peripheral nerves (Koliatsos et al. 1993; Griesbeck et al. 1995). This upregulation occurs in Schwann cells, beginning at the end of the first week after lesion and increasing continuously during the following 4 weeks (Meyer et al. 1992). At that time, levels of BDNF production are about 10-fold higher than the maximal levels of NGF which can be observed a few days after nerve lesion. This scenario would only make BDNF available to lesioned motoneurons later, when the nerve fibers regenerate to their original muscle fibers. Therefore, a decreased responsiveness of lesioned motoneurons to BDNF, within a few days after lesion, would not be compatible with a functional role of this factor during the long time period of axonal regrowth after nerve lesion.

In order to test the hypothesis that BDNF must be available continuously at physiological concentrations for lesioned motoneurons, recombinant adenoviruses were used for local overexpression of BDNF after motor nerve lesion in newborn rats (Gravel et al. 1997). Indeed, this procedure could lead to prolonged survival of motoneuron cell bodies. The molecular counterpart for the influence of concentration (Vejsada et al. 1994) and application mode (bolus vs continuous application) might reside in the regulation of high-affinity BDNF receptor expression on the cell surface of motoneurons. Cell culture experiments with cerebellar granula cells have shown that high levels of BDNF can lead to a dramatic decrease of trkB receptor expression on the cell surface, most probably due to a block in retransport of full-length trkB binding sites from intracellular compartments to the cell surface (Carter et al. 1995). Similar mechanisms could play a role in motoneurons when BDNF is administered pharmacologically.

BDNF protein and bioactivity have been detected in platelets obtained from human blood samples (Yamamoto and Gurney 1990). The absolute quantities of BDNF protein in platelets might be considerable, as BDNF concentrations in human serum have been found at levels of about 15 ng/ml (Rosenfeld et al. 1995), which would be sufficient for saturation of high-affinity receptors on motoneurons. It is not known whether these high levels of endogenous BDNF are available to degenerating motoneurons or whether they act on degenerating motoneurons in patients with ALS.

The daily subcutaneous injection of BDNF has been shown to slow down the disease progress in wobbler mice (Ikeda et al. 1995). However, other mouse mutants, such as the *pmn* mouse, do not show any positive effects after daily subcutaneous injection of the factor (HOLTMANN and SENDTNER, unpublished observation).

A recent phase-III study with recombinant BDNF in patients with ALS did not demonstrate any positive effect on the course of the disease (summarized in SENDTNER 1997a). BDNF was well tolerated but, on average, the disease progress was not different from that of placebo-treated control patients (THE BDNF STUDY GROUP 1995). Future studies are in progress to overcome pharmacological problems associated with the subcutaneous injection of BDNF. One of these strategies will be to apply recombinant BDNF, through electronic pumps, into the subarachnoidal space of the lumbar spinal cord, from where it can diffuse in the cerebrospinal fluid and reach motoneurons by retrograde transport after being taken up from axons. Indeed, intrathecal administration has been shown to be safe and effective in animals (DITTRICH et al. 1996), and this procedure provides means by which BDNF can reach the motoneurons and lead to measurable cellular effects (Fig. 2).

The pharmacological potential of NT-3 has been underestimated by the relatively small survival effect on lesioned motoneurons in vivo and in cell culture (SENDTNER et al. 1992a; HENDERSON et al. 1993; HUGHES et al. 1993; KOLIATSOS et al. 1993). After facial nerve lesion, NT-3 supports only 25%–30% of axotomized motoneurons in comparison with about 50% rescued by BDNF (SENDTNER et al. 1992a). Also, in cell culture, NT-3 is less potent than BDNF (HENDERSON et al. 1993; HUGHES et al. 1993). Indeed, some reports in which the efficacy of BDNF and NT-3 were compared in their ability to rescue lesioned facial motoneurons, missed the effect of NT-3, probably because only a very low number of animals were investigated and only three randomly selected brain-stem sections were evaluated to determine the number of surviving motoneurons (KOLIATSOS et al. 1993).

Recent data suggest that the overexpression of NT-3 in skeletal muscle by means of adenoviral gene transfer leads to significant treatment effects in *pmn* mice, most probably by induction of massive local sprouting at the muscle endplates (HAASE et al. 1997). The same experiment showed that NT-3 had a very small (if any) survival effect on motoneuron cell bodies in these animals. Nevertheless, this treatment led to significant functional and clinical improvement in these mice. Consistent with a potential effect of NT-3 at the muscle endplate is the finding that skeletal muscle contains about 20 times more NT-

Fig. 2A–D. Distribution and effect of intrathecally adminstered BDNF in adult sheep. After chronic intrathecal infusion of BDNF, the factor is taken up in axons within the ventral root (**A**) and is transported retrogradely to the motoneuron cell bodies where it can be detected in vesicle-like structures around the nucleus (**B**). c-fos immunoreactivity in spinal motoneurons of control saline-treated sheep (**C**) and in a sheep that was treated with BDNF for 7 weeks (**D**). Chronic infusion of BDNF led to an increase in c-fos immunoreactivity and a translocation to cellular compartments in or close to the nucleus (**D**) (DITTRICH et al. 1996)

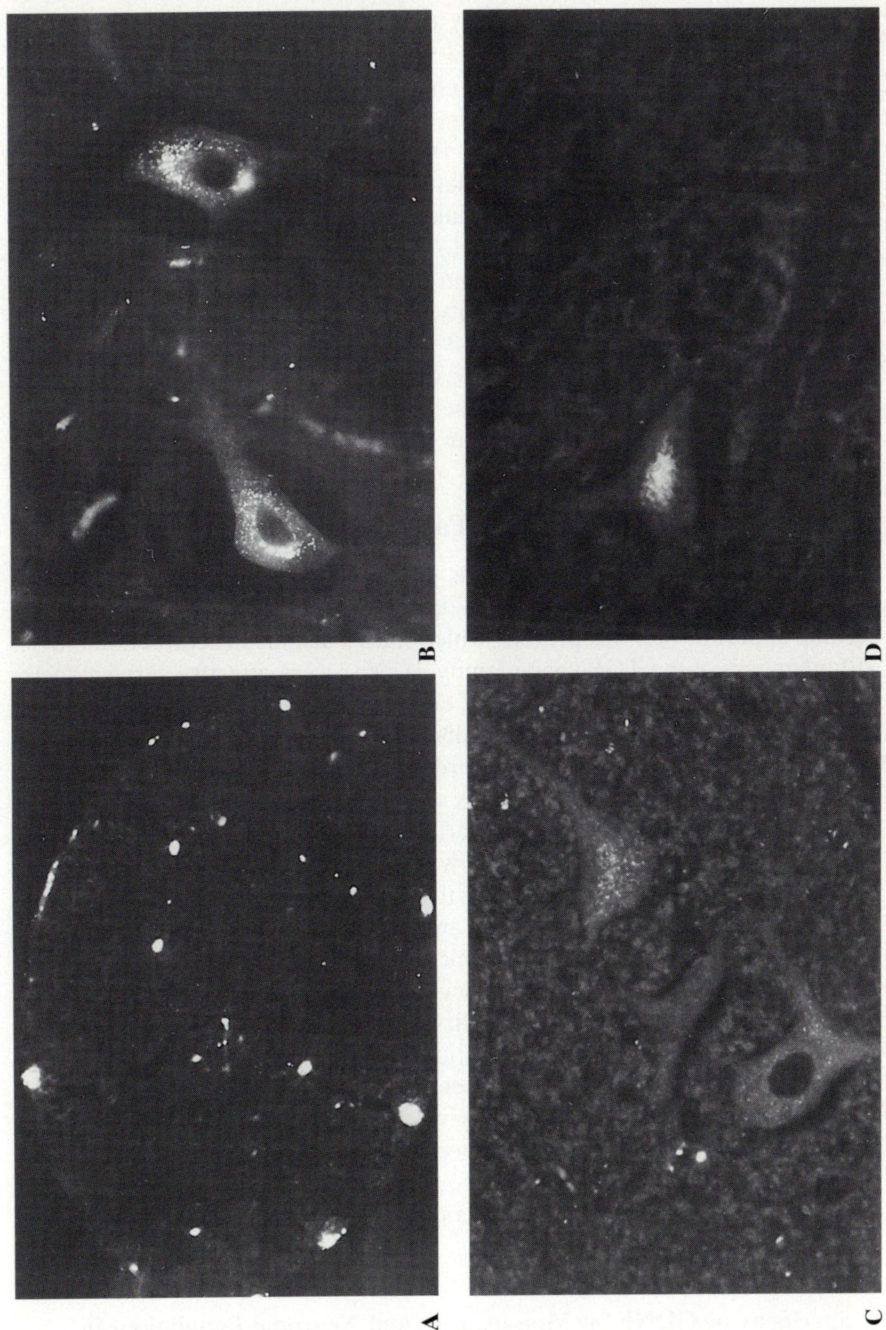

A B C D

3 than BDNF (GRIESBECK et al. 1995). Expression of NT-3 mRNA in skeletal muscle is also higher than that of NT-4/5; therefore, NT-3 might be physiologically available at the neuromuscular endplates.

NT-3 shows profound effects on synaptic efficacy in co-cultures of motoneurons and myocytes (LOHOFF et al. 1993). The increase in spontaneous and impulse-invoked synaptic currents detected in these cultures indicates that NT-3 is much more effective in modulating synaptic properties of motoneurons than in supporting their survival. This finding also explains the remarkable potentiating effect of NT-3 in *pmn* mice treated with CNTF (HAASE et al. 1997). Such data point to the possibility that co-treatment with specific combinations, involving, for example, NT-3 for increasing terminal sprouting and maintenance of muscle endplates, and other factors such as GDNF or BDNF for maintenance of the motoneuron cell bodies, could provide more effective treatment of motoneuron disease than treatment with each factor alone.

VI. Glial-Derived Neurotrophic Factor

Glial-derived neurotrophic factor was identified in 1993 as a potent survival factor for midbrain dopaminergic neurons (LIN et al. 1993). Very soon it became apparent that this protein, which shares distant structural homologies with members of the TGFβ gene family, is also a very effective survival factor for motoneurons. In cell cultures of embryonic rat motoneurons, 0.2 pg/ml, corresponding to 7 fM, supports half-maximal survival (HENDERSON et al. 1994a). Thus, GDNF was several orders of magnitude more potent than BDNF, CNTF or LIF. The same study showed no effect of GDNF on sensory, trigeminal or sympathetic neurons derived from embryonic or perinatal rats. Relatively high expression of GDNF was found in skeletal muscle, E15 hindlimb and Schwann cell cultures. Thus, it was concluded that GDNF represents a target-derived neurotrophic factor and is a strong candidate for regulating motoneuron survival during embryonic and postnatal development.

Experiments analyzing the potency of GDNF in rescuing facial motoneurons after nerve lesion showed that virtually all of the lesioned motoneurons could be rescued by local administration of the factor to the proximal nerve stump (HENDERSON et al. 1994a; YAN et al. 1995). Thus, GDNF was also more potent in rescuing motoneurons in vivo than CNTF or BDNF, which only supported about 50%–60% of lesioned motoneurons. Therefore, this factor was considered an excellent candidate to slow loss of function, degeneration and death of motoneurons in disorders such as ALS or SMA (HENDERSON et al. 1994a).

1. Specificity of GDNF for Motoneurons and Neuronal Populations in the Peripheral Nervous System

The original studies by HENDERSON et al. (1994a) did not show any efficacy of GDNF in supporting sensory or sympathetic neurons, arguing for a very specific role of GDNF for motoneurons and central dopaminergic neurons. However, follow-up studies showed that at high concentrations, GDNF also affected survival and neurite outgrowth of sympathetic neurons derived from newborn rat superior cervical ganglia (TRUPP et al. 1995). This study presented additional data which were apparently contradictory to the original report (HENDERSON et al. 1993). Analysis of developmental and tissue distribution of GDNF showed the highest levels of GDNF mRNA in testes and kidneys, followed by relatively high levels in skin and in the stomach, but only very little expression in skeletal muscle. Indeed, the levels in skeletal muscle were relatively low in 13-day-old rat embryos, decreased further until birth and were not detectable in adult rats. However, GDNF mRNA was found in Schwann cell lines, and nerve lesion increased GDNF mRNA expression, within 2 days, to maximal levels, which then decreased again. Therefore, a function of GDNF as an endogenous lesion factor for axotomized motoneurons (and probably other types of neurons) could be proposed, resembling very much the putative function of endogenous LIF and CNTF. It is possible that Schwann cells are not the only source of endogenous GDNF for motoneurons, as expression of GDNF mRNA has also been identified in the human spinal cord (SPRINGER et al. 1994) and in astrocytes in specific areas of the brain.

A potential effect of GDNF on peripheral sympathetic and sensory neurons was observed in studies with chick embryos (OPPENHEIM et al. 1995): The application of GDNF to the chorioallantoic membrane led to increased motoneuron survival during the critical period of physiological cell death, but also increased the number of surviving sympathetic and sensory neurons. Further support for the potential use of GDNF as a drug in the treatment of human ALS was provided by studies on the effect of GDNF in adult motoneurons (YAN et al. 1995). The local administration of 1 mg/ml GDNF could prevent lesion-induced atrophy, as measured by the loss of choline acetyltransferase activity in axotomized facial motoneurons in adult rats. Moreover, the subcutaneous administration of 5 mg/kg had the same effect, indicating that systemic application of GDNF in adult rats could prevent atrophy of motoneurons at the same high levels as the local administration.

2. Physiological Function of GDNF: Evidence from Gene Knockout Studies

Mice in which the GDNF gene was inactivated show renal agenesis and a complete lack of neurons in the autonomic ganglia of the gut forming the myenteric plexus (MOORE et al. 1996; PICHEL et al. 1996; SANCHEZ et al. 1996). Analysis of the nervous system identified deficits in several populations of sensory neurons, in particular from dorsal root, sympathetic and nodose ganglia. A small reduction in trigeminal and spinal lumbar motoneurons in the range of 20% was found, but not in facial motoneurons. Thus, a key role of GDNF in regulating survival of motoneurons during embryonic development can be excluded.

The GDNF-receptor complex involves a low-affinity binding component (GDNFRα) (JING et al. 1996), which is linked to the membrane via a GPI-anchor, comparable to the CNTFRα. In contrast to the CNTF/LIF-receptor complex, signal transduction of GDNF is mediated by a tyrosine kinase (c-ret) which associates with the GDNFRα after ligand binding and transmits the ligand-induced signal to the cell (DURBEC et al. 1996; TREANOR et al. 1996; TRUPP et al. 1996). Very similar defects in kidney development and development of the enteric nervous system were identified in c-ret-deficient mice.

3. The Pharmacological Potential of GDNF for Treatment of Human Motoneuron Disease

The original discovery of GDNF as a trophic factor for midbrain dopaminergic neurons has led its clinical propagation mainly into the direction of a drug candidate for treatment of Parkinson's disease. Indeed, it has been shown that GDNF treatment could lead to dramatic improvements in Parkinsonian monkeys (GASH et al. 1996). In perinatal rats, GDNF stimulates dopamine and serotonin synthesis after injection into the striatum (BECK et al. 1996). Tyrosine hydroxylase activity was also increased in the ventral mesencephalon, but GDNF did not induce sprouting of dopaminergic neurites; behavioral changes were observed as well in these newborn rodents. The GDNF-treated rats showed forelimb hyperflexure, dystonic changes in all limbs and a kinked tail (BECK et al. 1996). In adult rhesus monkeys, such strong behavioral effects were not observed after GDNF treatment (GASH et al. 1995). These monkeys experienced some weight loss, and dopamine levels in the substantia nigra and other areas of the brain were significantly increased. This was paralleled by an increase of dopamine-neuronal perikaryal size. Other animal models of Parkinson's disease, such as adult rats treated with a 6-hydroxydopamine (6-OHDA)-injection into the medial forebrain bundle, also showed positive effects (OPACKA-JUFFRY et al. 1995). Based on these data, phase-I clinical trials with GDNF in patients with Parkinson's disease have been started.

As GDNF injection into the brain is apparently well tolerated, clinical studies exploring its therapeutic potential for treatment of motoneuron disease could be started soon. On the one hand, GDNF is highly effective in supporting motoneuron survival in cell culture and in vivo. On the other hand, side-effects are expected after systemic injection of GDNF, as autonomic and cutaneous sensory neurons become highly responsive to GDNF with increased age (BUJ-BELLO et al. 1995; EBENDAL et al. 1995; MATHESON et al. 1997). Therefore, a strategy aiming at a more local delivery of the factor to degenerating motoneurons might have higher chances for positive effects. However, even if such conditions could be defined, it is not clear whether GDNF treatment can result in clinical improvement. Treatment studies in *pmn* mice have shown that GDNF has a marked effect in preventing the degeneration of motoneuron cell bodies in the facial nucleus and the spinal cord (SAGOT et al. 1996). However, the factor does not stimulate axonal regeneration, and thus, does not lead to any functional improvement or increased survival in these mouse mutants. Thus, GDNF differs completely from CNTF which affects both survival of motoneuron cell bodies and neurite outgrowth (SENDTNER et al. 1992b), and from NT-3 which shows little effect on the survival of cell bodies but a significant effect on axonal regeneration and sprouting (HAASE et al. 1997).

VII. Insulin-Like Growth Factors (IGF)

The insulin-like growth factors (IGF-I and IGF-II) are structurally related to insulin and more distantly to relaxin (LEROITH and ROBERTS 1993). They are derived from precursor proteins containing two domains that are homologous to the A and B chains of insulin. In contrast to insulin, the C domain of IGFs is not removed. Circulating IGF-I has originally been proposed to mediate the effect of growth hormone. However, the presence of IGF-I in multiple tissues, in particular the nervous system, has pointed to a more specific effect of this factor on neuronal functions (LEROITH et al. 1993). The IGF actions are modulated both positively and negatively by IGF-binding proteins. Six distinct IGF-binding proteins have been identified so far, and their role for modulating IGF so far, and function on motoneurons is still unclear. Among these binding proteins, IGFBP-5 is highly expressed in Schwann cells (CHENG et al. 1996) and it is to be expected that this and other IGF-binding proteins contribute in modulating IGF-I and IGF-II availability from skeletal muscle cells (NEFF et al. 1993) and from the circulation.

Due to the high levels of IGFs in body fluids, these factors were not originally considered as specific survival factors for motoneurons. The IGF-I receptor is widely expressed in the central nervous system (LEROITH et al. 1993), both in neuronal and glial cells. The level of the IGF-I receptor, which transduces cellular responses of IGF-I and IGF-II, is very high in the brain during embryonic development, but is then significantly downregulated after birth. Nevertheless, IGF-I-receptor expression is also detectable at significant levels in postnatal motoneurons, and many biological activities have been observed in motoneurons after pharmacological IGF-I injection into skeletal muscle of lesioned peripheral nerves.

1. Specific Function of IGF-I on Developing and Postnatal Motoneurons

After the demonstration that IGF-I is a specific survival factor for embryonic chick and rat motoneurons (ARAKAWA et al. 1990; HUGHES et al. 1993; NEFF et al. 1993), a series of experiments analyzing the pharmacological potential of this factor in the treatment of motoneuron degeneration in postnatal animals was initiated. Injection of IGF-II on the surface of the gluteus muscle of the adult rat induced nodal sprouting of innervating motor nerves and terminal sprouting at the endplates. In motoneurons, GAP-43 and tubulin-α-1 expression were increased. These findings indicated that IGF-I might play a physiological role in modulating postnatal motor-endplate stability and plasticity (CARONI and GRANDES 1990; CARONI and SCHNEIDER 1994; CARONI et al. 1994).

The original survival effects of IGF-I in cultures of purified motoneurons from chick embryos were underestimated (ARAKAWA et al. 1990), probably because of the presence of horse serum in these cultures (PROSSER and MCLAREN 1992). Embryonic rat motoneurons in serum-free cultures showed very potent survival effects of IGF-I in a range comparable to that of BDNF or GDNF (HUGHES et al. 1993). However, the local administration of IGF-I to axotomized facial motoneurons in newborn rats showed a survival effect which was much smaller (in a range of 30%) than that of BDNF (approximately 50%) or GDNF (approximately 90%–100%). It is not clear whether inhibitory binding protein or submaximal concentrations of these factors are responsible for the small effect in vivo. It would be interesting to know whether isoforms of IGF-I lacking the first three amino acids (Des1–3-IGF) or IGF-I-mutants with reduced affinity to IGFBPs differ from IGF-I in their potential to support lesioned motoneurons in newborn rodents. This would help to find out whether the presence of binding proteins inhibits IGF effects by restricting the availability to cellular receptors on motoneurons, or whether they concentrate the factor locally, and thus increase availability of IGFs to motoneurons.

2. Pharmacokinetics of IGF-I

IGF-I differs from neurotrophins and other neurotrophic factors by its ability to cross the blood–brain barrier (REINHARDT and BONDY 1994). Moreover, IGF-I is present in relatively high quantities as an endogenous protein that circulates in blood in association with its binding proteins. Clinical studies have shown that systemic injection of IGF-I leads to insulin-like responses when the factor is injected subcutaneously at doses of 0.06–0.12 mg/kg or intravenously at 0.03 mg/kg (STONG and RASKIN 1993). Under such conditions, levels of free IGF-I in serum increased significantly from 5 ng/ml to about 10–15 ng/ml, indicating that the pharmacologically applied IGF-I is only bound in low quantities to the binding proteins (STONG and RASKIN 1993). Thus, the factor could indeed be available to motoneurons, provided that the local environment at sites where IGF-I can be taken up, in particular the motor endplates, do not contain high levels of inhibitory binding proteins.

3. Effects of IGF-I in Animal Models of Motoneuron Degeneration

The specific retrograde transport of IGF-I in peripheral nerves and the upregulation of IGF-I production in lesioned sciatic nerves have suggested that IGF-I plays an important role in peripheral-nerve regeneration (summarized by HANSSON 1993). The daily injection of adult mice in which the peripheral nerve was lesioned with IGF-I showed an enhanced functional recovery, as measured by grip strength and other functional parameters (CONTRERAS et al. 1993). Moreover, IGF-I has been used for experimental treatment of the wobbler mouse mutant, an animal model of human motoneuron disease (HANTAI et al. 1995). Recombinant human IGF-I (1 mg/kg) was injected daily over a period of 6 weeks. This treatment led to a marked overall weight increase, improved muscle strength and an increase in the diameter of muscle fibers. However, the number of spinal-cord motoneurons and levels of choline acetyltransferase, which are reduced in these mouse mutants during the course of the disease, were unchanged. Therefore, it is still unclear whether the beneficial effects seen in this mouse mutant were caused by action on motoneurons or by an effect of IGF-I in preventing muscular atrophy and degeneration of the neuromuscular endplates.

Clinical trials with IGF-I have been initiated and a phase-III trial was finished in 1997. Although the results of this trial are not yet available, it has become evident that IGF-I does not stop the disease process, nor does the treatment lead to major improvements of muscle strength and overall survival in these patients. These results lead us back to the question whether inhibitory binding proteins in peripheral nerves and the spinal cord prevent IGF-I from accessing motoneurons, and whether the observed reactions in these patients are due to indirect effects on skeletal muscle cells. This question has to be answered and new strategies should be developed to improve the availability of the pharmacologically applied IGF-I to motoneurons.

VIII. Future Perspectives: Are Newest Clinical Trials in ALS Patients with Neurotrophic Factors Meaningful?

Previous clinical studies of the systemic administration of CNTF, BDNF or IGF-I did not fulfill the high expectations (Table 2). In the case of CNTF, major side-effects were observed, and the BDNF and IGF-I trials showed little, if any efficacy. This demonstrates potential restrictions in the usefulness of these factors for treatment of motoneuron disease. In all of these cases, it was not clear whether the factors given systemically had reached the motoneurons in sufficient quantities, or whether the disease mechanisms underlying sporadic ALS could be influenced at all by increasing the concentration of these factors beyond the levels available from endogenous sources. Nevertheless, the positive effects that these factors demonstrated in various animal models of human motoneuron disease, apparently caused by independent gene defects, and data that apoptotic mechanisms could play a role in human ALS indicate that treatment with neurotrophic factors should make sense. Cellular changes which are usually seen in lesion models where neurotrophic factors are active, such as the upregulation of p75 (KERKHOFF et al. 1991; SEEBURGER et al. 1993) or other changes resembling apoptotic cell death (HIRANO and IWATA 1979; CHOU 1992; TROOST et al. 1995; LO et al. 1995), which are generally observed in sporadic ALS, indicate that interfering with these mechanisms using neurotrophic factors is a promising strategy for treatment of this disease.

Table 2. Clinical trials with neurotrophic factors in patients with amyotrophic lateral sclerosis (ALS)

Factor	Status	Number of patients	Dose (μg/kg body weight)	Duration	Application	Result	Reference
CNTF	Phase I	57	0.5–30 every other day	2 weeks	Subcutaneous	Fever, weight loss	ACTS, 1995
CNTF	Phase I	22	2–200 daily	4 weeks	Subcutaneous	Herpes, stomatitis, skin reactions, fever, weight loss	ACTS, 1993 Miller et al. 1993
CNTF	Phase II/III	730	15, 30 every other day	9 months	Subcutaneous	Side effects, no statistically significant effect	ACTS, 1996
CNTF	Phase II	570	0.5, 2, 5 daily	6 months	Subcutaneous	Side effects, no effect on disease	Miller et al. 1996
CNTF	Phase I	6	ca 0.5 daily	<3 months	Encapsulated cells, intrathecal	Well tolerated	Aebischer et al. 1996
CNTF	Phase I	4	8–192 daily	2 weeks	Intrathecal	Leg cramping, CSF pleocytosis, rise in CSF protein	Penn et al. 1997
BDNF	Phase I/II	283	10–300 daily	6 months	Subcutaneous	Well tolerated	Bradley et al. 1995
BDNF	Phase III	1150	25–100 daily	9 months	Subcutaneous	Well tolerated, no significant effect	
BDNF	Phase I	ca 25		No data available	Intrathecal	No data available	
IGF-I	Phase III	266	50,100 daily	9 months	Subcutaneous	Well tolerated, ALS scores significantly different, no major effects	Lai et al. 1995
GDNF	Phase I		No data available		Intraventricular	No data available	

1. Strategies to Increase the Availability of Pharmacologically Applied Neurotrophic Factors to Degenerating Motoneurons

Usually, neurotrophic factors are released by muscle cells, Schwann cells or glial cells that interact closely with motoneurons. These cells release the factors at low, physiological concentrations. They are then taken up and transported retrogradely to the motoneuron cell bodies. In this way, these factors differ completely from hormones, such as erythropoetin or colony-stimulating factors, which are normally present in blood and act on responsive cells from the circulation. At this time, there is no means of administering these growth factors in a way resembling the physiological availability of their endogenous counterparts. Although adenoviral gene transfer in the *pmn* mouse mutants and in newborn rats could show high efficacy of virally overexpressed NT-3 (HAASE et al. 1997) or CNTF and BDNF (GRAVEL et al. 1997), these techniques are far from being applicable for treatment of human ALS because of the immunological reactions to infected cells and the lack of experience with long-term expression with such viral vectors (SENDTNER et al. 1997a). At present, intrathecal administration (DITTRICH et al. 1996), which makes the factor available continuously to ventral roots, where it can be taken up and retrogradely transported the short distance to the cell bodies in the spinal cord, is more feasible. The implantation of encapsulated cells continuously releasing these factors in low, but physiologically relevant concentrations (AEBISCHER et al. 1996) are, therefore, more promising than the systemic administration of these factors.

2. Development of Modified Factors with Increased Specificity and Improved Pharmacokinetic Properties

In the case of IGF-I, truncated forms of the protein have been identified that have reduced affinity to IGF-binding proteins (SARA et al. 1993). In addition, several mutants which are biologically active, but not inhibited by binding proteins, have been designed and expressed. This points to the possibility of designing pharmacologically applicable neurotrophic factors which might be available at higher levels to degenerating motoneurons after systemic application. Indeed, first steps have been made to modify neurotrophins so that these factors can cross the blood–nerve barrier (FRIDEN et al. 1993). The determination of the 3D protein structures of BDNF and NT-4, as well as their corresponding receptors, could help to design low-molecular weight receptor agonists or modified proteins with improved pharmacological properties. In the case of CNTF, mutants have been identified by phage-display technology which shows altered binding properties to individual receptor components (SAGGIO et al. 1995), without losing the biological activity. If CNTF homologues with increased stability could be designed that do not bind to soluble CNTFRα, causing side-effects in the liver or immune system (ECONOMIDES et al. 1995), such factors could have a significantly higher therapeutic potential, and reduce side-effects which currently limit the use of these factors for treatment of ALS.

3. Combinations of Neurotrophic Factors: The Better Strategy?

The large variety of growth factors that can support motoneuron survival and function indicates that they play together in a very complex manner to regulate survival and functional maintenance during development and the postnatal period. Therefore, it is unlikely that monotherapy with neurotrophic factors influences all the parameters necessary for functional improvement in the case of ALS. Experiments in *pmn* mice have shown that GDNF prevents the degeneration of motoneuron cell bodies, but does not stimulate axonal regrowth or reinnervation of muscle fibers, and thus the factor does not lead to any clinical improvement in these animal models of motoneuron disease (Sagot et al. 1996). Co-treatment with GDNF, CNTF, BDNF and NT-3 could possibly enhance the efficacy of this treatment (Arakawa et al. 1990; Zurn et al. 1996; see also Thoenen et al. 1993 for review).

Indeed, cell-culture experiments have shown that combinations of neurotrophic factors, for example CNTF and IGF-I, do not only lead to additive survival effects, but to supra-additive potentiating effects (Arakawa et al. 1990; Hughes et al. 1993). In mouse mutants, the combination of CNTF, BDNF and NT-3 is much more effective than any monotherapy (Mitsumoto et al. 1994b; Haase et al. 1997). These data indicate that treatment with suitable combinations of neurotrophic factors might be more beneficial than treatment with one factor alone. Therefore, the selection of combinations of neurotrophic factors with complementary effects on motoneuron survival, axonal regeneration and motor endplate function is a major challenge in this field. A better understanding of how these factors work together on a cellular and molecular level could even be of benefit in providing a better understanding of the molecular mechanisms underlying ALS.

References

Adler R, Landa KB, Manthorpe M, Varon S (1979) Cholinergic neurotrophic factors: intraocular distribution of trophic activity for ciliary neurons. Science 204:1434–1436

Aebischer P, Schluep M, Deglon N, Joseph JM, Hirt L, Heyd B, Goddard M, Hammang JP, Zurn AD, Kato AC, Regli F, Baetge EE (1996) Intrathecal delivery of CNTF using encapsulated genetically modified xenogeneic cells in amyotrophic lateral sclerosis patients. Nat Med 2:696–699

Ait Ikhlef A, Murawsky M, Blondet B, Hantaz Ambroise D, Martinou JC, Rieger F (1995) The motoneuron degeneration in the wobbler mouse is independent of the overexpression of a Bcl2 transgene in neurons. Neurosci Lett 199:163–166

ALS CNTF Treatment Study (ACTS) group (1993) Recombinant human ciliary neurotrophic factor (rhCNTF) in amyotrophic lateral sclerosis: Phase I–II safety, tolerability and pharmakokinetic studies. Neurology 43:A416 [Abstract]

The ALS CNTF Treatment Study (ACTS) Phase I-II Study Group (1995a) The pharmacokinetics of subcutaneously administered recombinant human ciliary neurotrophic factor (rhCNTF) in patients with amyotrophic lateral sclerosis: relation to parameters of the acute-phase response. Clin Neuropharmacol 18:500–514

ALS CNTF Treatment Study (ACTS) Phase I-II Study Group (1995b) A phase I study of recombinant human ciliary neurotrophic factor (rhCNTF) in patients with amyotrophic lateral sclerosis. Clin Neuropharmacol 18:515–532

The ALS CNTF Study Group (1996) A double-blind placebo-controlled clinical trial of subcutaneous recombinant human ciliary neurotrophic factor (rhCNTF) in amyotrophic lateral sclerosis. Neurology 46:1244–1249

ALS CNTF Treatment Study (ACTS) group (1996) A double-blind placebo-controlled clinical trial of subcutaneous recombinant human ciliary neurotrophic factor (rhCNTF) in amyotrophic lateral sclerosis. Neurology 46:1244–1249

Anand P, Parrett A, Martin J, Zeman S, Foley P, Swash M, Leigh PN, Cedarbaum JM, Lindsay RM, Williams Chestnut RE et al. (1995) Regional changes of ciliary neurotrophic factor and nerve growth factor levels in post mortem spinal cord and cerebral cortex from patients with motor disease. Nat Med 1:168–172

Arakawa Y, Sendtner M, Thoenen H (1990) Survival effect of ciliary neurotrophic factor (CNTF) on chick embryonic motoneurons in culture: Comparison with other neurotrophic factors and cytokines. J Neurosci 10:3507–3515

Barbin G, Manthorpe M, Varon S (1984) Purification of the chick eye ciliary neuronotrophic factor. J Neurochem 43:1468–1478

Barde Y-A (1990) The nerve growth factor family. Prog Growth Factor Res 2:237–248

The BDNF Study Group, Bradley We (1995) A phase I/II study of recombinant brain-derived neurotrophic factor (r-metHuBDNF) in patients with amyotrophic lateral sclerosis (abstract). 120th Annual Meeting of the American Neurological Association Washington

Beck KD, Irwin I, Valverde J, Brennan TJ, Langston JW, Hefti F (1996) GDNF induces a dystonia-like state in neonatal rats and stimulates dopamine and serotonin synthesis. Neuron 16:665–673

Bensimon G, Lacomblez L, Meininger V, ALS-Riluzole Study Group (1994) A controlled trial of riluzole in amyotrophic lateral sclerosis. N Engl J Med 330:585–591

Blondet B, Hantaz Ambroise D, Ait Ikhlef A, Cambier D, Murawsky M, Rieger F (1995) Astrocytosis in wobbler mouse spinal cord involves a population of astrocytes which is glutamine synthetase-negative. Neurosci Lett 183:179–182

Bradley WG, The BDNF Study Group (1995) A phase I/II study of recombinant human brain-derived neurotrophic factor in patients with amyotrophic lateral sclerosis. Ann Neurol 38:971

Bronson RT, Lake BD, Cook S, Taylor S, Davisson MT (1993) Motor neuron degeneration of mice is a model of neuronal ceroid lipofuscinosis (Batten's disease). Ann Neurol 33:381–385

Brooks BP, Fischbeck KH (1995) Spinal and bulbar muscular atrophy: a trinucleotide-repeat expansion neurodegenerative disease. Trends Neurosci 18:459–461

Brooks BR, Sanjak M, Mitsumoto H, Szirony K, Neville H, Ringel S, Brinkmann J, Pestronk A, Florence J, Cedarbaum J, Charatan M, Stambler N, Wittes J, Brittain E (1993) Recombinant human ciliary neurotrophic factor (rhCNTF) in amyotrophic lateral sclerosis (ALS) patients: dose selection strategy in phase I–II safety, tolerability and pharmakokinetic studies. Can J Neurol Sci 20 [Suppl 4]:83

Buj Bello A, Buchman VL, Horton A, Rosenthal A, Davies AM (1995) GDNF is an age-specific survival factor for sensory and autonomic neurons. Neuron 15:821–828

Camu W, Henderson CE (1992) Purification of embryonic rat motoneurons by panning on a monoclonal antibody to the low-affinity NGF receptor. J Neurosci Methods 44:59–70

Caroni P, Grandes P (1990) Nerve sprouting in innervated skeletal muscle induced by exposure to elevated levels of insulin-like growth factors. J Cell Biol 110:1307–1317

Caroni P, Schneider C (1994) Signaling by insulin-like growth factors in paralyzed skeletal muscle: rapid induction of IGF1 expression in muscle fibers and prevention of interstitial cell proliferation by IGF-BP5 and IGF-BP4. J Neurosci 14:3378–3388

Caroni P, Schneider C, Kiefer MC, Zapf J (1994) Role of muscle insulin-like growth factors in nerve sprouting: suppression of terminal sprouting in paralyzed muscle by IGF-binding protein 4. J Cell Biol 125:893–902

Carter BD, Zirrgiebel U, Barde YA (1995) Differential regulation of p21ras activation in neurons by nerve growth factor and brain-derived neurotrophic factor. J Biol Chem 270:21751–21757

Carter BD, Kaltschmidt C, Kaltschmidt B, Offenhauser N, Bohm Matthaei R, Baeuerle PA, Barde YA (1996) Selective activation of NF-kappa B by nerve growth factor through the neurotrophin receptor p75 (see comments). Science 272:542–545

Cheng HL, Randolph A, Yee D, Delafontaine P, Tennekoon G, Feldman EL (1996) Characterization of insulin-like growth factor-I and its receptor and binding proteins in transected nerves and cultured Schwann cells. J Neurochem 66:525–536

Chou SM (1992) Pathology-light microscopy of amyotrophic lateral sclerosis. In: Smith RA (ed) Handbook of amyotrophic lateral sclerosis. Marcel Dekker, New York, pp 133–182

Conover JC, Erickson JT, Katz DM, Bianchi LM, Poueymirou WT, McClain J, Pan L, Helgren M, Ip NY, Boland P, Friedman B, Wiegand S, Vejsada R, Kato AC, DeChiara TM, Yancopoulos GD (1995) Neuronal deficits, not involving motor neurons, in mice lacking BDNF and/or NT4. Nature 375:235–238

Contreras PC, Steffler C, Vaught JL (1993) rhIGF-I enhances functional recovery from sciatic crush: time-course and dose-response study. Ann NY Acad Sci 692:314–316

Curtis R, Adryan KM, Zhu Y, Harkness PJ, Lindsay RM, Distefano PS (1993) Retrograde axonal transport of ciliary neurotrophic factor is increased by peripheral nerve injury. Nature 365:253–255

Curtis R, Scherer SS, Somogyi R, Adryan KM, Ip NY, Zhu Y, Lindsay RM, Distefano PS (1994) Retrograde axonal transport of LIF is increased by peripheral nerve injury: correlation with increased LIF expression in distal nerve. Neuron 12:191–204

Davis S, Aldrich TH, Ip NY, Stahl N, Scherer S, Farruggella T, Distefano PS, Curtis R, Panayotatos N, Gascan H, Chevalier S, Yancopoulos GD (1993) Released form of CNTF receptor-alpha component as a soluble mediator of cntf responses. Science 259:1736–1739

DeChiara TM, Vejsada R, Poueymirou WT, Acheson A, Suri C, Conover JC, Friedman B, McClain J, Pan L, Stahl N, Ip NY, Kato A, Yancopoulos GD (1995) Mice lacking the CNTF receptor, unlike mice lacking CNTF, exhibit profound motor neuron deficits at birth. Cell 83:313–322

Dittrich F, Thoenen H, Sendtner M (1994) Ciliary neurotrophic factor: pharmakokinetics and acute phase response. Ann Neurol 35:151–163

Dittrich F, Ochs G, Grobe-Wilde A, Berweiler U, Yan Q, Miller JA, Toyka KV, Sendtner M (1996) Pharmakokinetics of intrathecally apllied BDNF and effects on spinal motoneurons. Exp Neurol 141:225–239

Duchen LW, Strich SJ, (with an Appendix by D.S.Falconer) (1968) An hereditary motor neurone disease with progressive denervation of muscle in the mouse: the mutant "wobbler". J Neurol Neurosurg Psychiat 31:535–542

Durbec P, Marcos Gutierrez CV, Kilkenny C, Grigoriou M, Wartiowaara K, Suvanto P, Smith D, Ponder B, Costantini F, Saarma M, Sariola H, Pachnis V (1996) GDNF signalling through the Ret receptor tyrosine kinase. Nature 381:789–793

Ebendal T, Tomac A, Hoffer BJ, Olson L (1995) Glial cell line-derived neurotrophic factor stimulates fiber formation and survival in cultured neurons from peripheral autonomic ganglia. J Neurosci Res 40:276–284

Economides AN, Ravetch JV, Yancopoulos GD, Stahl N (1995) Designer cytokines: targeting actions to cells of choice. Science 270:1351–1353

Eide FF, Lowenstein DH, Reichardt LF (1993) Neurotrophins and their receptors – current concepts and implications for neurologic disease. Exp Neurol 121:200–214

Eriksson NP, Lindsay RM, Aldskogius H (1994) BDNF and NT-3 rescue sensory but not motoneurones following axotomy in the neonate. Neuroreport 5:1445–1448

Ernfors P, Persson H (1991) Developmentally regulated expression of NDNF/NT-3 mRNA in rat spinal cord motoneurons and expression of BDNF mRNA in embryonic dorsal root ganglion. Eur J Neurosci 3:953–961

Ernfors P, Kucera J, Lee KF, Loring J, Jaenisch R (1995) Studies on the physiological role of brain-derived neurotrophic factor and neurotrophin-3 in knockout mice. Int J Dev Biol 39:799–807

Fink JK, Wu CB, Jones SM et al. (1995) Familial spastic paraplegia: tight linkage to chromosome 15q. Am J Hum Genet 56:188–192

Frade JM, Rodriguez Tebar A, Barde YA (1996) Induction of cell death by endogenous nerve growth factor through its p75 receptor. Nature 383:166–168

Friden PM, Walus LR, Watson P, Doctrow SR, Kozarich JW, Bäckman C, Bergman H, Hoffer B, Bloom F, Granholm A-C (1993) Blood-brain barrier penetration and in vivo activity of an NGF conjugate. Science 259:373–377

Friedman B, Scherer SS, Rudge JS, Helgren M, Morrisey D, McClain J, Wang, Wiegand SJ, Furth ME, Lindsay RM, Ip NY (1992) Regulation of ciliary neurotrophic factor expression in myelin-related Schwann cells in vivo. Neuron 9:295–305

Funakoshi H, Belluasdo N, Arenas E, Yamamoto Y, Casabona A, Persson H, Ibanez CF (1995) Muscle-derived neurotrophin-4 as an activity-dependent trophic signal for adult motor neurons. Science 268:1495–1499

Gash DM, Zhang Z, Cass WA, Ovadia A, Simmerman L, Martin D, Russell D, Collins F, Hoffer BJ, Gerhardt GA (1995) Morphological and functional effects of intranigrally administered GDNF in normal rhesus monkeys. J Comp Neurol 363:345–358

Gash DM, Zhang Z, Ovadia A, Cass WA, Yi A, Simmerman L, Russell D, Martin D, Lapchak PA, Collins F, Hoffer BJ, Gerhardt GA (1996) Functional recovery in parkinsonian monkeys treated with GDNF. Nature 380:252–255

Gearing DP, Bruce AG (1992) Oncostatin M binds the high-affinity leukemia inhibitory factor receptor. New Biol 4:61–65

Gearing DP, Thut CJ, VandeBos T, Gimpel SD, Delaney PB, King J, Price V, Cosman D, Beckmann MP (1991) Leukemia inhibitory factor receptor is structurally related to the IL-6 signal transducer, gp130. EMBO J 10:2839–2848

Gravel C, Götz R, Lorrain A, Sendtner M (1997) Adenoviral gene transfer of ciliary neurotrophic factor and brain-derived neurotrophic factor leads to longterm survival of axotomized motoneurons. Nat Med 3:765–770

Griesbeck O, Parsadanian AS, Sendtner M, Thoenen H (1995) Expression of neurotrophins in skeletal muscle: quantitative comparison and significance for motoneuron survival and maintenance of function. J Neurosci Res 42:21–33

Haase G, Kennel P, Pettmann B, Vigne E, Akli S, Revah F, Schmalbruch H, Kahn A (1997) Gene therapy of murine motor neuron disease using adenoviral vectors for neurotrophic factors. Nat Med 3:429–436

Hamburger V (1934) The effects of wing bud extirpation on the development of the central nervous system in chick embryos. J Exp Zool 68:449–494

Hamburger V (1958) Regression versus peripheral control of differentiation in motor hyperplasia. Am J Anat 102:365–410

Hansson H-A (1993) Insulin-like growth factors and nerve regeneration. Ann NY Acad Sci 692:161–171

Hantai D, Akaaboune M, Lagord C, Murawsky M, Houenou LJ, Festoff BW, Vaught JL, Rieger F, Blondet B (1995) Beneficial effects of insulin-like growth factor-I on wobbler mouse motoneuron disease. J Neurol Sci 129 [Suppl]:122–126

Hazan J, Lamy C, Melki J et al. (1993) Autosomal dominant familial spastic paraplegia is genetically heterogeneous and one locus maps to chromosome 14q. Nat Genet 5:163–167

Helgren ME, Friedman B, Kennedy M, Mullholland K, Messer A, Wong V, Lindsay RM (1992) Ciliary neurotrophic factor (CNTF) delays motor impairments in the mnd mouse, a genetic model of motor neuron disease (abstract). Neurosci Abstr 267.11:618

Henderson CE, Camu W, Mettling C, Gouin A, Poulsen K, Karihaloo M, Rullamas J, Evans T, McMahon SB, Armanini MP, Berkemeier L, Phillips HS, Rosenthal A (1993) Neurotrophins promote motor neuron survival and are present in embryonic limb bud. Nature 363:266–270

Henderson CE, Phillips HS, Pollock RA, Davies AM, Lemeulle C, Armanini M, Simpson LC, Moffet B, Vandlen RA, Koliatsos VE, et al. (1994a) GDNF: a potent survival factor for motoneurons present in peripheral nerve and muscle. Science 266:1062–1064

Henderson JT, Seniuk NA, Richardson PM, Gauldie J, Roder JC (1994b) Systemic administration of ciliary neurotrophic factor induces cachexia in rodents. J Clin Invest 93:2632–2638

Hentati A, Bejaoui K, Pericak-Vance MA, Hentati F, Speer MC, Hung W-Y, Figlewicz DA, Haines J, Rimmler J, Hamida CB, Hamida MB, Brown RH Jr, Siddique T (1994a) Linkage of recessive familial amyotrophic lateral sclerosis to chromosome 2q33-q35. Nature Genet 7:425–428

Hentati A, Pericak-Vance MA, Hung W-Y, Belal S, Laing N, Boustany R-M, Hentati F, Ben Hamida M, Siddique T (1994b) Linkage of "pure" autosomal recessive familial spastic paraplegia to chromosome 8 markers and evidence of genetic locus heterogeneity. Hum Mol Genet 3:1263–1267

Hentati A, Pericak-Vance MA, Lennon F, Wasserman B, Hentati F, Juneja T, Angrist MH, Hung W-Y, Boustany R-M, Bohlega S, Iqbal Z, Huether CH, Ben Hamida M, Siddique T (1994c) Linkage of a locus for autosomal dominant familial spastic paraplegia to chromosome 2p markers. Hum Mol Genet 3:1867–1871

Hirano A, Iwata M (1979) Pathology of motor neurons with special reference to amyotrophic lateral sclerosis and related diseases. In: Tsubaki T, Toyokura Y (eds) Amyotrophic lateral sclerosis. University Park Press, Baltimore, pp 107–134

Holliday M, Hamburger V (1975) Reduction of the naturally occurring motor neuron loss by enlargement of the periphery. J Comp Neurol 170:311–320

Huber J, Dittrich F, Phelan P (1993) Characterisation of high-affinity and low-affinity receptors for ciliary neurotrophic factor. Eur J Biochem 218:1031–1039

Hughes RA, Sendtner M, Thoenen H (1993) Members of several gene families influence survival of rat motoneurons in vitro and in vivo. J Neurosci Res 36(6):663–671

Ikeda K, Klinkosz B, Greene T, Cedarbaum JM, Wong V, Lindsay RM, Mitsumoto H (1995) Effects of brain-derived neurotrophic factor on motor dysfunction in wobbler mouse motor neuron disease. Ann Neurol 37:505–511

Ip NY, McClain J, Barrezueta NX, Aldrich TH, Pan L, Li YP, Wiegand SJ, Friedman B, Davis S, Yancopoulos GD (1993) The alpha component of the CNTF receptor is required for signaling and defines potential CNTF targets in the adult and during development. Neuron 10:89–102

Jackson M, Morrison KE, Al Chalabi A, Bakker M, Leigh PN (1996) Analysis of chromosome 5q13 genes in amyotrophic lateral sclerosis: homozygous NAIP deletion in a sporadic case. Ann Neurol 39:796–800

Jing S, Wen D, Yu Y, Holst PL, Luo Y, Fang M, Tamir R, Antonio L, Hu Z, Cupples R, Louis JC, Hu S, Altrock BW, Fox GM (1996) GDNF-induced activation of the ret protein tyrosine kinase is mediated by GDNFR-alpha, a novel receptor for GDNF. Cell 85:1113–1124

Jones CT, Brock DJH, Chancellor AM, Warlow CP, Swingler RJ (1993) Cu/Zn superoxide dismutase (SOD1) mutations and sporadic amyotrophic lateral sclerosis. Lancet 342:1050–1051

Kerkhoff H, Jennekens FGI, Troost D, Veldman H (1991) Nerve growth factor receptor immunostaining in the spinal cord and peripheral nerves in amyotrophic lateral sclerosis. Acta Neuropathol (Berl) 81:649–656

Klein R, Smeyne RJ, Wurst W, Long LK, Auerbach BA, Joyner AL, Barbacid M (1993) Targeted disruption of the trkB neurotrophin receptor results in nervous system lesions and neonatal death. Cell 75:113–122

Koliatsos VE, Shelton DL, Mobley WC, Price DL (1991) A novel group of nerve growth factor receptor-immunoreactive neurons in the ventral horn of the lumbar spinal cord. Brain Res 541:121–128

Koliatsos VE, Clatterbuck RE, Winslow JW, Cayouette MH, Price DL (1993) Evidence that brain-derived neurotrophic factor is a trophic factor for motor neurons in vivo. Neuron 10:359–367

Koliatsos VE, Cayouette MH, Berkemeier LR, Clatterbuck RE, Price DL, Rosenthal A (1994a) Neurotrophin 4/5 is a trophic factor for mammalian facial motor neurons. Proc Natl Acad Sci U S A 91:3304–3308

Koliatsos VE, Price WL, Pardo CA, Price DL (1994b) Ventral root avulsion: an experimental model of death of adult motor neurons. J Comp Neurol 342:35–44

Kostic V, Jackson-Lewis V, de Bibao F, Dubois-Dauphin M, Przedborski S (1997) Bcl-2: prolonging life in a transgenic mouse model of familial amyotrophic lateral sclerosis. Science 277:599–562

Kucera J, Ernfors P, Jaenisch R (1995) Reduction in the number of spinal motor neurons in neurotrophin-3-deficient mice. Neurosci 69:312–330

La Spada AR, Wilson EM, Lubahn DB, Harding AE, Fischbeck KH (1991) Androgen receptor gene mutations in X-linked spinal and bulbar muscular atrophy. Nature 352:77–79

Lai EC, Felice BW, Festoff BW et al (1995) A double-blind, placebo-controlled study of recombinant human insulin-like growth factor in the treatment of amyotrophic lateral sclerosis. Ann Neurol 38:971

Lefebvre S, Burglen L, Reboullet S, Clermont O, Burlet P, Viollet L, Benichou B, Cruaud C, Millasseau P, Zeviani M et al. (1995) Identification and characterization of a spinal muscular atrophy-determining gene (see comments). Cell 80:155–165

LeRoith D, Roberts CT Jr (1993) Insulin-like growth factors. Ann NY Acad Sci 692: 1–9

LeRoith D, Werner H, Faria TN, Kato H, Adamo M, Roberts CT Jr. (1993) Insulin-like growth factor receptors: implications for nervous system function. Ann NY Acad Sci 692:22–32

Levi-Montalcini R, Meyer H, Hamburger V (1954) In vitro experiments on the effects of mouse sarcomas 180 and 37 on the spinal and sympathetic ganglia of the chick embryo. Cancer Res 14:49–57

Li M, Sendtner M, Smith A (1995) Essential function of LIF receptor in motor neurons. Nature 378:724–727

Lin L-FH, Mismer D, Lile JD, Armes LG, Butler ET, III, Vannice JL, Collins F (1989) Purification, cloning, and expression of ciliary neurotrophic factor (CNTF). Science 246:1023–1025

Lin L-FH, Doherty DH, Lile JD, Bektesh S, Collins F (1993) GDNF: a glial cell line-derived neurotrophic factor for midbrain dopaminergic neurons. Science 260: 1130–1132

Lindsay RM (1996) Therapeutic potential of the neurotrophins and neurotrophin-CNTF combinations in peripheral neuropathies and motor neuron diseases. Ciba Found Symp 196:39–48

Liu X, Ernfors P, Wu H, Jaenisch R (1995) Sensory but not motor neuron deficits in mice lacking NT4 and BDNF. Nature 375:238–240

Lo AC, Houenou LJ, Oppenheim RW (1995) Apoptosis in the nervous system: morphological features, methods, pathology, and prevention. Arch Histol Cytol 58:139–149

Lohof AM, Ip NY, Poo M (1993) Potentiation of developing neuromuscular synapses by the neurotrophins NT-3 and BDNF. Nature 363:350–353

Longo FM, Manthorpe M, Varon S (1982) Spinal cord neurotrophic factors (SCNTFs). I. Bioassay of Schwannoma and other conditioned media. Dev Brain Res 3:277–294

Manthorpe M, Skaper S, Adler R, Landa K, Varon S (1980) Cholinergic neuronotrophic factors: fractionation properties of an extract from selected chick embryonic eye tissues. J Neurochem 34:69–75

Manthorpe M, Skaper SD, Williams LR, Varon S (1986) Purification of adult rat sciatic nerve ciliary neuronotrophic factor. Brain Res 367:282–286

Masu Y, Wolf E, Holtmann B, Sendtner M, Brem G, Thoenen H (1993) Disruption of the CNTF gene results in motor neuron degeneration. Nature 365:27–32

Matheson CR, Carnahan J, Urich JL, Bocangel D, Zhang TJ, Yan Q (1997) Glial cell line-derived neurotrophic factor (GDNF) is a neurotrophic factor for sensory neurons: comparison with the effects of the neurotrophins. J Neurobiol 32:22–32

Meyer M, Matsuoka I, Wetmore C, Olson L, Thoenen H (1992) Enhanced synthesis of brain-derived neurotrophic factor in the lesioned peripheral nerve: Different mechanisms are responsible for the regulation of BDNF and NGF mRNA. J Cell Biol 119:45–54

Miller RG, Bryan WW, Dietz M et al. (1993) Safety, tolerability and pharmakokinetics of recombinant human ciliary neurotrophic factor (rhCNTF) in patients with amyotrophic lateral sclerosis. Ann Neurol 34:304

Miller RG, Petajan JH, Bryan WW, Armon C, Barohn RJ, Goodpasture JC, Hoagland R, Parry GJ, Ross MA, Stromatt SC, the rhCNTF ALS Study Group (1996) A placebo-controlled trial of recombinant human ciliary neurotrophic (rhCNTF) factor in amyotrophic lateral sclerosis. Ann Neurol 39:256–260

Mitsumoto H, Ikeda K, Holmlund T, Greene T, Cedarbaum JM, Wong V, Lindsay RM (1994a) The effects of ciliary neurotrophic factor on motor dysfunction in wobbler mouse motor neuron disease. Ann Neurol 36:142–148

Mitsumoto H, Ikeda K, Klinkosz B, Cedarbaum JM, Wong V, Lindsay RM (1994b) Arrest of motor neuron disease in wobbler mice cotreated with CNTF and BDNF. Science 265:1107–1110

Miyata Y, Kashihara Y, Homma S, Kuno M (1986) Effects of nerve growth factor on the survival and synaptic function of Ia sensory neurons axotomized in neonatal rats. J Neurosci 6:2021–2018

Moore MW, Klein RD, Farinas I, Sauer H, Armanini M, Phillips H, Reichardt LF, Ryan AM, Carver Moore K, Rosenthal A (1996) Renal and neuronal abnormalities in mice lacking GDNF. Nature 382:76–79

Neff NT, Prevette D, Houenou LJ, Lewis ME, Glicksman MA, Yin Q-W, Oppenheim RW (1993) Insulin-like growth factors: putative muscle-derived trophic agents that promote motoneuron survival. J Neurobiol 24:1578–1588

O'Brien RJ, Fischbach GD (1986) Isolation of embryonic chick motoneurons and their survival in vitro. J Neurosci 6:3265–3274

Opacka Juffry J, Ashworth S, Hume SP, Martin D, Brooks DJ, Blunt SB (1995) GDNF protects against 6-OHDA nigrostriatal lesion: in vivo study with microdialysis and PET. Neuroreport 7:348–352

Oppenheim RW (1991) Cell death during development of the nervous system. Annu Rev Neurosci 14:453–501

Oppenheim RW, Qin-Wei Y, Prevette D, Yan Q (1992) Brain-derived neurotrophic factor rescues developing avian motoneurons from cell death. Nature 360:755–757

Oppenheim RW, Houenou LJ, Johnson JE, Lin LF, Li L, Lo AC, Newsome AL, Prevette DM, Wang S (1995) Developing motor neurons rescued from programmed and axotomy-induced cell death by GDNF. Nature 373:344–346

Panayotatos N, Radziejewska E, Acheson A, Pearsall D, Thadani A, Wong V (1993) Exchange of a single amino acid interconverts the specific activity and gel mobility of human and rat ciliary neurotrophic factors. J Biol Chem 268:19000–19003

Penn RD, Kroin JS, York MM, Cedarbaum JM (1997) Intrathecal ciliary neurotrophic factor delivery for treatment of amyotrophic lateral sclerosis. Neurosurgery 40:94–100

Pennica D, Shaw KJ, Swanson TA, Moore MW, Shelton DL, Zioncheck KA, Rosenthal A, Taga T, Paoni NF, Wood WI (1995) Cardiotrophin-1. Biological activities and binding to the leukemia inhibitory factor receptor/gp130 signaling complex. J Biol Chem 270:10915–10922

Pennica D, Arce V, Swanson TA, Vejsada R, Pollock RA, Armanini M, Dudley K, Phillips HS, Rosenthal A, Kato AC, Henderson CE (1996) Cardiotrophin-1, a cytokine present in embryonic muscle, supports long-term survival of spinal motoneurons. Neuron 17:63–74

Pichel JG, Shen L, Sheng HZ, Granholm AC, Drago J, Grinberg A, Lee EJ, Huang SP, Saarma M, Hoffer BJ, Sariola H, Westphal H (1996) Defects in enteric innervation and kidney development in mice lacking GDNF. Nature 382:73–76

Prosser CG, McLaren RD (1992) Insulin-like growth factor binding proteins of equine serum. Biochem Biophys Res Commun 189:1255–1260

Reinhardt RR, Bondy CA (1994) Insulin-like growth factors cross the blood–brain barrier. Endocrinology 135:1753–1761

Rosen DR, Siddique T, Patterson D, Figlewicz DA, Sapp P, Hentati A, Donaldson D, Goto J, O'Regan JP, Deng H-X, Rahmani Z, Krizus A, McKenna-Yasek D, Cayabyab A, Gaston SM, Berger R, Tanzi RE, Halperin JJ, Herzfeldt B, Van den Berg R, Hung W-Y, Bird T, Deng G, Mulder DW, Smyth C, Laing NG, Soriano E, Pericak-Vance MA, Haines J, Rouleau GA, Gusella JS, Horvitz HR, Brown Jr. RH (1993) Mutation in Cu/Zn superoxide dismutase gene are associated with familial amyotrophic lateral sclerosis. Nature 362:59–62

Rosenfeld RD, Zeni L, Haniu M, Talvenheimo J, Radka SF, Bennett L, Miller JA, Welcher AA (1995) Purification and identification of brain-derived neurotrophic factor from human serum. Protein Expr Purif 6:465–471

Roy N, Mahadevan MS, McLean M, Shutler G, Yaraghi Z, Farahani R, Baird S, Besner Johnston A, Lefebvre C, Kang X et al. (1995) The gene for neuronal apoptosis inhibitory protein is partially deleted in individuals with spinal muscular atrophy (see comments). Cell 80:167–178

Saggio I, Gloaguen I, Poiana G, Laufer R (1995) CNTF variants with increased biological potency and receptor selectivity define a functional site of receptor interaction. EMBO J 14:3045–3054

Sagot Y, Dubois Dauphin M, Tan SA, De Bilbao F, Aebischer P, Martinou -, JC, Kato AC (1995a) Bcl-2 overexpression prevents motoneuron cell body loss but not axonal degeneration in a mouse model of a neurodegenerative disease. J Neurosci 15:7727–7733

Sagot Y, Tan SA, Baetge E, Schmalbruch H, Kato AC, Aebischer P (1995b) Polymer encapsulated cell lines genetically engineered to release ciliary neurotrophic factor can slow down progressive motor neuronopathy in the mouse. Eur J Neurosci 7:1313–1322

Sagot Y, Tan SA, Hammang JP, Aebischer P, Kato AC (1996) GDNF slows loss of motoneurons but not axonal degeneration or premature death of pmn/pmn mice. J Neurosci 16:2335–2341

Sanchez MP, Silos Santiago I, Frisen J, He B, Lira SA, Barbacid M (1996) Renal agenesis and the absence of enteric neurons in mice lacking GDNF. Nature 382:70–73

Sara VR, Carlsson-Skwirut C, Drakenberg K, Giacobini MB, Håkansson L, Mirmiran M, Nordberg A, Olson L, Reinecke M, Ståhlbom PA, Sandberg Nordqvist AC (1993) The biological role of truncated insulin-like growth factor-1 and the tripeptide GPE in the central nervous system. Ann NY Acad Sci 692:183–191

Schmalbruch H (1984) Motoneuron death after sciatic nerve section in newborn rats. J Comp Neurol 224:252–258

Schmalbruch H, Jensen HJS, Bjaerg M, Kamieniecka Z, Kurland L (1991) A new mouse mutant with progressive motor neuronopathy. J Neuropathol Exp Neurol 50:192–204

Schnell L, Schneider R, Kolbeck R, Barde Y-A, Schwab ME (1994) Neurotrophin-3 enhances sprouting of corticospinal tract during development and after spinal cord lesion. Nature 367:170–173

Seeburger JL, Tarras S, Natter H, Springer JE (1993) Spinal cord motoneurons express $p75^{NGFR}$ and $p145^{trkB}$ mRNA in amyotrophic lateral sclerosis. Brain Res 621:111–115

Sendtner M (1997) Gene therapy for motoneuron disease. Nat Med 3:380–381
Sendtner M, Kreutzberg GW, Thoenen H (1990) Ciliary neurotrophic factor prevents the degeneration of motor neurons after axotomy. Nature 345:440–441
Sendtner M, Holtmann B, Kolbeck R, Thoenen H, Barde Y-A (1992a) Brain-derived neurotrophic factor prevents the death of motoneurons in newborn rats after nerve section. Nature 360:757–758
Sendtner M, Schmalbruch H, Stöckli KA, Carroll P, Kreutzberg GW, Thoenen H (1992b) Ciliary neurotrophic factor prevents degeneration of motor neurons in mouse mutant progressive motor neuronopathy. Nature 358:502–504
Sendtner M, Stöckli KA, Thoenen H (1992c) Synthesis and location of ciliary neurotrophic factor in the rat sciatic nerve of the adult rat after lesion and during regeneration. J Cell Biol 118:139–148
Sendtner M, Carroll P, Holtmann B, Hughes RA, Thoenen H (1994a) Ciliary neurotrophic factor. J Neurobiol 25:1436–1453
Sendtner M, Dittrich F, Hughes RA, Thoenen H (1994b) Actions of CNTF and neurotrophins on degenerating motoneurons: preclinical studies and clinical implications. J Neurol Sci 124 [Suppl]:77–83
Sendtner M, Götz R, Holtmann B, Escary J-L, Masu Y, Carroll P, Wolf E, Brehm G, Brulet P, Thoenen H (1996) Cryptic physiological trophic support of motoneurons by LIF disclosed by double gene targeting of CNTF and LIF. Curr Biol 6:686–694
Sendtner M, Götz R, Holtmann B, Thoenen H (1997). Endogenous ciliary neurotrophic factor is a lesion factor for axotomized motoneurons in adult mice. J Neurosci 17:6999–7006
Siddique T, Nijhawan D, Hentati A (1996) Molecular genetic basis of familial ALS. Neurology 47[Suppl 2]:S27–S35
Smith RA (1992) Handbook of amyotrophic lateral sclerosis. Marcel Dekker, New York
Snider WD, Thanedar S (1989) Target dependence of hypoglossal motor neurons during development and in maturity. J Comp Neurol 279:489–498
Sobue G, Hashizume Y, Mukai E, Hirayama M, Mitsuma T, Takahashi A (1989) X-linked recessive bulbospinal neuronopathy. A clinicopathological study. Brain 112:209–232
Springer JE, Mu X, Bergmann LW, Trojanowski JQ (1994) Expression of GDNF mRNA in rat and human nervous tissue. Exp Neurol 127:167–170
Stahl N, Yancopoulos GD (1994) The tripartite CNTF receptor complex: activation and signaling involves components shared with other cytokines. J Neurobiol 25:1454–1466
Stöckli KA, Lottspeich F, Sendtner M, Masiakowski P, Carroll P, Götz R, Lindholm D, Thoenen H (1989) Molecular cloning, expression and regional distribution of rat ciliary neurotrophic factor. Nature 342:920–923
Stoeckel K, Thoenen H (1975) Retrograde axonal transport of nerve growth factor: specificity and biological importance. Brain Res 85:337–341
Stong DB, Raskin R (1993) Effects of multiple subcutaneous doses of rhIGF-1 on total and free IGF-1 levels and blood glucose in humans. Ann NY Acad Sci 692:317–320
Strohmaier C, Carter BD, Urfer R, Barde YA, Dechant G (1996) A splice variant of the neurotrophin receptor trkB with increased specificity for brain-derived neurotrophic factor. EMBO J 15:3332–3337
Thoenen H, Barde Y-A (1980) Physiology of nerve growth factor. Physiol Rev 60:1284–1335
Thoenen H, Hughes RA, Sendtner M (1993) Trophic support of motoneurons: physiological, pathophysiological, and therapeutic implications. Exp Neurol 124:47–55
Treanor JJ, Goodman L, de Sauvage F, Stone DM, Poulsen KT, Beck CD, Gray C, Armanini MP, Pollock RA, Hefti F, Phillips HS, Goddard A, Moore MW, Buj Bello A, Davies AM, Asai N, Takahashi M, Vandlen R, Henderson CE, Rosenthal A (1996) Characterization of a multicomponent receptor for GDNF. Nature 382:80–83

Troost D, Aten J, Morsink F, de Jong JM (1995) Apoptosis in amyotrophic lateral sclerosis is not restricted to motor neurons. Bcl-2 expression is increased in unaffected post-central gyrus. Neuropathol Appl Neurobiol 21:498–504

Trupp M, Ryden M, Jornvall H, Funakoshi H, Timmusk T, Arenas E, Ibanez CF (1995) Peripheral expression and biological activities of GDNF, a new neurotrophic factor for avian and mammalian peripheral neurons. J Cell Biol 130:137–148

Trupp M, Arenas E, Fainzilber M, Nilsson AS, Sieber BA, Grigoriou M, Kilkenny C, Salazar Grueso E, Pachnis V, Arumae U, Sariola H, Saarma M, Ibanez CF (1996) Functional receptor for GDNF encoded by the c-ret proto-oncogene. Nature 381:785–788

Vejsada R, Sagot Y, Kato AC (1994) BDNF-mediated rescue of axotomized motor neurones decreases with increasing dose. Neuroreport 5:1889–1892

Vejsada R, Sagot Y, Kato AC (1995) Quantitative comparison of the transient rescue effects of neurotrophic factors on axotomized motoneurons in vivo. Eur J Neurosci 7:108–115

Wayne DB, Heaton MB (1990) The ontogeny of specific retrograde transport of nerve growth factor by motoneurons of the brainstem and spinal cord. Dev Biol 138:484–498

Wilhelmsen KC, Lynch T, Pavlou E, Higgins M, Nygaard TG (1994) Localization of disinhibition-dementia-parkinsonism-amyotrophy complex to 17q21–22. Am J Hum Genet 55:1159–1165

Williams LR, Manthorpe M, Barbin G, Nieto-Sampedro M, Cotman CW, Varon S (1984) High ciliary neuronotophic specific activity in rat peripheral nerve. Int J Dev Neurosci 2:177–180

Wong V, Pearsall D, Arriaga R, Ip NY, Stahl N, Lindsay RM (1995) Binding characteristics of ciliary neurotrophic factor to sympathetic neurons and neuronal cell lines. J Biol Chem 270:313–318

Yamamoto H, Gurney ME (1990) Human platelets contain brain-derived neurotrophic factor. J Neurosci 10:3469–3478

Yan Q, Snider WD, Pinzone JJ, Johnson EM Jr (1988) Retrograde transport of nerve growth factor (NGF) in motoneurons of developing rats: assessment of potential neurotrophic effects. Neuron 1:335–343

Yan Q, Elliott J, Snider WD (1992) Brain-derived neurotrophic factor rescues spinal motor neurons from axotomy-induced cell death. Nature 360:753–755

Yan Q, Elliott JL, Matheson C, Sun J, Zhang L, Mu X, Rex KL, Snider WD (1993) Influences of neurotrophins on mammalian motoneurons in vivo. J Neurobiol 24:1555–1577

Yan Q, Matheson C, Lopez OT (1995) In vivo neurotrophic effects of GDNF on neonatal and adult facial motor neurons. Nature 373:341–344

Yoshida K, Taga T, Saito M, Suematsu S, Kumanogoh A, Tanaka T, Fujiwara H, Hirata M, Yamagami T, Nakahata T, Hirabayashi T, Yoneda Y, Tanaka K, Wang WZ, Mori C, Shiota K, Yoshida N, Kishimoto T (1996) Targeted disruption of gp130, a common signal transducer for the interleukin 6 family of cytokines, leads to myocardial and hematological disorders. Proc Natl Acad Sci USA 93:407–411

Zurn AD, Winkel L, Menoud A, Djabali K, Aebischer P (1996) Combined effects of GDNF, BDNF, and CNTF on motoneuron differentiation in vitro. J Neurosci Res 44:133–141

CHAPTER 5

Neuropharmacology of Insulin-Like Growth Factors

D.N. Ishii and S.-F. Pu

Abbreviations

ALS	amyotrophic lateral sclerosis
BBB	blood–brain barrier
BDNF	brain-derived neurotrophic factor
CNS	central nervous system
CSF	cerebrospinal fluid
CNTF	ciliary neurotrophic factor
GABA	γ-aminobutyric acid
IGF	insulin-like growth factor
IGFBP	insulin-like growth factor binding protein
IDDM	insulin-dependent diabetes mellitus
NGF	nerve growth factor
NIDDM	non-insulin-dependent diabetes mellitus
RGD	Arg-Gly-Asp sequence for binding to extracellular matrix proteins
SOD	superoxide dismutase
ZDF	Zucker diabetic fatty

A. Introduction

The past decade has brought an explosion of neurobiological discoveries, and, with it, elevated hopes for the development of new treatments for diseases and disorders of the nervous system. The cost of treating trauma and neurodegenerative disorders is staggering. For example, the annual expenditure in the United States for CNS trauma is US $4.7 billion, for stroke $11.3 billion, for Parkinson's disease and other movement disorders $2.5 billion, for Alzheimer's disease and other dementias $50 billion, and for neuromuscular disorders $5 billion. These CNS disorders involve 6.5 million cases and peripheral neuropathy involves millions of additional cases. These disorders have been targeted in the development of new neuropharmacological agents. Neurotrophic factors, such as neurotrophins and insulin-like growth factors (IGFs), are among the leading drug candidates.

This article is focused particularly on the neuropharmacology of IGFs. It will be discussed that IGFs differ in fundamental ways from the classic neurotrophins. IGFs are, whereas neurotrophins are not, circulating neurotrophic factors. IGFs are, whereas neurotrophins are not, ubiquitous with respect to capacity to act on diverse neuronal populations. These differences have profound implications for the design of clinical trials to treat neurological disorders.

Pharmacokinetic parameters helpful in the design of routes of administration are discussed, as well as dose and dose schedules for the therapeutic use of IGFs. As is true for other hormones, the emergence of side-effects will be influenced by the route of administration, patient's age, physiological condition, disease state, and whether treatment doses are intended for physiological replacement or pharmacological enhancement.

Although it would be desirable to discover small lipophilic drug agonist molecules that may be taken orally, particularly to treat CNS disorders, decades of pharmaceutical-industry experience suggest that agonists of neurotrophic factors may be indeed difficult to come by. This may be because neurotrophic factors are fairly large molecules that have many contact sites on their receptors which are dispersed across large molecular distances. Therefore, small molecules may not be able to span these distances and form the numbers of contacts necessary to activate the receptors. Thus, the neurotrophic factors themselves are likely, at least in the near future, to remain the best drug agonist candidates. Small molecule antagonists, by contrast, are generally much easier to design.

B. Background

The IGF-I and IGF-II genes are large; each unique gene gives rise to multiple transcripts, and the IGF proteins are complexed to an array of binding proteins. The receptors for IGFs in the nervous system differ from those in peripheral tissues. IGF-I is under growth-hormone regulation, whereas IGF-II is not. A large body of literature shows that IGFs are neurotrophic growth factors.

I. IGF Genes and Transcripts

The nomenclature for IGF genes, transcripts and binding proteins was revised at the 2nd International Symposium on IGFs in San Francisco, CA, in 1991 (Holthuizen et al. 1991). The purpose of multiple IGF transcripts is unclear.

1. IGF-I

The mammalian IGF-I gene spans approximately 50–80 kb and contains six exons. Alternative leader exon 1 or exon 2 can be spliced to exon 3. Exon 5 is retained in some transcripts, but spliced out of others. There are seven poly(A) sites in human, but three in rat exon 6. Transcripts are generally referred to by size; those containing exon 1 are called class-1 transcripts and those containing exon 2 are called class-2 transcripts.

Mature IGF-I is a basic polypeptide of 70 amino acids. It mediates many, but not all of the actions of growth hormone. Transgenic mice overexpressing IGF-I have enlarged body and organ size (MATHEWS et al. 1988). Interestingly, there is a disproportionate increase in brain size (CARSON et al. 1993).

2. IGF-II

The IGF-II gene spans 30–36 kb of nucleotide sequence and has three independent promoters in the rat and mouse, and four promoters in humans. Rodent genes have six exons, and exons 1–3 act as alternative leader exons. The human gene has nine exons, and exons 1, 4, 5 or 6 act as alternative leader exons. Because the IGF-II coding sequence is found in exons 7–9 (or exons 4–6 in rodents), all IGF-II transcripts encode pre-pro-IGF-II. The first promoter in humans is absent in rats and mice, and is a liver-specific promoter. Circulating IGF-II is produced predominantly by liver, hence, IGF-II levels are elevated in humans but extremely low in rodents.

Gene inactivation by homologous recombination shows that the IGF-II gene increases prenatal, but not postnatal growth (DECHIARA et al. 1990). Circulating IGF-II levels do not increase during puberty and remain high in humans long after the growth spurt, indicating that its major postnatal role is not as a growth factor.

One observation which suggests a selective role for IGF-II in the nervous system is that the IGF-II mRNAs are much more abundant in brain and spinal cord than in other tissues of the adult rat (SOARES et al. 1985, 1986; ROTWEIN et al. 1988). The choroid plexus and leptomeninges are enriched in IGF-II mRNAs (HYNES et al. 1988; ICHIMIYA et al. 1988; STYLIANOPOULOU et al. 1988) and may be the main production source of IGF-II in cerebrospinal fluid (HASELBACHER and HUMBEL 1982). IGF-II is the predominant IGF in brain. IGF-II gene expression in muscle is closely correlated with polyneuronal innervation during synaptogenesis in embryonic rats (ISHII 1989) and during re-establishment of neuromuscular synapses in adult rats (GLAZNER and ISHII 1995). Mature IGF-II is a neutral protein of 67 amino acids.

The IGF-II gene is subject to parental imprinting (DECHIARA et al. 1991). Only the paternal allele is expressed, whereas the maternal allele is repressed in peripheral tissues and in the leptomeninges. By contrast, the maternal allele is expressed in regions of the brain, such as the cerebellum and the cortex (HU et al. 1995). The reason for maternal influence in brain, but paternal influence in peripheral tissues is unknown. Imprinting also occurs in the type-II IGF receptor which selectively binds IGF-II. In this case, the maternal allele is expressed and the paternal allele is silent (BARLOW et al. 1991).

II. IGF Receptors

1. Type-I Receptors

The type-I IGF receptor is structurally similar to the insulin receptor. The heterotetrameric receptor is comprised of two alpha extracellular subunits and two membrane-spanning beta subunits. The beta subunit is a tyrosine kinase. There is a preference for binding IGF-I, but IGF-II also binds with relatively high affinity. Most of the actions of both IGFs are believed to be mediated through the type-I receptor. However, it is unexplained why transgenic mice overexpressing IGF-I have a much greater growth response than mice overexpressing IGF-II.

Posttranslational modification includes glycosylation of the alpha subunit. The neuronal is smaller than the peripheral tissue type-I IGF receptor due to reduced glycosylation (Heidenreich and Brandenberg 1986; Burgess et al. 1987). It is possible that selective effects on the nervous system may be obtained by IGF binding to this receptor which is distributed to neurons of the peripheral as well as central nervous system.

Binding of IGF-I and IGF-II to type-I IGF receptors is correlated with neurite outgrowth (Recio-Pinto and Ishii 1988) and capacity to increase the expression of genes encoding axonal cytoskeletal proteins such as tubulin (Mill et al. 1985). The K_d of IGF-I binding to high affinity receptors is about 0.1–0.3 nM on neurons. Receptors are found in nerve terminals, along the axon shaft and on the cell bodies.

2. Type-II Receptors

The type-II IGF receptor is comprised of a single polypeptide chain and does not contain intrinsic tyrosine-kinase activity. It may be linked to a G-protein. This receptor is also the mannose-6-phosphate receptor and is implicated in lysosomal trafficking. The precise role of the type-II IGF receptor remains somewhat mysterious. It has a much higher affinity for IGF-II than IGF-I.

III. IGF Binding Proteins

There are at least six members of an IGF-binding protein (IGFBP) gene family (for review, see Clemmons et al. 1993). IGFBP-3 is the predominant IGFBP in the circulation and binds to both IGF-I and IGF-II. Together with the acid labile subunit, a 1:1:1 complex of 150 kDa is produced. A serine protease can cleave IGFBP-3, resulting in loss of binding to the acid-labile subunit. The IGFBP-3 fragment forms a 30 kDa complex with IGFs which has reduced affinity compared with the 150 kDa complex. IGFBP-3 and -4 are glycosylated. IGFBP-1 and -2 contain RGD sequences, which may facilitate binding to the extracellular matrix. These various IGFBPs have differential affinity for IGF-I and IGF-II. Mainly, they sequester and inhibit IGF activity, but in some cases increase in activity is reported. Emerging data suggest there may be a family of proteases, each specific for a particular IGFBP.

C. Neurotrophic Relationships

IGFs have been found to act on virtually all, if not all, of the many types of neurons in mammals. IGFs seem to provide ubiquitous neurotrophic support for the central and peripheral nervous system, which is consistent with the wide distribution of IGFs throughout the nervous system. The neurobiology has been reviewed elsewhere (DEVASKAR 1991; DE PABLO and DE LA ROSA 1995; ISHII et al. 1996), hence only a brief overview is provided here.

I. Peripheral Nervous System

Physiological concentrations of highly purified preparations of IGF-I and IGF-II can support neurite outgrowth in cultured sensory, sympathetic, neuroblastoma (RECIO-PINTO and ISHII 1984; MILL et al. 1985; RECIO-PINTO et al. 1986; ISHII and RECIO-PINTO 1987) and motor (CARONI and GRANDES 1990) neurons. Survival is also supported (RECIO-PINTO et al. 1986). Unlike, NGF, which is not a mitogen, IGFs stimulate mitosis in sympathetic neuroblasts (DICICCO-BLOOM and BLACK 1988).

Following nerve crush in adult rats, IGF gene expression is increased in nerve Schwann cells (GLAZNER et al. 1994; PU et al. 1995). Administration of IGF-II increases, whereas anti-IGF antiserum reduces the regeneration of motor axons in nerves (NEAR et al. 1992). IGF-I (KANJE et al. 1989) and IGF-II (GLAZNER et al. 1993) administration increases sensory-nerve regeneration rate as well. Axotomy in neonatal rats results in death of motoneurons, and such death is prevented by IGF-II administration (PU et al. 1995). Moreover, the administration of anti-IGF antibodies or IGFBP, locally to the nerve stump, increases the death of motoneurons, showing that endogenous nerve IGF is essential for survival. IGF-I and IGF-II treatment of chick embryos prevents the developmentally programmed death of motoneurons (NEFF et al. 1993).

II. Central Nervous System

Primary cell cultures of various central-nervous-system tissues have been studied. DNA synthesis is stimulated in cultured brain neurons (LENOIR and HONEGGER 1983). IGF-I treatment enhances the survival of mesencephalon, spinal cord, cerebral cortex, retina, cerebellum and basal forebrain neurons (DECHIARA et al. 1991; DEVASKAR 1991; BOZYCZKO-COYNE et al. 1993; MASTERS and RAIZADA 1993). However, IGFs ability to increase motoneuron survival seems to require the presence of astrocytes in culture (ANG et al. 1992). GABA, glutamate, acetylcholine, dopamine and other neurotransmitter systems are modulated. IGF-I treatment can increase Ca^{2+}-current density in cultured cells (EL-BADRY et al. 1989). Under conditions of hypoglycemic stress, IGFs can protect cultured hippocampal and septal neurons (CHENG and MATTSON 1992). Strains of mice deficient in IGF-I show poor development of certain brain regions, such as the suprachiasmatic nucleus, pineal body and cerebrum (NOGUCHI et al. 1983, 1986). Myelination is reduced as well (NOGUCHI et al. 1982), which complements the observation that IGF-I induces oligodendrocyte development in culture (MCMORRIS et al. 1986). In a single case of an infant with megalencephaly, IGF-II content was elevated in CSF (SCHOENLE et al. 1986).

D. Neurological Disorders Targeted for IGF Therapy

I. Diabetic Neuropathy

1. Pathophysiology

The clinical manifestations and pathophysiology of diabetic neuropathy has been reviewed (Dyck et al. 1987; Ward 1989; Vinik et al. 1992; Thomas and Tomlinson 1993). Approximately 39%–66% of the estimated 13 million diabetic patients in the USA have neuropathy that is detectable using recent definitions and methods of measurement (The DCCT Research Group 1988; Dyck et al. 1993). Clinically symptomatic neuropathy, however, is evident in 13%–15% of all patients with type-I (insulin-dependent diabetes mellitus; juvenile onset) and type-II (non-insulin-dependent diabetes mellitus; adult onset) disorder. Only 7% of children have symptomatic neuropathy, but this value reaches 50% in patients in the later decades of life. More than half of all diabetic males (>3 million cases) are impotent. A slowing of conduction velocity is observed almost universally in patients, but its relationship to the progression towards symptomatic neuropathy is unclear.

The sensory, sympathetic and motor systems may be afflicted, and the most prevalent form of this heterogeneous disease is symmetrical polyneuropathy. Pain, paresthesia, defective thermoregulation, loss of bladder control, gastroparesis, impotence and cardiac denervation are but a few of the consequences. Symptomatic autonomic neuropathy is associated with an increased risk of mortality: as high as 50% within 5–10 years of diagnosis (Ewing et al. 1980). Secondary consequences of denervation include the diabetic foot and more than 50000 limb amputations annually.

The longest nerves are generally afflicted first in polyneuropathy. The main pathological features include a dwindling of axonal diameters, loss of synapses, and a dying back axonopathy which involves both non-myelinated and myelinated nerves (Archer et al. 1983; Said et al. 1983). Segmental demyelination may be observed in the latter. The structural lesions are more severe in type-I than type-II diabetes (Sima et al. 1988; Yagihashi 1995). A major contributor to denervation and loss of neurons may be a failure of nerves to regenerate properly (Longo et al. 1986; Ekstrom and Tomlinson 1989). Ultimately, a progressive but variable loss of sensory, sympathetic and motor neurons may result in permanent loss of function.

The pathogenesis of diabetic neuropathy remains a subject of intense debate. Risk factors include age, duration of disease, height (probably due to longer nerve fibers) and consumption of alcohol and tobacco. Multi-factorial, weak genetic risk factors may be operative. Hyperglycemia and increased production of polyols together with non-enzymatic glycation of proteins is believed to contribute to neuropathy. On the other hand, it remains unexplained why hyperglycemia does not correlate with any of the major risk factors. Beyond a small increase in conduction velocity, aldose-reductase inhibitors, designed to inhibit polyol production have not lived up to expectations in extensive clinical trials, albeit a few trials are ongoing. The possibility that inhibitors of protein glycation may be useful is under preclinical consideration. The normalization of glucose, for example by pancreatic transplantation, has not been found to reverse existing neuropathy, but may retard progression. Microvascular disease with ischemia may be another contributing factor. Cause and effect become difficult to dissociate, because neural disturbances may contribute to microvascular disease. Vascular tone is regulated by sympathetic and sensory C-fibers (FLEMING et al. 1989; AHLUWALIA and VALLANCE 1997). Further study is needed to determine the relative contribution of microvascular disease, hyperglycemia, non-enzymatic glycation or the combination of these factors to axonopathy and the pathogenesis of neuropathy.

More recently, it has been proposed that a decline in IGF activity contributes significantly to the causation of diabetic neuropathy (ISHII 1993, 1995). This theory suggests that: (a) IGF-I, IGF-II and, possibly, insulin provide redundant neurotrophic support under normal conditions; (b) IGF activity is reduced in diabetes; and (c) the age-dependent decline in IGF activity is, at least in part, responsible for the age-dependent risk of neuropathy. Loss of IGF neurotrophic support could cause myriad deleterious effects. The expression of many genes regulated by IGFs in neurons and supporting glial or Schwann cells may be abnormal. For example, the expression of genes encoding axonal cytoskeletal proteins would be reduced, leading to dwindling of axonal diameters, loss of synapses and loss of axons. There would be an increased risk of neuron death. The loss of circulating IGF activity and decreased IGF gene expression throughout most of the nervous system would lead to polyneuropathy. However, individual differences in gene expression and local differences in autocrine/paracrine activity of IGFs, together with other neurotrophic factors, may partially explain heterogeneous neuropathies. A complex clinical picture emerges when one begins to consider other exacerbating factors, such as autoimmune attack on the nervous system and environmental factors such as alcohol.

The complex IGF-regulatory and signaling system may contribute to multi-factorial genetic risk. The relationship to other predisposing factors, such as height, is considered. Redundant but age-dependent neurotrophic support might explain the observation that younger IDDM patients have a lower risk of neuropathy because their residual IGF levels would be higher than older patients. Risk would continually increase with age due to the progressive rundown of IGF activity. Indeed, neuropathy in elderly non-diabetic individuals is qualitatively similar to diabetic neuropathy (JACOBS and LOVE 1985). Chronic hyperglycemia and/or microvascular disease may further aggravate a weakened nervous system and contribute to duration-dependent risk; however, other possibilities are not excludable. Various predictions of this theory have been tested, as discussed below.

2. Experimental Observations in Non-Primates

a) *IGF Activity in Experimental IDDM*

The alterations in IGF gene expression and neural disturbances in type-I and type-II diabetic rats are summarized in Table 1. Streptozotocin was administered to adult rats in order to reduce the capacity of the pancreas to produce insulin. In this type-I model of diabetes, it is known that circulating IGF-I levels are reduced (Phillips and Young 1976; Baxter et al. 1979; Maes et al. 1983) and that IGF-I gene expression is reduced in liver, the primary source of circulating IGF-I (Bornfeldt et al. 1989; Fagin et al. 1989). The rate of decline in IGF-I gene expression (Ishii et al. 1994) precedes the development of neuropathy (Carsten et al. 1989). Unlike in humans, IGF-II mRNA content is developmentally downregulated in rat liver, circulating IGF-II levels are very low and redundant circulating neurotrophic support is more quickly lost in

Table 1. Insulin-like Growth Factor (IGF) and neural disturbances in diabetic rats

	Type I (IDDM)	Type II (NIDDM)
Diabetic Profile		
Cause of diabetes	Streptozotocin	Spontaneous
Insulin	Hypoinsulinemic	Hyperinsulinemic
Glucose	Hyperglycemic	Hyperglycemic
Body weight	Loss	Obese
IGF and Neural Disturbances		
Circulation		
IGF-I	Decreased	Decreased
IGF BP-1	Increased	?
IGF BP-3	Decreased	?
Liver		
IGF-I mRNA	Decreased	Decreased
IGF-II mRNA[a]		
Sciatic nerve		
IGF-I mRNA	Decreased	Normal
IGF-II mRNA	Decreased	Decreased
Hyperalgesia	Yes	Yes
Impaired regeneration	Yes	No
Conduction velocity	Decreased	Decreased
Spinal cord		
IGF-I mRNA	Decreased	Normal
IGF-II mRNA	Decreased	Decreased
Myelopathy[b]	Yes	?
Brain		
IGF-II mRNA	Decreased	Decreased
Brain weight	Normal	Reduced
Encephalopathy[b]	Yes	Yes

[a] IGF-II gene expression is developmentally downregulated in rat but not human liver, which is the main source of circulating neurotrophic IGF activity.
[b] For diabetic myelopathy and encephalopathy see Mooradian 1988; McCall 1991; Wuarin et al. 1996.

diabetes; this species-dependent biochemical difference may explain, at least in part, why neuropathy develops more quickly in rats than in humans. A useful piece of information when planning IGF treatment in rats is that the daily production of circulating IGF-I is 31 μg/day/rat (Schwander et al. 1983; Scott et al. 1985).

IGFs are paracrine as well as endocrine factors, and IGF gene expression was examined in the nervous system of diabetic rats. IGF-I mRNA content is selectively reduced in the spinal cord (Ishii et al. 1994), the sciatic nerve (Wuarin et al. 1994) and the adrenal gland (Ishii et al. 1994). In addition, IGF-II mRNA content is selectively reduced in nerve (Wuarin et al. 1994), spinal cord and brain (Wuarin et al. 1996). These are among the earliest known biochemical lesions in the nervous system and precede the onset of diabetic neuropathy, myelopathy and encephalopathy.

Insulin administration incompletely restores IGF mRNA content in liver (Ishii et al. 1994), nerves (Wuarin et al. 1994), brain and spinal cord (Wuarin et al. 1996). This might explain why insulin is only partially effective in protecting against neuropathy in clinical trials.

IGFBP-1 is increased in serum from diabetic rats and humans (Brismar et al. 1988; Unterman et al. 1989), but IGFBP-3 is decreased (Zapf et al. 1980). Both IGFBP-1 and IGFBP-2 mRNAs (Ooi et al. 1990) and immunoreactivity (Gelato et al. 1992) are increased in liver, and IGFBP-2 mRNA is increased in the pituitary (Gelato et al. 1992) from IDDM rats. In contrast, IGFBP-3 is decreased in liver, and IGFBP-1 and IGFBP-2 are increased in kidney (Gelato et al. 1992). There seems to be a reciprocal relationship between circulating IGF-I and IGFBP-1 levels (Hall et al. 1988).

b) IGF Activity in Experimental NIDDM

The Zucker diabetic fatty rat has been used extensively as a model of type-II diabetes. The ZDF (*fa/fa*) rat is obese, hyperinsulinemic and spontaneously diabetic. In contrast, the +/+ littermates are lean and have normal insulin and glucose levels. As in type-I rats, IGF-I and -II mRNA contents are reduced in liver, nerve, spinal cord and brain of *fa/fa* vs. +/+ rats (Wuarin et al. 1996; Zhuang et al. 1997).

An interesting biochemical difference is that sciatic nerve IGF-I mRNA content is reduced in rats with type-I, but not type-II, disease. This tissue-selective difference is difficult to reconcile on the basis of a dissimilarity in glycemic state. Moreover, nerve regeneration is impaired to a greater degree in type-I than type-II diabetic rats (unpublished observation). These inequalities might be related to the observation that nerve-fiber atrophy and loss is more severe in type-I than type-II rats and patients (Sima et al. 1988; Yagihashi 1995). As the protection offered by circulating IGFs is lost with age, nerve damage may become greater in type-I than type-II disease because of the greater loss of paracrine IGF-I activity within the nerves of IDDM patients.

c) IGF Treatment Prevents Neuropathy

Theory predicts that IGF replacement therapy should prevent neuropathy (Ishii 1995). The subcutaneous implantation of osmotic mini pumps that continuously release IGF-I or IGF-II (15 μg/kg/day), in fact, prevents the impairment of nerve regeneration in type-I diabetic rats (Ishii and Lupien 1995). A longer duration of treatment can reverse this impairment (Zhuang et al. 1996). Single, daily subcutaneous injections are also effective. Furthermore, diabetic pain or hyperalgesia can be arrested by the subcutaneous administration of IGF-I or IGF-II in type-I diabetic rats (Zhuang et al. 1996). This treatment is also effective in type-II diabetic rats (Zhuang et al. 1997).

d) Relationship of Disturbances in IGF Axis to Hyperglycemia, Hyperinsulinemia and Weight Loss

These data show that in type-I and type-II diabetic rats, there is a profound loss of the major sources of endocrine and paracrine IGF activity which normally supports neurons. The decrease in IGF gene expression in neural tissues is independent of weight loss (type I) or gain (type II), as well as of hypo- (type I) or hyperinsulinemia (type II) (Ishii et al. 1994; Wuarin et al. 1994, 1996; Zhuang et al. 1997).

Circulating IGF-I levels do not correlate with glucose levels in diabetic patients (Tan and Baxter 1986) or diabetic rhesus monkeys (Bodkin et al. 1991). Urinary IGF-I output levels do not correlate with glucose levels in IDDM children (Quattrin et al. 1992). Moreover, insulin, rather than glucose, regulates serum IGFBP-1 levels in humans, as shown by glucose-clamp studies (Suikkari et al. 1988).

The lack of a direct relationship between disturbances in the IGF axis and hyperglycemia in diabetes is not unexpected, because hyperglycemia does not correlate with any of the risk factors for neuropathy. In contrast, a decrease in IGF activity correlates with neuropathy.

Despite the best advice of physicians, diabetic patients often find it difficult to adequately control hyperglycemia and obesity. It might be considered very encouraging news that IGF treatment prevents or reverses neuropathy independently of unabated hyperglycemia in type-I and type-II diabetic rats (Ishii and Lupien 1995; Zhuang et al. 1996, 1997).

It is noted that the administration of much larger supraphysiological doses of IGF-I (300 μg/rat/day) can prevent weight loss in diabetic rats (Scheiwiller et al. 1986). Similarly, large doses can reduce hyperglycemia. However, such doses are much larger than the 15 μg/kg/day physiological replacement doses sufficient to prevent neuropathy. The neurotrophic actions of IGFs may be selectively achieved through the higher affinity neural, rather than peripheral, tissue IGF receptors.

3. IGF Activity in Primates

a) Diabetic Monkeys

Rhesus monkeys, like many humans, progress with age from young, lean and normoglycemic to obese, hyperinsulinemic and glucose-intolerant individuals. Eventually they convert to hyperglycemia and full-blown diabetes. It is interesting that in every stage of disease there is a decrease in IGF-I levels (Bodkin et al. 1991) and diabetic neuropathy is observed (Cornblath et al. 1989).

b) Clinical Diabetes

After the second decade of life, there is a slow and incessant decrease in circulating IGF levels (Hall and Sara 1984). Type-I and type-II diabetic patients are found to have an approximate 50% reduction in IGF-I levels, relative to age-matched non-diabetic subjects, that is superimposed on the age-dependent decrease (Tan and Baxter 1986). Moreover, circulating IGF-I levels are reduced to a greater extent in those diabetic patients with neuropathy than those without (Migdalis et al. 1995). Other factors which may reduce IGF activity include the presence of antibodies to type-I IGF receptors which are detected in sera from some diabetic patients (Tappy et al. 1988).

II. Chemotherapy-Induced Neuropathy

The emergence of neuropathy can limit the dose and duration of chemotherapy. If neuropathy could be prevented, a more aggressive treatment may benefit patients. For example, vinca alkaloids, such as vincristine, cause depolymerization of microtubules and induce peripheral neuropathy. In a preliminary report, IGF-I administration appears to prevent loss of grip strength and sustain motor amplitude in mice treated with vincristine (Apfel et al. 1993). This was observed at the very high dose of 1 mg/kg/day.

Certain neoplasms may exhibit accelerated growth in response to IGFs, and careful evaluation would be needed. For example, neuroblastoma, the most-common childhood solid tumor, responds to insulin and IGFs with increased protein content, thymidine incorporation and proliferation, at least in culture (Recio-Pinto and Ishii 1984; Ishii and Recio-Pinto 1987). Autocrine production of IGF may support neuroblastoma cells (El-Badry et al. 1989) and small cell lung cancer (Jaque et al. 1988).

III. Amyotrophic Lateral Sclerosis (ALS)

Popularly known as Lou Gehrig's Disease, ALS involves loss of upper and lower motor neurons, with onset often in the fourth decade of life.

Mild sensory and sub-clinical autonomic abnormalities are sometimes less appreciated. This disease also involves non-neural tissues, and abnormalities are found in the ultrastructure of liver mitochondria (Nakano et al. 1987). The incidence is approximately 1 per 100000, and about 10% of cases are familial. A defect in the Cu/Zn SOD1 gene is found in some familial cases, and introduction of this mutant human gene into trangenic mice can cause loss of motor neurons (Gurney et al. 1994; Wong et al. 1995). Since the wild-type mouse SOD gene remains functional, it appears that the mutant human gene results in an enzyme with an acquired deleterious function. It is curious to see that the mutant gene is not immediately deadly to motoneurons, suggesting that ALS emerges partially as a consequence of an age-dependent loss of neuroprotective activity. The defect in the more common sporadic cases of ALS remains unknown.

Because neurotrophic factors can protect normal neurons, clinical trials have been undertaken to determine whether neurotrophic factors may protect against ALS. The axons of spinal motoneurons lie in peripheral nerves, and subcutaneously administered neurotrophic factors may act on motor axons and nerve terminals. Sprouting can be induced from motor terminals by injecting IGF over muscle (Caroni and Grandes 1990). CNTF, BDNF and IGF-I have been tested in ALS patients, but significant improvements have not been reported in the scientific literature. The clinical trial for IGF-I was reported in the popular press, but is unpublished in a medical journal, and it is impossible to evaluate how robust the treatment or end-point analyses were. It might be noted that neurotrophic factors are not reported to be depleted in ALS patients or transgenic SOD mice. Thus, the progression of disease occurs despite normal levels of neurotrophic factors. The decision to test neurotrophic factors clinically is based on the assumption that supraphysiological doses may be protective. Bell-shaped dose response curves can be obtained with neurotrophic factors, and it is not known whether optimum doses were tested. It would be useful to test whether IGFs can prevent motor-neuron death in transgenic SOD mice, and the pharmacological conditions needed for a positive outcome, if any. As discussed in Sect. VI, certain neuromuscular diseases, such as myotonic dystrophy, do appear to be responsive to IGF treatment.

IV. Stroke

Unilateral carotid ligation, together with inhalation hypoxia, causes widespread death of neurons and infarct within the hippocampus, striatum, thalamus and lateral and pyriform cortices. Experimental intracranial administration of IGF-I can prevent the loss of neurons provoked by hypoxic-ischemic injury in rats (Gluckman et al. 1992). A single injection of IGF-I into the lateral ventricles, 2 h after hypoxic-ischemic injury was observed to reduce the secondary death of neurons.

V. Alzheimer's Disease

Alzheimer's disease is characterized by widespread loss of neurons in various parts of the brain, as well as by accumulation of neurofibrillary tangles, increased deposition of extracellular beta-amyloid plaques and progressive memory loss (Katzman 1986; Price 1986). There is atrophy of the hippocampus, substantia nigra, amygdala, parietal lobe, frontal lobe and caudate/putamen, which shows the wide variety of different types of neurons at risk (Mann 1991). Recent advances have focused on the familial forms of disease. For example, early-onset disease is positively associated with an increased dose of the apoE4 allele of the apolipoprotein-E gene in certain families. The Presenilin-1 and -2 genes are mutated in about half of familial cases, causing early onset of the syndrome in the fifth decade. Likewise, mutations in the beta-amyloid precursor protein is linked with early onset Alzheimer's disease. All of these mutations are associated with an increase in production of amyloid beta protein or density of plaques containing this protein. As a caveat, the correlation of plaque density is not as strong as the correlation of loss of synapses in the neocortex with the Alzheimer's syndrome (Terry et al. 1991), and much remains to be learned about the pathogenesis of disease, particularly in the more-common sporadic form of the syndrome. It is particularly encouraging that the human mutant amyloid precursor-protein gene has been introduced into transgenic mice, causing plaques and cognitive impairment.

Despite the presence of the genetic defect, the familial forms of Alzheimer's disease are not usually phenotypically displayed until the fifth decade or later in life. This suggests that protective factors are lost with aging, or that defects are accumulated, permitting the phenotype to emerge. Aging rats, like humans, show memory deficits, and this is associated with loss of IGF activity. IGF-II mRNA content is reduced in the hippocampus, hypothalamus, striatum, cerebral cortex and cerebellum of old rats, and is associated with increased methylation at the IGF-II gene locus (Kitraki et al. 1993). Binding to type-I IGF receptors is also reduced in the cortex and hippocampus of aged rats (Thornton et al. 1996). Osmotic mini pumps were used to infuse IGF-I into the ventricles of rats, and this was found to reduce the age-related decrement in memory acquisition tasks (Mooney et al. 1996). Taken together with the hypoxic-ischemic injury example (Gluckman et al. 1992), these data show that intracranial administration of IGFs can support a variety of different brain neurons. This is encouraging when considering Alzheimer's disease, because the pathology shows that many different types of neurons are afflicted. Thus, IGFs may be more protective than neurotrophic factors such as NGF which has actions that are confined to the cholinergic neurons of the brain. Also, cocktails of IGFs and NGF may be particularly helpful to provide generalized support for the brain as well as specific support for the hippocampal cholinergic neurons.

VI. Myotonic Dystrophy

Insulin resistance is observed in patients with myotonic dystrophy. When IGF-I (70μg/kg) was administered, there was an increase in muscle strength as well as neuromuscular function in patients with myotonic dystrophy (Vlachopapadopoulou et al. 1995). Dramatic improvement was reported in two patients. Animal studies show that IGF treatment reduces muscle protein degradation and increases hind-limb utilization in mice with muscular dystrophy (Zdanowicz et al. 1995).

E. Pharmacological Considerations

I. Routes of Administration

The pharacokinetics of IGFs suggest that the most likely route for many clinical indications would continue to be subcutaneous parenteral administration, particularly to treat the peripheral nervous system. The relatively long half-lives of IGFs readily permit single, daily subcutaneous injections to achieve desirable steady-state plasma concentrations. There are fenestrated capillaries at the ganglia which allow molecules the size of IGFs to easily reach sensory and sympathetic neurons. Circulating IGFs can also act on motor nerve terminals and possibly nodes of Ranvier. Retrograde axonal transport of IGFs, or their second messengers, would permit circulating IGFs to act on central neurons, the axons of which lie in peripheral nerves. Subcutaneous injection of recombinant human (rh) IGF-I does not cause pain, although attention needs to be given to pH and buffer concentration (Fransson and Espander-Jansson 1996).

Extended-duration IGF preparations may emerge either from formulations that control the rate of drug dissolution and absorption or from devices that slowly release IGFs from a subcutaneously implanted pump. For example, an osmotic mini pump might be implanted to continuously release IGFs for several months. Oral or nasal administration may also become feasible if better methods to control the rate and extent of absorption were developed.

The intravascular route of administration is riskier for drugs, in general, and preference would be lower particularly where drugs are intended to be distributed for self-administration, as in chronic neurodegenerative disorders. Nevertheless, there are situations in which acute onset of drug action may be desired following, for example, trauma, where there may be a brief time window for the prevention of secondary death of neurons.

The BBB and blood–spinal cord barrier are generally considered to be significant impediments to the use of neurotrophic polypeptides for treating the central nervous system. Lipophilic molecules can cross these barriers, but polar or ionized molecules ordinarily cannot, excepting those compounds with specific-transport carriers, such as glucose or amino acids. The therapeutic potential of IGFs was initially explored in diseases of the peripheral nervous system, where investigators are not immediately faced with the daunting problem of the BBB. Clinical trials for central nervous system disorders face difficult, albeit not insurmountable, challenges. The recruitment of patients is more difficult when faced with the prospect of having an access hole drilled through the skull to permit intracranial administration of a neurotrophic agent, yet this has been considered due to the desperate situation of patients with Alzheimer's or Parkinson's diseases. Safety is also an issue.

Various technologies are being developed, such as implantation of cells expressing transfected genes into the brain, or encapsulation of neurotrophic factors in lipophilic carriers, in the hope of overcoming the BBB. Another interesting approach involves the production of fusion proteins which bind to the transferrin receptor for transport into the brain. Obviously, patient preference as well as the ability to conduct clinical trials for polypeptide neurotrophic factors would be profoundly influenced by new procedures to defeat the BBB, and this remains a research priority.

There are suggestions that IGFs may be transported across the BBB. For example, IGF receptors are present on endothelial cells lining brain microvessels (Frank et al. 1986; Duffy et al. 1988). Silver-grain counts are observed in brain parenchyma following intravenous infusion of ^{125}I-labeled IGFs in rats (Reinhardt and Bondy 1994). In contrast, *N*-Met IGF-I is not found in CSF of sheep, following an intravenous infusion (Hodgkinson et al. 1991). These are highly provocative findings for basic neuroscience. However, insulin and IGFs can be substantially degraded during infusion, and there is a need to demonstrate that, in autoradiograms, the grain counts represent intact ligand rather than radiolabeled fragments.

Even if intact IGF reaches brain parenchyma, it might be considered that the BBB is not absolute. For example, 1% of circulating penicillin is found in the CSF, and this value may be increased in response to infections that cause inflammation of the meninges. IGF gene expression is particularly high at the choroid plexus and leptomeninges, which are widely believed to be the main sites for synthesis of IGFs found in CSF. What is the relative ratio of IGF in CSF derived from choroid plexus/leptomeninges vs the circulation? Thus, the clinical issue is not only whether circulating neurotrophic factors can cross the BBB, but whether they enter the brain in amounts sufficient to alter the biochemistry and function of the central nervous system. A brain-stem lesion caused by intracisternal injection of 6-hydroxydopamine normally results in loss of the hind-limb reflex. Such a reflex is spared when IGF is administered subcutaneously after the lesion (Pulford et al. 1997).

II. Volume of Distribution and Daily Production

The volume of distribution of rhIGF-I is approximately 160–180 ml/kg (Lieberman et al. 1992) or 200–360 ml/kg (Grahnen et al. 1993) and is reduced somewhat after daily treatment for 5 days to 154 ml/kg (Lieberman et al.

1992). In contrast, it is reported to increase from 183 ml/kg to 266 ml/kg following IGF-I treatment in patients with growth hormone-receptor deficiency (Vaccarello et al. 1993). The volume is reduced in dialysis patients (Fouque et al. 1995). The volume for IGF-II is likely to be quite similar, albeit differences in affinity for IGFBPs may modify its volume somewhat.

The daily production in a 73-kg male was reported to be 136 μg/kg/day for IGF-I and 179 μg/kg/day for IGF-II (Guler et al. 1989b). In six patients with an average age of 36 years, Fouque et al. (1995) report an IGF-I production rate of 49 μg/kg/day. This value is similar to the 38 μg/kg/day reported by Wilton et al. (1991), and 50 μg/kg/day by Grahnen et al. (1993).

III. Bound and Free IGF Pools

Circulating IGF-I and IGF-II are found primarily in a 150-kDa complex of IGF, IGFBP-3 and the acid-labile subunit (1 : 1 : 1): approximately 70% of IGFs are in this complex (Gargosky et al. 1994). IGFBP-3 comprises about a third of the circulating IGFBPs and IGF blood levels correlate positively and more closely with this BP than with other IGFs (Blum et al. 1993). The 150-kDa complex is undetectable outside of the vascular compartment.

Smaller IGF complexes of approximately 44 kDa are formed from truncated IGFBP-3 as well as lesser amounts of IGFBP-6, IGFBP-2, IGFBP-1 and IGFBP-4. These are found in the vascular and extracellular compartments. The predominant complex in CSF is comprised of IGF-II and IGFBP-2.

Infusion of IGF-I in amounts exceeding daily production rates can rapidly decrease circulating IGF-II concentrations (Guler et al. 1989a; Zenobi et al. 1992; Bach et al. 1994). This might occur because of displacement of IGF-II bound to IGFBPs, by IGF-I, keeping in mind the shorter half-life of free IGF-II. It seems unlikely that this would occur with lower physiological replacement doses of IGF-I, but this needs to be studied.

IV. Elimination Half-Time

The half-life of free IGF-I is approximately 10–20 min (Guler et al. 1989b; Zenobi et al. 1992), and of free IGF-II approximately 10 min (Guler et al. 1989b). These values are similar to that for insulin. However, because IGFs are bound to serum IGFBP, the half-time of the 150-kDa bound form is 8–20 h for IGF-I (Guler et al. 1989b; Grahnen et al. 1993; Vaccarello et al. 1993) and 13.5 h for IGF-II (Guler et al. 1989a). The half-life is reduced to 6 h (Grahnen et al. 1993), but unchanged by IGF-I infusion, in patients with growth hormone-receptor deficiency (Vaccarello et al. 1993). It is also reduced in dialysis patients (Fouque et al. 1995).

The clearance of IGF-I is estimated at about 0.20 ml/min/kg in normal subjects (Grahnen et al. 1993). It is not markedly altered in diabetic subjects (Bach et al. 1994). Clearance also remains unchanged in subjects with chronic renal failure, although the volume of distribution can be reduced due to an increase in serum IGFBP-3 as a consequence of IGF-I infusion (RABKIN et al. 1996). Thus, lower urinary excretion rates in IDDM patients (QUATTRIN et al. 1992) may primarily reflect decreased serum IGF-I levels. The serum half-life of IGF-I is not increased, but rather decreased, in patients with renal failure, suggesting kidney clearance does not contribute substantially to the half-life and that IGF-I may not accumulate during chronic administration in such patients (FOUQUE et al. 1995). The clearance is increased to 0.6 ml/min/kg in growth hormone-receptor deficiency (GRAHNEN et al. 1993).

IGF-I renal excretion rate is estimated to be 0.1–1.4 μg/kg/day (HIZUKA et al. 1991), and 1.2 μg/kg/day and 0.3 μg/kg/day in normal and IDDM children, respectively (QUATTRIN et al. 1992). Young, healthy IDDM patients without albuminuria have a reduced renal excretion of both growth hormone and IGF-I. Renal excretion seems to account for loss of between 3% and 10% of the daily production rate.

V. Clinical Effects of Recombinant Human IGF-I

1. Normal Subjects

The doses discussed herein are mainly subcutaneous doses and refer to the total daily dose which, in some studies, was administered in multiple divided doses. There is a dose-dependent emergence of various responses. Many of these responses in normal subjects might be considered side-effects because they emerge at supraphysiological doses of IGF-I. For example, the preponderance of studies cited in this and the next section have been conducted with doses which are several fold greater than the daily production rate (38–50 μg/kg/day). In general, chronic doses below 40 μg/kg/day appear to be well tolerated. Consideration should be given to the physiological state in interpreting these data.

Hypoglycemia was observed with a subcutaneous continuous-infusion of 768 μg/kg/day rhIGF-I, but not with 480 μg/kg/day, although glucose levels fell from 4.4 mmol/l to 2.6 mmol/L (GULER et al. 1989a). During this 6-day study, the blood pressure, pulse rate and body temperature were stable, and the two adult male subjects felt normal throughout the experiment. Circulating IGF-II levels were reduced and creatinine clearance was increased secondary to an increase in glomerular filtration rate. Plasma uric acid and urea levels were reduced, and there was no increase in body weight, indicating that fluid retention did not occur. Under a euglycemic clamp, it was shown that glucose consumption was increased by IGF-I (TURKALJ et al. 1992). In addition, there was a decrease in triglycerides, free fatty acids, leucine and whole-body protein breakdown. Insulin and C-peptide were also reduced. IGF-I infusion at 24 μg/kg/hour causes an increase in glomerular filtration rate and renal plasma flow (GIORDANO and DEFRONZO 1995). A more complete discussion of the effects of IGF-I on glucose disposition, lipid levels and general metabolism may be found elsewhere (FROESCH and HUSSAIN 1994; KOLACZYNSKI and CARO 1994).

Doses less than 100μg/kg/day caused no change in pulse rate, blood pressure, hematology or urinalysis after 9 days of treatment, and transient hypoglycemia was observed at 100μg/kg/day (Stong and Raskin 1993). This same dose, when administered 30 min after breakfast, did not produce hypoglycemia (Hizuka et al. 1991). IGFBPs are believed to be present to protect the body from the hypoglycemic actions of circulating IGFs, and a considerable excess of IGF appears to be necessary to produce a decline in glucose concentrations.

An extensive dose–response study was conducted in 18 normal postmenopausal women (Ebeling et al. 1993). Doses below 60μg/kg/day produced minimal or no side effects. Side-effects began to emerge within 6 days at doses above 120μg/kg/day. These included sinus tachycardia with palpitations, parotid discomfort, weight gain and edema. At the highest dose of 180μg/kg/day, orthostatic hypotension and dizziness occurred following the subcutaneous injections. All of these effects were reversible on withdrawal. Hypoglycemia was not observed at any of these doses.

2. Patient Populations

Swelling and tenderness of the parotid gland was observed in diabetic patients treated with 240μg/kg/day rhIGF-I after 1 week, and this was reversible following cessation of treatment (Zenobi et al. 1992). Younger diabetic subjects appear better able than older patients to tolerate high IGF-I doses (Bach et al. 1994). Large chronic IGF-I doses can cause arthralgia, myalgia, hypophosphatemia (treatable with potassium phosphate), edema, dyspnea, tachycardia, orthostatic hypotension, bilateral jaw tenderness and cranial-nerve palsies in diabetic patients with and without severe insulin resistance (Schalch et al. 1993; Jabri et al. 1994; Usala et al. 1994). Microalbuminuria was unchanged in a 5-day study (Schalch et al. 1993). The side effects associated with the high doses of IGF-I needed to control hyperglycemia makes this an unacceptable therapy to Jabri et al (1994) as well as to others.

The heart rate was increased with IGF-I doses between 80μg/kg/day and 240μg/kg/day in patients with growth hormone-receptor deficiency (Vasconez et al. 1994). A case of reversible Bell's Palsy is reported in a 2-year study with 31 such patients (Ranke et al. 1995). Glomerular filtration rate and renal plasma flow was increased, but without effect on kidney volume in patients with end-stage renal disease by 200μg/kg/day IGF-I treatment (Miller et al. 1994). Chronic administration of high doses of IGF-I results in downregulation of IGF receptors on red blood cells in patients with Laron syndrome (Eshet et al. 1993). Clinical evidence of side effects was not observed in two children with the Laron syndrome after 17 months of treatment with 80μg/kg/day IGF-I (Heinrichs et al. 1993). Likewise, side-effects were mild in 17 similar children treated with 120μg/kg/day IGF-I for 12 months (Guevara-Aguirre et al. 1995). Resistance to side effects may be due to the younger age, the Laron syndrome or both.

Low doses of 30μg/kg/day IGF-I, administered to elderly women for 4 weeks, were well tolerated (THOMPSON et al. 1995), as was 40μg/kg/day for 8 weeks in adolescent males with IDDM (CHEETHAM et al. 1995). There was no change in hematological tests, glomerular filtration rate or albuminuria.

Clinical results have not implicated IGF treatment in the exacerbation of diabetic retinopathy or nephropathy. Patients with acromegaly have elevated growth hormone and IGF-I levels, but are not reported to have increased incidence of renal failure or glomerular sclerosis. Renal hypertrophy can be produced in diabetic rats, but this was observed when extremely large doses of IGF-I, greater than the daily production, were administered. When IGF replacement doses (15μg/kg/day) were administered to IDDM rats, renal enlargement was not observed (unpublished observation). Glomerular sclerosis does not develop in transgenic mice overexpressing IGF-I (MATHEWS et al. 1988), but does in mice overexpressing growth hormone, implicating a greater pathological role for the latter (DOI et al. 1988). Nevertheless, it would be important to monitor these complications in any long-term clinical study.

It might be considered that IGFs are mitogens, and may exacerbate growth of pre-existing tumors. Use of IGF is likely to be contraindicated in patients with known or suspected malignancies. However, the risk in normal subjects would probably be no greater than for insulin, also a mitogen yet a relatively safe drug.

VI. Effects of Recombinant Human IGF-II

IGF-II has been administered to a few subjects to determine its pharmacokinetics (GULER et al. 1989). At high doses, IGF-II, like IGF-I, can cause hypoglycemia (HIZUKA et al. 1991). However, rising-dose studies to determine side-effects have not been published. The side effects of IGF-II may differ somewhat from those of IGF-I, because these ligands have overlapping but non-identical actions. It was discussed earlier that transgenic mice overexpressing the IGF-I gene show much greater growth than those overexpressing the IGF-II gene. IGF-I causes greater muscle differentiation, whereas IGF-II greater neuronal differentiation in cultured explanted tissues (CHENG and MATTSON 1992). IGF-I, but not IGF-II, causes mitosis in cultured Schwann cells (SCHUMACHER et al. 1993).

F. Concluding Comments

The IGFs are found to differ in several important ways from the "classic" neurotrophic factors exemplified by neurotrophins, such as NGF. For example, IGFs provide ubiquitous neurotrophic support for virtually all, if not all, peripheral and central neurons. IGFs therefore have the possibility of treating disorders in which diverse populations of neurons are at risk, such as diabetic neuropathy, Alzheimer's disease and trauma. In contrast, neurotrophins are restricted in their actions to discrete populations of neurons. For example, the classic neurotrophin, NGF, binds to TrkA receptors which are limited in distribution in the brain to cholinergic neurons. Therefore, NGF may be particularly useful in treating cholinergic neurons in the hippocampus, but would not be expected to protect other types of neurons afflicted, for example, in Alzheimer's disease. A cocktail might be optimum, whereby IGFs are administered to provide general protection for the nervous system and other neurotrophic factors enhance protection for specific classes of neurons at risk in particular patients or diseases.

Another difference is that IGFs are circulating factors. They are present both in the circulation and in the CSF, which might be expected for ubiquitous neurotrophic factors. Subcutaneous IGF administration would result in a distribution similar to normal endogenously produced IGFs. In contrast, neurotrophins are compartmentalized by virtue of their production in target tissues and are not found in appreciable quantities in the circulation. Subcutaneous administration would result in loss of compartmentalization; neurotrophins may reach inappropriate targets, and this may possibly provoke undesirable responses, such as the hyperalgesia observed after NGF treatment. Once again, cocktails may be useful; IGFs could be added in combination, not only to further support neurons, but also to potentially reduce NGF hyperalgesia.

IGF-I and IGF-II produce many overlapping and non-overlapping actions. Thus, distinct products may emerge for these ligands, each with slightly different actions and side-effects. It seems probable that the first neurotrophic therapeutic agent will be developed for peripheral neuropathy. The subcutaneous route of administration is tried and true, and not dependent on as extensive research and development as would be needed for CNS treatment. However, this picture may rapidly change if efficient methods were discovered to deliver neurotrophic factors across the BBB.

Acknowledgements. This work was supported in part by grant RO1 DK53922-09 from the National Institute of Diabetes and Digestive and Kidney Diseases, and grant R49/CCR811509 from the Centers for Disease Control.

References

Ahluwalia A, Vallance P (1997) Evidence for functional responses to sensory nerve stimulation of rat small mesenteric veins. J Pharmacol Exp Ther 281:9–14

Ang LC, Bhaumick B, Munoz DG, Sass J, Juurlink BHG (1992) Effects of astrocytes, insulin and insulin-like growth factor I on the survival of motoneurons in vitro. J Neurol Sci 109:168–172

Apfel SC, Arezzo JC, Lewis ME, Kessler JA (1993) The use of insulin-like growth factor I in the prevention of vincristine neuropathy in mice. Ann NY Acad Sci 692:243–245

Archer AG, Watkins PJ, Thomas PK, Sharma AK, Payan J (1983) The natural history of acute painful neuropathy in diabetes mellitus. J Neurol Neurosurg Psychiatry 46:491–499

Bach MA, Chin E, Bondy CA (1994) The effects of subcutaneous insulin-like growth factor-I infusion in insulin-dependent diabetes mellitus. J Clin Endocrinol Metab 79:1040–1045

Barlow DP, Stoger R, Herrmann BG, Saito K, Schweifer N (1991) The mouse insulin-like growth factor type 2 receptor is imprinted and closely linked to the Tme locus. Nature 349:84–87

Baxter RC, Brown AS, Turtle JR (1979) Decrease in serum receptor-reactive somatomedin in diabetes. Horm Metab Res 11:216–220

Black MM, Greene LA (1982) Changes in the colchicine susceptibility of microtubules associated with neurite outgrowth: studies with nerve growth factor-responsive PC12 pheochromocytoma cells. J Cell Biol 95:379–386

Blum WF, Hall K, Ranke MB, Wilton P (1993) Growth hormone insensitivity syndromes: a preliminary report on changes in insulin-like growth factors and their binding proteins during treatment with recombinant insulin-like growth factor I. Acta Paediatr 82 [Suppl]:15–19

Bodkin NL, Sportsman R, DiMarchi RD, Hansen BC (1991) Insulin-like growth factor-I in non-insulin-dependent diabetic monkeys: basal plasma concentrations and metabolic effects of exogenously administered biosynthetic hormone. Metabolism 40:1131–1137

Bornfeldt KE, Arnqvist HJ, Enberg B, Mathews LS, Norstedt G (1989) Regulation of insulin-like growth factor-I and growth hormone receptor gene expression by diabetes and nutritional state in rat tissues. J Endocrinol 122:651–656

Bozyczko-Coyne D, Glickman MA, Prantner JE, McKenna B, Connors T, Friedman C, Dasgupta M, Neff NT (1993) IGF-I supports the survival and/or differentiation of multiple types of central nervous system neurons. Ann NY Acad Sci 692:311–313

Brismar K, Gutniak M, Povoa G, Werner S, Hall K (1988) Insulin regulates the 35 kDa IGF binding protein in patients with diabetes mellitus. J Endocrinol Invest 11:599–602

Burgess SK, Jacobs S, Cuatrecasas P, Sahyoun N (1987) Characterization of a neuronal subtype of insulin-like growth factor I receptor. J Biol Chem 262:1618–1622

Caroni P, Grandes P (1990) Nerve sprouting in innervated adult skeletal muscle induced by exposure to elevated levels of insulin-like growth factors. J Cell Biol 110:1307–1317

Carson MJ, Behringer RR, Brinster RL, McMorris FA (1993) Insulin-like growth factor I increases brain growth and central nervous system myelination in transgenic mice. Neuron 10:729–740

Carsten RE, Whalen LR, Ishii DN (1989) Impairment of spinal cord conduction velocity in diabetic rats. Diabetes 38:730–736

Cheetham TD, Holly JM, Clayton K, Cwyfan-Hughes S, Dunger DB (1995) The effects of repeated daily recombinant human insulin-like growth factor I administration in adolescents with type 1 diabetes. Diabet Med 12:885–892

Cheng B, Mattson MP (1992) IGF-I and IGF-II protect cultured hippocampal and septal neurons against calcium-mediated hypoglycemic damage. J Neurosci 12:1558–1566

Clemmons DR, Jones, JI, Busby WH, Wright G (1993) Role of insulin-like growth factor binding proteins in modifying IGF actions. Ann NY Acad Sci 692:10–21

Cornblath DR, Dellon AL, MacKinnon SE (1989) Spontaneous diabetes mellitus in a rhesus monkey: neurophysiological studies. Muscle Nerve 12:233–235

The DCCT Research Group (1988) Factors in development of diabetic neuropathy: baseline analysis of neuropathy in feasibility phase of Diabetes Control and Complications Trial (DCCT). Diabetes 37:476–481

de Pablo F, de la Rosa EJ (1995) The developing CNS: a scenario for the action of proinsulin, insulin and insulin-like growth factors. Trends Neurosci 18:143–150

DeChiara TM, Efstratiadis A, Robertson EJ (1990) A growth-deficiency phenotype in heterozygous mice carrying an insulin-like growth factor II gene disrupted by targeting. Nature 345:78–80

DeChiara TM, Robertson EJ, Efstratiadis A (1991) Parental imprinting of the mouse insulin-like growth factor II gene. Cell 64:849–859

Devaskar SH (1991) A review of insulin/insulin-like peptide in the central nervous system. In: Raizada MK, LeRoith D (eds) Molecular biology and physiology of insulin and insulin-like growth factors. Plenum Press, New York, pp 385–396

DiCicco-Bloom E, Black IB (1988) Insulin growth factors regulate the mitotic cycle in cultured rat sympathetic neuroblasts. Proc Natl Acad Sci. USA 85:4066–4070

Doi T, Pardridge WM, Quaife C, Conti FG, Palmiter RD, Behringer RR, Brinster RL, Striker GE (1988) Progressive glomerulosclerosis develops in transgenic mice chronically expressing growth hormone and growth hormone releasing factor but not in those expressing insulin-like growth factor-1. Am J Pathol 131:398–403

Duffy KR, Pardridge WM, Rosenfeld RG (1988) Human blood–brain barrier insulin-like growth factor receptor. Metabolism 37:136–140

Dyck PJ, Thomas PK, Asbury AK, Winegrad AI, Porte D, Jr (1987) Diabetic neuropathy. WB Saunders, Philadelphia

Dyck PJ, Kratz KM, Karnes JL, Litchy WJ, Klein R, Pach JM, Wilson DM, O'Brien PC, Melton LJ 3rd, Service FJ (1993) The prevalence by staged severity of various types of diabetic neuropathy, retinopathy, and nephropathy in a population-based cohort: the Rochester diabetic neuropathy study. Neurology 43:817–824

Ebeling PR, Jones JD, O'Fallon WM, Janes CH, Riggs BL (1993) Short-term effects of recombinant human insulin-like growth factor I on bone turnover in normal women. J Clin Endocrinol Metab 77:1384–1387

Ekstrom PAR, Tomlinson DR (1989) Impaired nerve regeneration in streptozotocin-diabetic rats. Effects of treatment with an aldose reductase inhibitor. J Neurol Sci 93:231–237

El-Badry OM, Romanus JA, Helman LJ, Cooper MJ, Rechler MM, Israel MA (1989) Autonomous growth of a human neuroblastoma cell line is mediated by insulin-like growth factor II. J Clin Invest 84:829–839

Eshet R, Klinger B, Silbergeld A, Laron Z (1993) Modulation of insulin like growth factor I (IGF-I) binding sites on erythrocytes by IGF-I treatment in patients with Laron syndrome (LS). Regul Pept 48:233–239

Ewing DJ, Campbell IW, Clarke BF (1980) The natural history of diabetic autonomic neuropathy. Q J Med 49:95–108

Fagin JA, Roberts CT, Jr, LeRoith D, Brown AT (1989) Coordinate decrease of tissue insulin-like growth factor I posttranscriptional alternative mRNA transcripts in diabetes mellitus. Diabetes 38:428–434

Fleming BP, Biggins IL, Morris JL, Gannon BJ (1989) Noradrenergic and peptidergic innervation of the extrinsic vessels and microcirculation of the rat cremaster muscle. Microvasc Res 38:255–268

Fouque D, Peng SC, Kopple JD (1995) Pharmacokinetics of recombinant human insulin-like growth factor-1 in dialysis patients. Kidney Int 47:869–875

Frank HJL, Pardridge WM, Morris WL, Rosenfeld RG, Choi TB (1986) Binding and internalization of insulin and insulin-like growth factors by isolated brain microvessels. Diabetes 35:654–661

Fransson J, Espander-Jansson A (1996) Local tolerance of subcutaneous injections. J Pharm Pharmacol:1012–1015

Froesch ER Hussain M (1994) Recombinant human insulin-like growth factor-I: a therapeutic challenge for diabetes mellitus. Diabetologia 37 suppl:S179–S185

Gargosky SE, Wilsin KF, Fielder PJ, Vaccarello MA, Diamond FB, Baxter RC, Rosenbloom AL, Guevara-Aguirre J, Rosenfeld RG (1994) Effects of insulin-like growth factor I treatment on the molecular distribution of insulin-like growth factors among different binding proteins. Acta Paediatr 399 suppl:159–162

Gelato MC, Alexander D, Marsh K (1992) Differential tissue regulation of insulin like growth factor binding proteins in experimental diabetes mellitus in the rat. Diabetes 41:1511–1519

Giordano M, DeFronzo RA (1995) Acute effect of human recombinant insulin-like growth factor I on renal function in humans. Nephron 71:10–15

Glazner GW, Ishii DN (1995) Insulin-like growth factor gene expression in rat muscle during reinnervation. Muscle Nerve 18:1433–1442

Glazner GW, Lupien S, Miller JA, Ishii DN (1993) Insulin-like growth factor-II increases the rate of sciatic nerve regeneration in rats. Neuroscience 54:791–797

Glazner GW, Morrison AE, Ishii DN (1994) Elevated insulin-like growth factor (IGF) gene expression in sciatic nerves during IGF-supported nerve regeneration. Mol Brain Res 25:265–272

Gluckman P, Klempt N, Guan J, Mallard C, Sirimanne E, Dragunow M, Klempt M, Singh K, Williams C, Nikolics K (1992) A role for IGF in the rescue of CNS neurons following hypoxic-ischemic injury. Biochem Biophys Res Commun 182:593–599

Grahnen A, Kastrup K, Heinrich U, Gourmelen M, Preece MA, Vaccarello MA, Guevara-Aguirre J, Rosenfeld RG, Sietnieks A (1993) Pharmacokinetics of recombinant human insulin-like growth factor I given subcutaneously to healthy volunteers and to patients with growth hormone receptor deficiency. Acta Paediatr 82 [Suppl]:9–13

Guevara-Aguirre J, Vasconez O, Martinez V, Martinez AL, Rosenbloom AL, Diamond FBJ, Gargosky SE, Nonoshita L, Rosenfeld RG (1995) A randomized, double blind, placebo-controlled trial on safety and efficacy of recombinant human insulin-like growth factor-I in children with growth hormone receptor deficiency. J Clin Endocrinol Metab 80:1393–1398

Guler HP, Eckardt KU, Zapf J, Bauer C, Froesch ER (1989a) Insulin-like growth factor I increase glomerular filtration rate and renal plasma flow in man. Acta Endocrinol (Copenh) 121:101–106

Guler HP, Zapf J, Schmid C, Froesch ER (1989b) Insulin-like growth factors I and II in healthy man. Estimations of half-lives and production rates. Acta Endocrinol (Copenh) 121:753–758

Gurney ME, Pu H, Chiu AY, Dal Canto MC, Polchow CY, Alexander DD, Caliendo J, Hentati A, Kwon YW, Deng H-X, Chen W, Zhai P, Sufit RL, Siddique T (1994) Motor neuron degeneration in mice that express a human Cu, Zn superoxide dismutase mutation. Science 264:1772–1775

Hall K, Sara VR (1984) Somatomedin levels in childhood, adolescence and adult life. Clin Endocrinol Metab 13:91–112

Hall VK, Lundin G, Povoa G (1988) Serum levels of the low molecular weight form of insulin-like growth factor binding protein in healthy subjects and patients with growth hormone deficiency, acromegaly and anorexia nervosa. Acta Endocrinol (Copenh) 118:321–326

Haselbacher GK, Humbel RE (1982) Evidence for two species of insulin-like growth factor II (IGF-II and big IGF-II) in human spinal fluid. Endocrinology 110:1822–1824

Heidenreich KA, Brandenberg D (1986) Oligosaccharide heterogeneity of insulin receptors. Comparison of N-linked glycosylation of insulin receptors in adipocytes and brain. Endocrinology 118:1835–1842

Heinrichs C, Vis HL, Bergmann P, Wilton P, Bourguignon JP (1993) Effects of 17 months treatment using recombinant insulin-like growth factor-I in two children with growth hormone insensitivity (Laron) syndrome. Clin Endocrinol 38:647–651

Hizuka N, Takano K, Asakawa K, Fukuda I, Ohta T, Shizume K, Demura H (1991) Administration of insulin-like growth factors in normal adults, patients with growth hormone deficiency and rats. In: Spencer EM (ed) Modern concepts of insulin-like growth factors. Elsevier, New York, pp 607–615

Hodgkinson SC, Spencer GSG, Bass JJ, Davis SR, Gluckman PD (1991) Distribution of circulating insulin-like growth factor-I (IGF-I) into tissues. Endocrinology 129:2085–2093

Holthuizen E, LeRoith D, Lund PK, Roberts C, Rotwein P, Spencer EM, Sussenbach JS (1991) Revised nomenclature for the insulin-like growth factor genes and transcripts. In: Spencer EM (ed) Modern concepts of insulin-like growth factors. Elsevier, New York, pp 733–736

Hu J-F, Vu TH, Hoffman AR (1995) Different biallelic activation of three insulin-like growth factor II promoters in the mouse central nervous system. Mol Endocrinol 9(5):628–636

Hynes MA, Brooks PJ, Van Wyk JJ, Lund PK (1988) Insulin-like growth factor II messenger ribonucleic acids are synthesized in the choroid plexus of the rat brain. Mol Endocrinol 2:47–54

Ichimiya Y, Emson PC, Northrop AJ, Gilmour RS (1988) Insulin-like growth factor II in the rat choroid plexus. Mol Brain Res 4:167–170

Ishii DN (1989) Relationship of insulin-like growth factor II gene expression in muscle to synaptogenesis. Proc Natl Acad Sci USA 86:2898–2902

Ishii DN (1993) Insulin and related neurotrophic factors in diabetic neuropathy. Diabet Med 10 [Suppl. 12]:14S–15S

Ishii DN (1995) Implication of insulin-like growth factors in the pathogenesis of diabetic neuropathy. Brain Res Rev 20:47–67

Ishii DN, Lupien SB (1995) Insulin-like growth factors protect against diabetic neuropathy: effects on sensory nerve regeneration in rats. J Neurosci Res 40:138–144

Ishii DN, Recio-Pino E (1987) Role of insulin, insulin-like growth factors, and nerve growth factor in neurite formation. In: Raizada MK, Phillips MI, LeRoith D (eds) Insulin, insulin-like growth factors, and their receptors in the central nervous system. Plenum Press, New York, pp 315–348

Ishii DN, Guertin DM, Whalen LR (1994) Reduced insulin-like growth factor I mRNA content in liver, adrenal glands and spinal cord of diabetic rats. Diabetologia 37:1073–1081

Ishii DN, Pu S-F, Glazner GW, Zhuang H-X, Marsh DJ (1996) Roles of insulin-like growth factors in peripheral nerve regeneration and motor neuron survival. In: Bell C (ed) Chemical factors in neural growth, degeneration and repair. Elsevier, New York, pp 399–421

Jabri N, Schalch DS, Schwartz SL, Fischer JS, Kipnes MS, Radnik BJ, Turman NJ, Marcsisin VS, Guler H-P (1994) Adverse effects of recombinant human insulin-like growth factor I in obese insulin-resistant type II diabetic patients. Diabetes 43:369–374

Jacobs JM, Love S (1985) Qualitative and quantitative morphology of human sural nerve at different ages. Brain 108:897–924

Jaque G, Rotsch M, Wegmann C, Worsch U, Maasberg M, Havemann K (1988) Production of immunoreactive insulin-like growth factor I and response to exogenous IGF in small cell lung cancer cell lines. Exp Cell Res 176:336–343

Kanje M, Skottner A, Sjöberg J, Lundborg G (1989) Insulin-like growth factor I (IGF-I) stimulates regeneration of the rat sciatic nerve. Brain Res 486:396–398

Katzman R (1986) Alzheimer's disease. N Engl J Med 314:964–973

Kitraki E, Bozas E, Philippidis H, Stylianopoulou F (1993) Aging-related changes in IGF-II and c-fos gene expression in the rat brain. Int J Dev Neurosci 11:1–9

Kolaczynski JW, Caro JF (1994) Insulin-like growth factor-therapy in diabetes: physiologic basis, clinical benefits, and risks. Ann Intern Med 120:47–55

Lenoir D, Honegger P (1983) Insulin-like growth factor I (IGF I) stimulates DNA synthesis in fetal rat brain cell cultures. Dev Brain Res 7:205–213

Lieberman SA, Bukar J, Chen SA, Celniker AC, Compton PG, Cook J, Albu J, Perlman AJ, Hoffman AR (1992) Effects of recombinant human insulin-like growth factor-I (rhIGF-I) on total and free IGF-I concentration, IGF-binding proteins, and glycemic response in humans. J Clin Endocrinol Metab 75:30–36

Longo FM, Powell HC, Lebeau J, Gerrero MR, Heckman H, Myers RR (1986) Delayed nerve regeneration in streptozotocin diabetic rats. Muscle Nerve 9:385–393

Maes M, Ketelslegers J-M, Underwood LE (1983) Low plasma somatomedin-C in streptozotocin-induced diabetes mellitus. Correlation with changes in somatogenic and lactogenic liver binding sites. Diabetes 32:1060–1069

Mann DMA (1991) The topographic distribution of brain atrophy in Alzheimer's disease. Acta Neuropathol 83:81–86

Masters BA, Raizada MK (1993) Insulin-like growth factor I receptors and IGF-I actions in neuronal cultures from the brain. Ann NY Acad Sci 692:89–101
Mathews LS, Hammer RE, Behringer RR, D'Ercole AJ, Bell GI, Brinster RL, Palmiter RD (1988) Growth enhancement of transgenic mice expressing human insulin-like growth factor I. Endocrinology 123:2827–2833
McCall AL (1991) The impact of diabetes on the CNS. Diabetes 41:557–570
McMorris FA, Smith TM, DeSalvo S, Furlanetto RW (1986) Insulin-like growth factor I/somatomedin C: a potent inducer of oligodendrocyte development. Proc Natl Acad Sci USA 83:822–826
Migdalis IN, Kalogeropoulou K, Kalantzis L, Nounopoulos C, Bouloukos A, Samartzis M (1995) Insulin-like growth factor-I and IGF-I receptors in diabetic patients with neuropathy. Diabet Med 12:823–827
Mill JF, Chao MV, Ishii DN (1985) Insulin, insulin-like growth factor II, and nerve growth factor effects on tubulin mRNA levels and neurite formation. Proc Natl Acad Sci USA 82:7126–7130
Miller SB, Moulton M, O'Shea M, Hammerman MR (1994) Effects of IGF-I on renal function in end-stage chronic renal failure. Kidney Int 46:201–207
Mooney M, Sonntag WE, Barra M, Xu X, Bennett S, Ingram R, Poe B, Markowska AL (1996) Insulin-like growth factor-(IGF-) increases working memory in aged animals. Soc Neurosci Abstr 22:1237
Mooradian AD (1988) Diabetic complications of the central nervous system. Endocr Rev 9:346–356
Nakano Y, Hirayama K, Terao K (1987) Hepatic ultrastructural changes and liver dysfunction in amyotrophic lateral sclerosis. Arch Neurol 44:103–106
Near SL, Whalen LR, Miller JA, Ishii DN (1992) Insulin-like growth factor-II stimulates motor nerve regeneration. Proc Natl Acad Sci USA 89:11716–11720
Neff NT, Prevette D, Houenou LJ, Lewis ME, Glicksman MA, Yin QW, Oppenheim RW (1993) Insulin-like growth factors: putative muscle-derived trophic agents that promote motoneuron survival. J Neurobiol 24:1578–1588
Noguchi T, Sugisaki T, Takamatsu K, Tsukada Y (1982) Factors contributing to the poor myelination in the brain of the Snell dwarf mouse. J Neurochem 39:1693–1699
Noguchi T, Sekiguchi M, Sugisaki T, Tsukada Y, Shimai K (1983) Faulty development of cortical neurons in the Snell dwarf cerebrum. Dev Brain Res 10:125–138
Noguchi T, Sugisaki T, Kudo M, Sato I (1986) Retarded growth of suprachiasmatic nucleus and pineal body in dw and lit dwarf mice. Dev Brain Res 26:161–172
Ooi GT, Orlowski CC, Brown AL, Becher RE, Unterman TG, Rechler MM (1990) Different tissue distribution and hormonal regulation of messenger RNAs encoding rat insulin-like growth factor-binding proteins 1 and 2. Mol Endocrinol 4:321–328
Phillips LS, Young HS (1976) Nutrition and somatomedin. II. Serum somatomedin activity and cartilage growth activity in streptozotocin-diabetic rats. Diabetes 25:516–527
Price DL (1986) New perspectives on Alzheimer's disease. Annu Rev Neurosci 9:489–512
Pu S-F, Zhuang H-X, Ishii DN (1995) Differential spatio-temporal expression of the insulin-like growth factor genes in regenerating sciatic nerve. Mol Brain Res 34:18–28
Pulford BE, Whalen LR, Ishii DN (1997) Subcutaneous IGF administration spares loss of the limb withdrawal reflex in 6-OHDA lesioned rats. Soc Neurosci Abstr 23:1705
Quattrin T, Albini CH, Reiter EO, Mills BJ, MacGillivray MH (1992) Urinary excretion of IGF-I and growth hormone in children with IDDM. Diabetes Care 15:490–494
Rabkin R, Fervenza FC, Maidment H, Ike J, Hintz R, Liu F, Bloedow DC, Hoffman AR, Gesundheit N (1996) Pharmacokinetics of insulin-like growth factor in advanced chronic renal failure. Kidney Int 49:1134–1140

Ranke MB, Savage MO, Chatelain P, Preece MA, Rosenfeld RG, Blum WF, Wilton P (1995) Insulin-like growth factor I improves height in growth hormone insensitivity: two years' results. Hormone Res 44:253–264

Recio-Pinto E, Ishii DN (1984) Effects of insulin, insulin-like growth factor-II and nerve growth factor on neurite outgrowth in cultured human neuroblastoma cells. Brain Res 302:323–334

Recio-Pinto E, Ishii DN (1988) Insulin and insulin-like growth factor receptors regulating neurite formation in cultured human neuroblastoma cells. J Neurosci Res 19:312–320

Recio-Pinto E, Rechler MM, Ishii DN (1986) Effects of insulin, insulin-like growth factor-II, and nerve growth factor on neurite formation and survival in cultured sympathetic and sensory neurons. J Neurosci 6:1211–1219

Reinhardt RR, Bondy CA (1994) Insulin-like growth factors cross the blood–brain barrier. Endocrinology 135:1753–1761

Rotwein P, Burgess SK, Milbrandt JD, Krause JE (1988) Differential expression of insulin-like growth factor genes in rat central nervous system. Proc Natl Acad Sci USA 85:265–269

Said G, Slama G, Selva J (1983) Progressive centripetal degeneration of axons in small fibre diabetic polyneuropathy. A clinical and pathological study. Brain 106:791–807

Schalch DS, Turman NJ, Marcsisin VS, Heffernan M, Guler HP (1993) Short-term effects of recombinant human insulin-like growth factor I on metabolic control of patients with type II diabetes mellitus. J Clin Endocrinol Metab 77:1563–1568

Scheiwiller E, Guler H-P, Merryweather J, Scandella C, Maerki W, Zapf J, Froesch ER (1986) Growth restoration of insulin-deficient diabetic rats by recombinant human insulin-like growth factor I. Nature 323:169–171

Schoenle EJ, Haselbacher GK, Briner J, Janzer RC, Gammeltoft S, Humbel RE, Prader A (1986) Elevated concentration of IGF II in brain tissue from an infant with megaencephaly. J Pediatr 108:737–740

Schumacher M, Jung-Testas I, Robel P, Baulieu E-E (1993) Insulin-like growth factor I: a mitogen for rat Schwann cells in the presence of elevated levels of cyclic AMP. Glia 8:232–240

Schwander JC, Hauri C, Zapf J, Froesch ER (1983) Synthesis and secretion of insulin-like growth factor and its binding protein by the perfused rat liver: dependence on growth hormone status. Endocrinology 113:297–305

Scott CD, Martin JL, Baxter RC (1985) Production of insulin-like growth factor I and its binding protein by adult rat hepatocytes in primary culture. Endocrinology 116:1094–1101

Sima AAF, Nathaniel V, Bril V, McEwen TAJ, Greene DA (1988) Histopathological heterogeneity of neuropathy in insulin-dependent and non-insulin dependent diabetes, and demonstration of axo-glial dysjunction in human diabetic neuropathy. J Clin Invest 81:349–364

Soares MB, Ishii DN, Efstratiadis A (1985) Developmental and tissue-specific expression of a family of transcripts related to rat insulin-like growth factor II mRNA. Nucleic Acids Res 13:1119–1134

Soares MB, Turken A, Ishii DN, Mills L, Episkopou V, Cotter S, Zeitlin S, Efstratiadis A (1986) Rat insulin-like growth factor II gene: a single gene with two promoters expressing a multitranscript family. J Mol Biol 192:737–752

Stong DB, Raskin R (1993) Effects of multiple subcutaneous doses of rhIGF-1 on total and free IGF-1 levels and blood glucose in humans. Ann NY Acad Sci 692:317–320

Stylianopoulou F, Herbert J, Soares MB, Efstratiadis A (1988) Expression of the insulin-like growth factor II gene in the choroid plexus and the leptomeninges of the adult rat central nervous system. Proc Natl Acad Sci USA 85:141–145

Suikkari A-M, Koivisto VA, Rutanen E-M, Yki-Jarvinen H, Karonen S-L, Seppala M (1988) Insulin regulates the serum levels of low molecular weight insulin-like growth factor-binding protein. J Clin Endocrinol Metab 66:266–272

Tan K, Baxter RC (1986) Serum insulin-like growth factor I levels in adult diabetic patients: the effect of age. J Clin Endocrinol Metab 63:651–655

Tappy L, Fujita-Yamaguchi Y, LeBon TR, Boden G (1988) Antibodies to insulin-like growth factor I receptors in diabetes and other disorders. Diabetes 37:1708–1714

Terry RD, Masliah E, Salmon DP, Butters N, Deteresa R, Hill R, Hansen LA, Katzman R (1991) Physical basis of congnitive alterations in Alzheimer's disease: synapse loss is the major correlate of cognitive impairment. Ann Neurol 30:572–580

Thomas PK, Tomlinson DR (1993) Diabetic and hypoglycemic neuropathy. In: Dyck PJ, Thomas PK, Griffin JW, Low PA, Poduslo JF (eds) Peripheral neuropathy. Saunders, Philadelphia, pp 1219–1250

Thompson JL, Butterfield GE, Marcus R, Hintz RL, Van Loan M, Ghiron L, Hoffman AR (1995) The effects of recombinant human insulin-like growth factor-I and growth hormone on body composition. J Clin Endocrinol Metab 80:1845–1852

Thornton P, Bennett S, Cooney P, Ingram R, Sonntag WE (1996) Decreases in type 1 insulin-like growth factor receptors in cortex and hippocampus of aged rats. Soc Neurosci Abstr 22:1234

Turkalj I, Keller U, Ninnis R, Vosmeer S, Stauffacher W (1992) Effect of increasing doses of recombinant human insulin-like growth factor-I on glucose, lipid, and leucine metabolism in man. J Clin Endocrinol Metab 75:1186–1191

Unterman TG, Oehler DT, Becker RE (1989) Identification of a type I insulin-like growth factor binding protein (IGF-BP) in serum from rats with diabetes mellitus. Biochem Biophys Res Commun 163:882–887

Usala AL, Madigan T, Burguera B, Cefalu W, Sinha MK, Powell JG, Usala SJ (1994) High dose intravenous, but not low dose subcutaneous, insulin-like growth factor-I therapy induces sustained insulin sensitivity in severely resistant type I diabetes mellitus. J Clin Endocrinol Metab 79:435–440

Vaccarello MA, Diamond FB, Guevara-Aguirre J, Rosenbloom AL, Fielder PJ, Gargosky S, Cohen P, Wilson K, Rosenfeld RG (1993) Hormonal and metabolic effects and pharmacokinetics of recombinant insulin-like growth factor-I in growth hormone receptor deficiency/Laron syndrome. J Clin Endocrinol Metab 77:273–280

Vasconez O, Martinez Z, Martinez AL, Hidalgo F, Diamond FB, Rosenbloom AL, Rosenfeld RG, Guevara-Aguirre J (1994) Heart rate increases in patients with growth hormone receptor deficiency treated with insulin-like growth factor I. Acta Paediatr 399 [Suppl]:137–139

Vinik AI, Holland MT, Le Beau JM, Liuzzi FJ, Stansberry KB, Colen LB (1992) Diabetic neuropathies. Diabetes Care 15:1926–1975

Vlachopapadopoulou E, Zachwieja JJ, Gertner JM, Manzione D, Bier DM, Matthews DE, Slonim AE (1995) Metabolic and clinical response to recombinant human insulin-like growth factor I in myotonic dystrophy – a clinical research center study. J Clin Endocrinol Metab 80:3715–3723

Ward JD (1989) Diabetic neuropathy. Br Med Bull 45:111–126

Wilton P, Sietnieks A, Gunnarsson R, Berger L, Grahnen A (1991) Pharmacokinetic profile of recombinant human insulin-like growth factor 1 given subcutaneously in normal subjects. Acta Paediatr 377 [Suppl]:S111–S114

Wong PC, Pardo CA, Borchelt DR, Lee MK, Copeland MG, Jenkins NA, Sisodia SS, Cleveland DW, Price DL (1995) An adverse property of a familial ALS-linked SOD1 mutation causes motor neuron disease characterized by vacuolar degeneration of mitochondria. Neuron 14:1105–1116

Wuarin L, Guertin DM, Ishii DN (1994) Reduction in insulin-like growth factor (IGF) gene expression in nerves precedes the onset of diabetic neuropathy. Exp Neurol 130:106–114

Wuarin L, Namdev R, Burns JG, Fei Z-J, Ishii DN (1996) Brain insulin-like growth factor-II mRNA content is reduced in insulin-dependent and non-insulin-dependent diabetes mellitus. J Neurochem 67:742–751

Yagihashi S (1995) Pathology and pathogenetic mechanisms of diabetic neuropathy. Diabetes Metab Rev 11:193–226

Zapf J, Morell B, Walter H, Laron Z, Froesch ER (1980) Serum levels of insulin-like growth factor (IGF) and its carrier protein in various metabolic disorders. Acta Endocrinol (Copenh) 95:505–517

Zdanowicz MM, Moyse J, Wingertzahn MA, O'Connor M, Teichberg S, Slonim AE (1995) Effect of insulin-like growth factor I in murine muscular dystrophy. Endocrinology 136:4880–4886

Zenobi PD, Graf S, Ursprung H, Froesch ER (1992) Effects of insulin-like growth factor-I on glucose tolerance, insulin levels, and insulin secretion. J Clin Invest 89:1908–1913

Zhuang H-X, Snyder CK, Pu S-F, Ishii DN (1996) Insulin-like growth factors reverse or arrest diabetic neuropathy: effects on hyperalgesia and impaired nerve regeneration in rats. Exp Neurol 140:198–205

Zhuang H-X, Wuarin L, Fei Z-J, Ishii DN (1997) Insulin-like growth factor (IGF) gene expression is reduced in neural tissues and liver from rats with non-insulin-dependent diabetes mellitus, and IGF treatment ameliorates diabetic neuropathy. J Pharmacol Exp Ther 283: 366–374

CHAPTER 6

Neurotrophic Factors in Peripheral Nerve Injury and Regeneration

N.M.J. Rupniak, J.M.A. Laird, S. Boyce, and R.G. Hill

A. Introduction

Damage to the human peripheral nervous system can result from many types of insult; examples are diabetes, traumatic injury, cytotoxic drugs, radiotherapy, infection, environmental pollutants such as organophosphates, and idiopathic neurodegenerative diseases such as amyotrophic lateral sclerosis. The consequences of peripheral nerve damage depend on the locus of the insult and are therefore also wide ranging (hearing loss, incontinence, persistent pain, respiratory complications, paralysis). Collectively, these conditions represent a major medical challenge because of the spectrum and severity of the resulting disability. Presently, there are few, if any, palliative treatments available and no curative therapy able to halt disease progression or restore normal function.

The proposed development of drug therapies for peripheral nerve damage highlights a number of medical and basic science issues. The ultimate goal of such therapeutic intervention must be to produce regeneration, appropriate re-innervation and, thus, functional recovery. In order to achieve this, early (and accurate) diagnosis of the disease is essential. However, in practice, patients are often not referred to a clinical neurologist until extensive damage to the nervous system has already been incurred. This may be because there is sufficient reserve capacity and plasticity in the nervous system to permit tolerance of damage, sometimes substantial, with only mild symptomatic impairment. This intrinsic capacity for functional recovery may be regarded as an encouraging sign in that even a modest retardation in the rate of neurodegeneration or the ability to enhance the function of surviving neurons with a neurotrophic agent might be sufficient to bring about a dramatic clinical improvement. The therapeutic reality, however, is that patients with advanced nervous-system damage also require substantial palliative support. The possibility of using drugs to reverse nervous-system damage and fully restore functional reinnervation of damaged tissues is, presently, a remote prospect.

The practical implementation of drug therapy aimed at repairing nerve damage is not a simple undertaking, since the regenerative process may be maladaptive. For example, aberrations in the course of regenerating sensory neurons can give rise to neuromas associated with persistent, intractable pain, and therapy with agents that enhance sprouting in such fibers could actually exacerbate the clinical consequences of certain types of nerve injury.

There are a number of endogenous neurotrophic factors that, when given exogenously, enhance peripheral nerve regeneration or reduce the extent of neurodegeneration in animal models of nerve injury. Because these are large protein molecules that penetrate the central nervous system poorly, diseases affecting the peripheral nervous system are widely acknowledged to be the most readily addressable clinical targets. In the following sections, we shall review recent preclinical and clinical experience with neurotrophic factors and assess their clinical potential.

B. Causes of Peripheral Nerve Damage

Peripheral neuropathy is a syndrome of sensory loss, muscle weakness and atrophy, vasomotor alterations and autonomic symptoms, either singly or in any combination, and can be distinguished from other neurodegenerative conditions as it represents a symptom complex, with many possible etiologies rather than a separate disease entity. Degeneration of peripheral neurons is seen as the result of idiopathic processes (hereditary neuropathies, Guillain-Barré syndrome) or as sequelae of systemic disease, exposure to toxins or trauma. Peripheral nerve damage may present as disease of a single nerve (mononeuropathy), in several nerves in separate locations (multiple mononeuropathy) or in many nerves simultaneously (polyneuropathy; Table 1).

Trauma is the most common cause of damage to a single nerve and may occur as a result of direct mechanical trauma (limb amputation, joint replacement surgery), or by compression or entrapment (trigeminal neuralgia, carpal tunnel syndrome, solid tumors). Hemorrhage into a nerve, or exposure to cold or radiation may also cause mononeuropathy. Infectious diseases (leprosy, HIV, Lyme disease, diphtheria toxin, herpes zoster) may cause single or multiple mononeuropathy. A variety of metabolic diseases may also cause neuropathy. The most common is diabetes mellitus, which most frequently results in a progressive distal polyneuropathy. Nutritional deficiencies, especially those involving vitamin-B deficiency, such as alcoholism and pernicious anemia and a wide range of xenobiotics (heavy metals, organophosphate insecticides, plasticizing agents) can cause neuropathy. Guillain-Barré Syndrome is an acute, rapidly progressing inflammatory polyneuropathy that generally arises within a few weeks of an infection, surgery or immunization, and results in muscle weakness, mild sensory loss and, in one third of patients, pain. Autonomic dysfunction, sufficient to be life-threatening, occurs in some patients. The majority of patients show considerable improvement after a few months, but some (10%) relapse into a chronic state. The cause of Guillain-Barré Syndrome is unknown.

Different conditions produce degeneration in different neuronal groups; thus, lead toxicity, porphyria and Guillain-Barré Syndrome primarily affect

Table 1. Comparison of the neuronal populations affected by peripheral neuropathies

	Neuronal population condition		
	Motor	Sensory	
		Large	Small
Diabetes	X	X	X
Traumatic injury	X	X	X
Cisplatin	X	X	
Taxol	X		
Motor Neuron Disease	X		
Post herpetic neuralgia	X		

motor neurones, whereas leprosy, AIDS and diabetes primarily affect sensory neurons. This may, in part, be ascribed to the differences in anatomy of the neurons that make up peripheral nerves. Motoneuron cell bodies are located in the CNS, protected by the blood–brain barrier, whereas sensory neuron cell bodies are found in the dorsal root ganglia, which do not have a barrier equivalent to the blood–brain or blood–nerve barrier (DISTEPHANO et al. 1992).

Hereditary neuropathies may involve either motor neurons or sensory neurons alone, or both motor and sensory neurons. Hereditary sensory neuropathies are rare and usually involve distal pain and temperature loss. The most common hereditary sensory-motor neuropathies are Charcot-Marie-Tooth disease and neurofibromatosis. Charcot-Marie-Tooth disease is characterized by distal weakness and atrophy, and a stocking-glove distribution loss of temperature and pain sensibility, due to demyelination and remyelination and degeneration in the distal nerves. Neurofibromatosis is characterized by skin lesions and neurofibromas (tumors of Schwann cells and nerve fibroblasts). The underlying cellular disorder is unknown. There are a number of hereditary motor neuropathies, clinical variants of motor neuron disease (MND or amyotrophic lateral sclerosis), including classical MND, progressive muscular atrophy, progressive bulbar palsy and pseudobulbar palsy. The incidence of MND is extremely rare, affecting about 1 in 100000 of the population, and it is a late-onset disorder. Most patients are aged over 50 years when they become aware of symptoms. About 5% of cases are familial with an autosomal dominant inheritance and with an earlier age of onset.

C. Symptoms and Pathophysiology of Peripheral-Nerve Damage

The degeneration of peripheral neurons is associated with loss of the function that they subserve. Autonomic neuropathy may lead to incontinence, postural hypertension or impotence. Variable vasomotor and sudomotor abnormalities may also be seen. The loss of large sensory fibers leads to deficits in proprioception and to loss of vibration and light touch sensation, resulting in gait abnormalities and clumsiness. The involvement of small sensory fibers results in alterations in pain and temperature sensation. Motor fiber loss is associated with muscle weakness and atrophy and loss of reflexes.

I. Sensory Neuropathies

Sensory neuropathies often result in abnormal sensations, which may be non-painful (tingling, buzzing; parasthesias) or painful. Abnormal sensations may be spontaneous, that is, occurring in the absence of external stimuli. Spontaneous pain is usually encountered as continuous burning pain, or as paroxysmal, lancinating pains occurring intermittently, and both may co-exist in the same patient. Abnormal painful responses to external stimuli applied to the affected area may be seen, such that normally innocuous stimuli (such as light brushing or objects at room temperature) provoke pain (allodynia), or that stimuli that normally evoke mildly painful sensations evoke intense pain (hyperalgesia).

The negative symptoms (loss of sensory, motor or autonomic function) are conceptually easy to understand as the functional consequences of interruption of connections between the CNS and the peripheral sensory receptors or effector organs. However, the positive symptoms that accompany many neuropathies require more explanation. Positive motor or autonomic symptoms are often the result of abnormalities in sensory fibers, as abnormal sensory input produces aberrant reflex responses (e.g., contractures or intense sudomotor and vasomotor activity). The most distressing positive symptoms are those associated with spontaneous pain. Two groups of mechanisms probably account for this: pathological changes in the peripheral neurons, as a result of injury, and CNS changes in response to nociceptive (damage-related) afferent input and the loss of portions of the normal afferent input.

Damage to the axons of peripheral neurons is followed by regeneration, with the formation of sprouts which attempt to grow back towards their innervation target. This re-innervation may be thwarted by the presence of obstructions or scar tissue, or a cycle of repeated degeneration followed by attempted regeneration may occur in the presence of metabolic or nutritional disease or toxicity. Electrophysiological recordings from animals have shown that the regenerating sprouts and also the cell bodies of damaged primary afferent neurons become spontaneously active, producing ectopic discharges. They may also acquire abnormal sensitivity to local mechanical, thermal and chemical stimuli, including circulating catecholamines (see Devor 1994).

In animal experiments, more than 70% of nociceptive neurons in the area of the spinal cord receiving input from a sciatic nerve with a partial neuroma responded to stimulation of the neuroma site by tapping or gentle movement, and abnormally high spontaneous activity was seen in a proportion of these

(LAIRD and BENNETT 1993). This abnormal activity would be expected to evoke the sensation of spontaneous pain following stimulation of sensitive sprouts. This expectation was confirmed in studies recording from transected nerves in patients with limb amputation, where the nerves that previously innervated the severed limb had formed a neuroma close to the point of amputation (NYSTROM and HAGBARTH 1981). Tapping of the neuroma evoked activity in the primary afferent fibers and painful or dyesthetic sensations. Injection of catecholamines around nerve-end neuromas in humans has also been found to be extremely painful (CHABAL et al. 1992). An acquired sensitivity to circulating catecholamines occurs after nerve damage (SATO and PERL 1991). In addition, sympathetic neurons may sprout, following nerve damage, and form new catecholamine-containing, basket-like connections around dorsal root ganglion cell bodies (MCLACHLAN et al. 1993).

Pathological activity in nociceptors as a result of nerve injury (ectopic discharge or responses to stimulation of sensitive nerve sprouts) also produces a variety of changes in the anatomy and neurochemistry of the spinal cord, including sprouting of the central processes of damaged primary afferents, degeneration of spinal neurons and changes in the expression of a variety of neurochemical markers (see BENNETT 1993), which may contribute to abnormal sensory processing after peripheral-nerve damage. The consequence is that activity in large myelinated afferents connected to low-threshold mechanoreceptors provokes painful sensations rather than tactile sensations (allodynia; TOREBJORK et al. 1992), and input from nociceptors evokes enhanced pain sensations (hyperalgesia; CERVERO et al. 1994).

II. Motor Neuronopathies

Motor-fiber loss is associated with muscle weakness and atrophy, and loss of reflexes. The symptoms are well illustrated by the hereditary motor-neuron diseases such as MND. The onset of MND is usually subtle and initial symptoms of fatigue, cramps and fasciculations of muscles are often overlooked. The patient's first complaint is usually of asymmetric muscle weakness and atrophy. The site of onset is random, but is more common in the hands and arms than in the legs or bulbar muscles (hips, tongue or throat). The partial weakness occurs in adjacent muscles and later spreads to muscles within the same limb or distant sites. These symptoms are often accompanied by spasticity and hyperactive reflexes. When the bulbar muscles are affected, patients have difficulty chewing and swallowing and speech is severely compromised. With time, the progressive muscle weakness leads to severe disability and eventually to death as a result of respiratory paralysis.

MND is characterized pathologically by progressive loss of pyramidal motor system efferents of the motor cortex, brainstem and spinal cord. The adjacent ascending sensory system is usually spared. In the brain, there is selective degeneration of Betz cells and the large pyramidal neurons from layer V of the motor cortex. In the spinal cord, there is degeneration of the corticospinal tracts in the white matter, whilst in the gray-matter degeneration is confined to motor neurons in lamina IX of the anterior horn. As a result of motor-neuron degeneration, the muscle fibers become denervated and atrophy.

Many etiological and pathological mechanisms have been proposed for MND. There is increasing evidence that abnormal excitatory amino-acid metabolism may be involved in the pathogenesis of MND (HUGON et al. 1989; PLAITAKIS 1990). It has been speculated that the combination of increased release of excitatory amino acids, together with reduced clearance in the ventral horn, leads to extremely high concentrations within the synaptic cleft, rendering these neurons vulnerable to excitotoxic damage. Oxidative mechanisms involving the activity of monoamine oxidase and free-radical formation have also been proposed to play a role in the etiology of MND. Mutations on the Cu/Zn superoxide dismutase (SOD-1) gene on chromosome 21 have been detected in some families with the autosomal dominant form of motor-neurone disease. These mutations result in structural deficits and decreased SOD-1 enzyme activity, leading to accumulation of free-oxygen or -hydroxyl radicals which are capable of inducing oxidative stress with subsequent neuronal damage. Antioxidants, such as vitamin E and *N*-acetylcysteine have been shown to prevent neuronal death caused by chronic inhibition of SOD-1 in cultured PC12 cells and spinal neurons in vivo (ROTHSTEIN et al. 1994; TROY and SHELANSKI 1994). Protection against free-radical toxicity may form a basis for future clinical trials.

Evidence linking MND with an autoimmune pathogenesis has also emerged. Elevated serum immunoglobulins (IgG) have been reported in as many as 60% of patients with MND (MEININGER et al. 1990). Autopsy findings have demonstrated IgG reactivity in motor neurons within anterior horn and in motor cortex of patients with MND (ENGELHARDT and APPEL 1990).

D. Current Approaches to Therapy

I. Sensory Neuropathies

In the case of neuropathies caused by metabolic disorders or nutritional deficiency, control of the precipitating causes usually halts progression. The symptoms may improve, presumably as a result of successful regeneration, but recovery is slow. There are no currently accepted therapies that assist or enhance the regeneration of damaged nerves or the re-innervation of denervated tissues.

1. Surgery

Surgery is often indicated to improve the chances of successful regeneration and re-innervation after traumatic injury of a nerve, and is also used to relieve compression or distortion of individual nerves, as in carpal tunnel syndrome. Resection of a painful nerve-end neuroma usually provides only temporary relief, since a new neuroma forms, but a number of techniques have been proposed to prevent the formation of a neuroma by providing a path for re-innervation of an alternative target. Such strategies may relieve phantom limb pain.

2. Analgesic Drugs

Palliative therapy for painful sensory neuropathies most commonly involves analgesic medication; the major limitation of such drugs is that they do not alter the underlying nerve damage. Opiates are generally the first-line treatment for severe pain, and there is no theoretical reason why they should not be effective in treating pain of neuropathic origin (Hill 1994). However, their usefulness in neuropathic-pain patients is the subject of some debate (Arnér and Meyerson 1988; Portenoy et al. 1990). It has been suggested that the dose-response curve for opiates in these patients may be shifted to the right, such that high doses are required to provide significant relief (Portenoy et al. 1990). This problem is compounded by the fact that neuropathic pain may be very severe. Thus, the side-effects produced by an effective analgesic dose may well be intolerable, especially for long-term use.

A range of other centrally acting drugs are employed for neuropathic pain, with varying success. Tricyclic antidepressants are the most commonly used and are reported to be effective analgesics in patients who are not clinically depressed (Max et al. 1991; McQuay et al. 1996), although their efficacy is variable. Certain anticonvulsants (especially lamotrigine and carbamazepine) and orally administered local anesthetics (such as lidocaine) are used to treat spontaneous neuropathic pain, especially that with a lancinating component (Tanelian and Brose 1991). NMDA receptor antagonists, such as ketamine and the antitussive medicine dextromethorphan, have also been found to relieve neuropathic pain in man. However, the psychotomimetic and motor side-effects of currently available NMDA receptor antagonists preclude their widespread clinical use.

Finally, sympathectomy, using ganglion-blocking drugs or local infusions of phentolamine, is sometimes undertaken in cases of severe, intractable pain. Sympatholytic therapy has a theoretical basis in that peripheral nerve damage causes acquired sensitivity of sprouts in neuromas to catecholamines. However, the identification of patients whose neuropathic pain may be sympathetically maintained is by virtue of their responsiveness to sympatholytic treatments (Raja et al. 1991).

II. Motor Neuronopathies

In the case of hereditary diseases, such as MND, symptom progression is extremely aggressive and, until recently, this disorder was considered to be untreatable; from diagnosis, the mean life expectancy for patients with sporadic MND is just 3 years, although a minority of patients may survive longer (Mulder and Howard 1976). Physiotherapy is often used to help maintain muscle function, whilst spasticity and muscle cramps may be reduced by treatment with anticonvulsants, such as baclofen or phenytoin. Tricyclic antidepressants may be useful to decrease saliva production. However, development of an effective drug to alleviate the symptoms or retard the progression of this disease has remained elusive, despite a number of clinical trials. Some progress has been made with the recent introduction of riluzole, a glutamate antagonist, which is the first agent shown to retard symptom progression and prolong survival (Bensinon et al. 1994; Lacomblez et al. 1996). Riluzole is now approved for the treatment of MND in the U.S.A. and Europe. Side-effects associated with riluzole include elevations in serum alanine aminotransferase levels, abdominal cramps and nausea.

MND is an important clinical target for neurotrophic agents. Since motor-neuron axons and their terminals lie outside the blood–brain barrier they are, therefore, accessible to agents delivered into the circulation. This provides a route into the motor neuron by retrograde transport (Di Stefano et al. 1992).

E. Methods for the Study of Peripheral Nerve Damage in Laboratory Animals

The development of new strategies for the treatment of peripheral neuropathies is dependent on the predictive validity of animal models in which trophic agents are evaluated. Peripheral neuropathy in man has a wide variety of causes, but the animal assays used to test the efficacy of potential treatments are generally models of damage produced by trauma, neurotoxins and diabetes, in young and previously healthy animals. Showing true functional recovery after nerve damage can be problematic, and often surrogate endpoints are used. The choice of both an appropriate model and a relevant endpoint is clearly crucial for the predictive value of any animal test.

I. Mechanical Injury

Mechanical damage of a single nerve, performed under anesthesia, is the classical method used to study the regeneration of both sensory and motor axons in vivo. One such method involves nerve transection, where the continuity of the axons themselves is interrupted, and there is also damage to the surrounding endoneurial sheaths and to Schwann-cell basal laminal tubes, so that appropriate axonal regrowth and functional re-innervation of the target tissue can often no longer be achieved. In this situation, regeneration is usually assessed morphologically several days after placing the transected nerve stumps in a silicone cuff filled with an inert polymer matrix (Madison et al.

1985). Neurotrophic factors may then be applied either directly at the site of nerve injury (in the silicon guide tube or topically via gel foam or osmotic mini pump), or by intravenous injection or infusion for a period of several days prior to assessment of the nerve regeneration distance.

Less-severe nerve damage can be achieved using a freeze lesion, which has the advantage of completely lesioning all fibers without disrupting the guidance channels formed by the Schwann cell tubes (FUGLEHOLM et al. 1994). Surgical crush injuries, typically of the sciatic nerve in rats, are the most commonly used form of mechanical trauma in studies of functional nerve regeneration. The degree of nerve damage and the time course for recovery from this varies considerably, depending on the duration, force, location and instrument employed to apply the crush (CHEN et al. 1992). Care therefore needs to be taken to calibrate the method used in order to achieve consistent results.

II. Neurotoxins

A number of toxins can produce damage to peripheral nerves. Toxins are usually delivered systemically to produce a polyneuropathy, but local delivery to a single nerve (usually using osmotic mini pumps) produces mononeuropathy; although technically more demanding, this method has the advantage of preserving the general health of the experimental animals. Different types of chemical toxins damage distinct sensory fiber afferents and this enables particular neuronal populations that are of most relevance to the clinical condition of interest to be targeted relatively specifically. Probably, the most widely used models of toxic neuropathies are those caused by cancer chemotherapeutic agents, since neuropathy is a dose-limiting side-effect of their use in man. Cisplatin produces a large sensory fiber neuropathy, accompanied by abnormalities in proprioception, whereas taxol produces a small sensory-fiber neuropathy and consequent insensitivity to noxious thermal stimulation (APFEL et al. 1991, 1992). A third cytotoxic drug, vincristine, produces a mixed motor and sensory neuropathy, with effects on both large- and small-diameter axons (see MCMAHON and PRIESTLEY 1995).

Exposure to toxic metals and other xenobiotics can induce MND-like syndromes in animals and man. Administration of aluminum or manganese to cynomolgus monkeys can cause degeneration of motor neurons in the spinal cord (GARRUTO et al. 1989). Similarly, plasticizing agents, such as *N*-butylbenzenesulphamide can induce a syndrome clinically and histologically resembling MND in rabbits (STRONG et al. 1990). Administration of cyclasin and β-*N*-methylamino-L-alanine (BMAA), neurotoxins isolated from cyclad seeds, to animals also induced motor neuron deficits similar to those observed in MND (SPENCER et al. 1986), and may explain the incidence of MND–Parkinsonism/dementia complex that occurs in certain Western Pacific islands where cyclad seeds are ingested in the diet.

III. Diabetes

Diabetic neuropathy is one of the most common causes of peripheral neuropathy. Acute diabetes may be induced in laboratory animals by administration of the toxin streptozotocin, which destroys the insulin-producing cells in the pancreas. This is the most commonly used method to study peripheral nerve function in diabetic animals, often by examination of changes in nerve conduction velocity and alterations in nociceptive thresholds. The rate of regeneration of peripheral nerves following mechanical trauma, such as transection, is also markedly retarded in experimentally induced diabetes (LONGO et al. 1986).

A major difference between most studies of neuropathy in diabetic laboratory animals and the situation in diabetic patients is that experimental studies generally use animals with full-blown, uncontrolled diabetes (hence hyperglycemia) whereas, in patients, the diabetes is controlled with insulin and by dietary measures. Thus, the changes in peripheral nerve function observed in laboratory animals, especially following acute exposure to streptozotocin, may differ significantly from the neuropathy that typically appears after several years of controlled diabetes in patients. Although several types of spontaneously diabetic animals, such as the *Ob/Ob* mouse (see CORTEIX et al. 1993; BREWSTER et al. 1994) are now available, studies of peripheral nerve function and the effects of neurotrophic factors have not yet been reported.

IV. Hereditary Motor Neuronopathies in Mice

There are several spontaneously occurring mutations in mice (designated *wobbler*, *pmn* and *Mnd*) that lead to selective degeneration of motor neurons. These differ in their symptoms and rate of progression of disease. The *wobbler* mouse has been the most widely used to evaluate neurotrophic factors (see Sect. E.IV). *Wobbler* mice develop motor-neuron degeneration mainly affecting the forelimbs. Clinical abnormalities are apparent at 3–4 weeks, when the mutants show retarded weight gain and forelimb weakness, muscle atrophy, tremor and abnormal gait. Disease progression is rapid up to 16 weeks of age, when some mice die as a result of severe muscle weakness; in others, disease progression may slow down or stop (DUCHEN and STRICH 1968).

The *pmn* mice develop paralysis of the hindlimbs and pelvic-girdle muscles within 3 weeks and die within 6–7 weeks of age; unlike *Mnd*, *pmn* is characterized pathologically by distal axonopathy, whilst the axons and cell bodies are relatively spared (LUDOLPH 1996). Unlike the *wobbler* and *pmn* mutants, the *Mnd* mouse has a late-onset neurodegenerative disease characterized by progressive deterioration in motor function from 5–6 months of age, moving from the hindlimbs to forelimbs, leading to eventual paralysis and premature death at 10–12 months of age (CALLAHAN et al. 1991; BOYCE et al. 1998).

F. Endpoints Used to Assess Peripheral Nerve Regeneration In Vivo

I. Quantitative Morphometric Analysis

The classical techniques for the study of peripheral-nerve regeneration are morphological. Such methods allow quantitative assessment of cell survival, fiber elongation and associated processes like myelination. An example of this approach is shown in Fig. 1, where the regeneration of large myelinated fibers is traced using a monoclonal antibody to intact neurofilaments in transverse sections of the sciatic nerve 5 days after crush injury in rats. Analysis of the number of positive fibers shows a clear difference in neurofilament number and organization in sections proximal and distal to the crush (Fig. 2).

Histochemical methods also enable examination of the re-innervation of specific targets, such as motor end-plates for example, by combined staining for acetylcholinesterase activity and silver staining to reveal the proximity of terminal neurites to the sole plate of the muscle fiber. Assessment of the status of unmyelinated fibres requires electron microscopy. The use of immuno-histochemical tracing techniques [e.g., to identify substance P or calcitonin

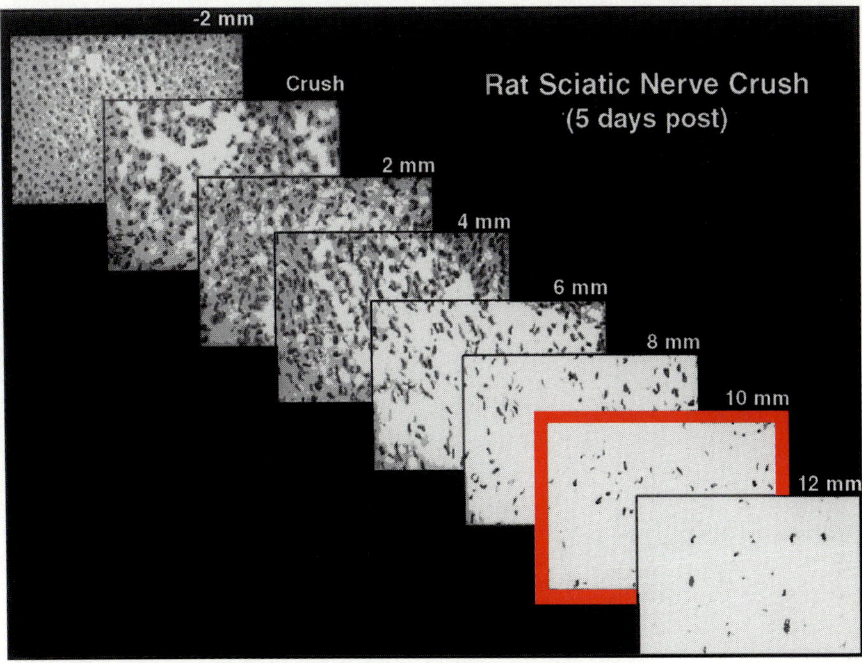

Fig. 1. Transverse sections through a sciatic nerve following nerve crush injury showing immunostaining of regenerating myelinated axons using an antibody to neurofilament (M. Rigby and D. Smith, unpublished observation)

gene-related peptide (CGRP)-containing sensory afferents] or neurochemical markers (e.g., choline acetyltransferase as a marker for motor neurons) is required to differentiate between motor, sensory and autonomic fibers traveling in peripheral nerve trunks. Axonal elongation of sensory fibers may also be assessed by measuring, in small segments of the nerve, the presence of ^{3}H-leucine-labeled amino acids applied to the cell bodies in the spinal ganglia. The labeled amino acid is incorporated into proteins and is transported along the regenerating fibers by fast axonal transport (Bisby and Chen 1990). However, the sensitivity of these methods may themselves be affected by both the pathophysiology of nerve damage and repair and by the neurotrophic agent under study. Furthermore, morphological techniques alone provide little insight into the recovery of function as a result of nerve regeneration and re-

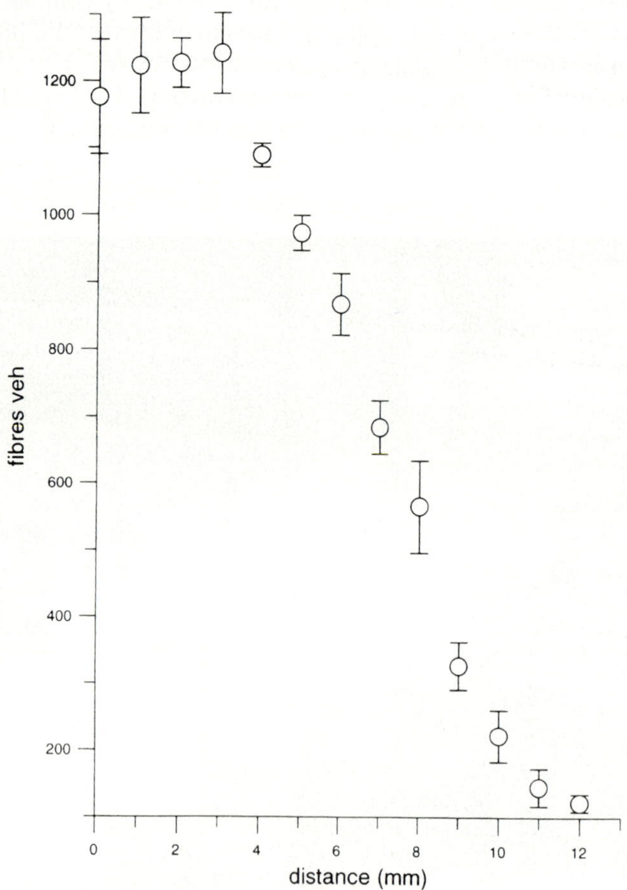

Fig. 2. Neurofilament counts showing the progress of regenerating axons distal to sciatic nerve crush injury (M. Rigby and D. Smith, unpublished observations) *veh* vehicle treatment

innervation and are, therefore, best used in conjunction with assays of functional recovery described below.

II. Functional Assays of Nerve Regeneration Distance

Several *in vivo* techniques using anesthetized animals allow measurement of the extent of axonal elongation of regenerating motor and sensory fibers several days after sciatic nerve crush injury, and permit the distinction between large- and small-diameter sensory fiber regeneration distances. Recording the compound action potential evoked by stimulating the spinal ventral roots (in which the axons of motor neurons run) along the length of a crushed nerve allows the identification of the point at which conduction fails and, thus, the point which motor fibers capable of sustaining action potentials have reached (NEAR et al. 1992; LAIRD et al. 1995; Fig. 3). The length of nerve between the crush injury and the regeneration front can then be measured with calipers and recorded as the regeneration distance in millimeters. The

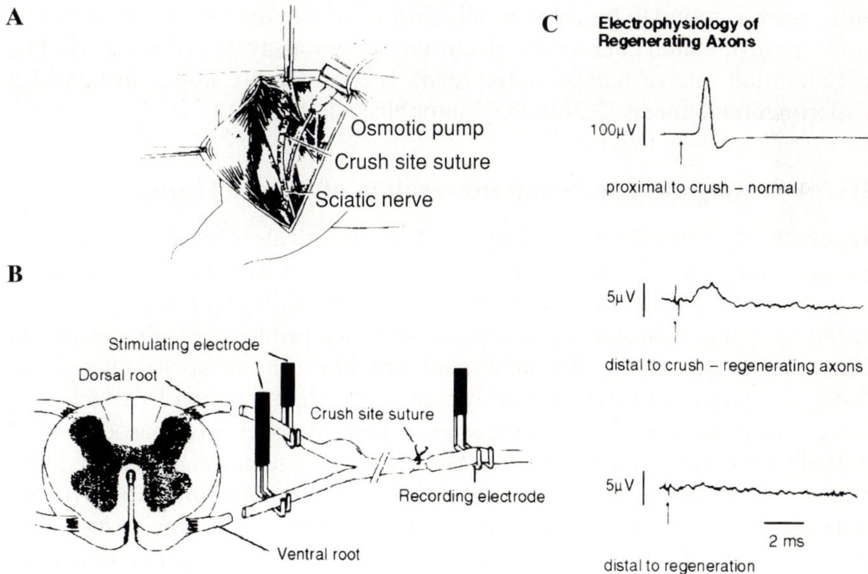

Fig. 3A–C. Diagram showing (**A**) the surgical preparation for sciatic nerve crush in anesthetized animals, and (**B**) experimental arrangement of stimulating and recording electrodes when determining nerve regeneration distance in vivo. Examples of the compound action potential (**C**) recorded in an injured sciatic nerve after stimulation of the ventral root (motor neurones activated) are shown. Note the different scale of the upper trace (recording approximately 3 mm proximal to the crush injury) compared with the center and lower traces (recordings made approximately 0.5 and 9 mm distal to the crush injury, respectively). Adapted with permission of the authors from LAIRD et al (1995)

same measurement made while stimulating spinal dorsal roots (which carry sensory axons) allows the identification of the point which functional large myelinated sensory fibers have reached. The time course for regeneration of sensory and motor axons after crush injury in normal rats is similar using this assay (2.4–2.5 mm/day; LAIRD et al. 1995).

The progress of fine unmyelinated fibers is difficult to measure using this technique since the compound action potential they evoke is much smaller and difficult to identify accurately in the regenerated portion of the nerve. However, the elongation of nociceptive fibers (unmyelinated or fine myelinated fibers) in a crushed nerve may be easily measured using the pinch reflex test (KANJE et al. 1989). In this assay, the distance that the axons have regenerated is determined by pinching the nerve with fine forceps, starting at the distal end and moving in 0.5-mm increments progressively closer to the site of crush injury. When the regenerating tips of the sensory axons are pinched, an injury discharge is evoked and this activates a nociceptive reflex response, causing a change in blood pressure and a contraction of muscles of the back. The regeneration distance is recorded in millimeters as the difference between this point and the location of the crush injury. In a study using this assay to examine the time course for regeneration of unmyelinated fibers in normal rats, this was found to be considerably faster (3.2 mm/day) than that observed for large myelinated fibers in the electrophysiology assay described above. The regeneration rate of unmyelinated fibers is considerably slower in rats with experimental diabetes (2.2 mm/day; unpublished observations).

III. Assessing the Functional Innervation of Target Tissues

Innervation of muscle may be assessed quantitatively with a nerve–muscle preparation either *in vitro* or *in vivo* (VERGARA et al. 1993). The nerve is stimulated electrically, and either the isometric tension generated or the electromyograph is measured and compared with that produced by direct stimulation of the muscle. A population of small sensory (primarily nociceptive) fibers have, in addition to their afferent function, an efferent action by which they release neuropeptides from their peripheral terminals, evoking vasodilatation and plasma extravasation, a process known as neurogenic inflammation. Measuring neurogenic inflammation provoked by electrical stimulation of the nerve, or by application of irritants such as mustard oil to the tissue, thus, provides a relatively simple quantitative method to assess functional re-innervation by this class of fibers (DONNERER et al. 1996).

Recovery of function following nerve damage may also be assessed by a variety of behavioral tests, which involve some measure of both motor and sensory integrity. A particularly useful and simple method for assessment of motor function is by analysis of the animals' walking pattern and toe-spread index (DE MEDINACELI et al. 1982; CHEN et al. 1992). Here, the paws are painted with dye and the animal is encouraged to walk on paper so that toe spread (the distance between the first and last digits) and the intra- and inter-step distances can be measured from the resulting footprints. Immediately after a sciatic nerve-crush injury, the toe spread of the ipsilateral paw becomes more narrow and gradually spreads out to the normal width as functional reinnervation proceeds (Fig. 4). Mice with hereditary motor neuronopathy develop marked abnormalities in walking pattern. *Mnd* mice exhibit a marked reduction in the distance between left and right hind paws (intra-step distance), but have a normal stride length (BOYCE et al. 1997). Sensorimotor

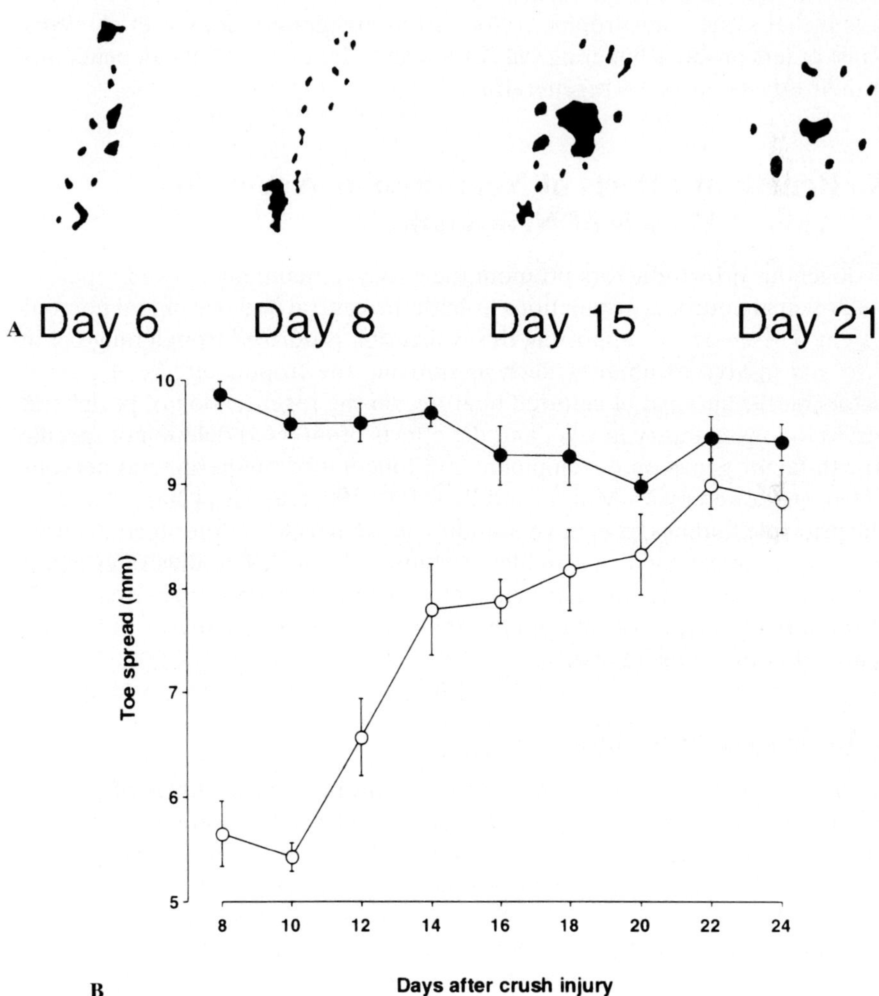

Fig. 4 A,B. Assessment of functional recovery following sciatic nerve crush injury in mice using measurement of toe spread. (**A**) Paw prints of mice at various times after nerve crush, and (**B**) time-course for recovery. -o-, ipsilateral limb; -•-, contralateral limb

coordination can also be assessed by the ability of animals to balance and walk along narrow dowels, climb ladders and remain on a revolving treadmill (Apfel et al. 1992; Boyce et al. 1997). Measurement of grip strength (Contreras et al. 1993) gives some indication of the degree of muscle denervation/re-innervation and is less affected by deficits in proprioception.

The function of sensory fibers may be tested by evoking spinal reflexes: stepping or placing reflexes for large fibers connected to mechanoreceptors and proprioceptors, and nociceptive withdrawal reflexes for small fibers connected to nociceptors (Apfel et al. 1991, 1992), although these tests may also reflect motor function. Another confounding factor when using nociceptive tests is that some neurotrophic factors act as analgesics (Cuevas et al. 1996), whilst others produce hyperalgesia (Lewin and Mendell 1993), independently of their effects on nerve regeneration.

G. Beneficial Effects of Neurotrophic Agents in Animal Models of Neuropathy

Endogenous growth factors promote the survival, maintenance and repair of the principal neuronal populations in both the central and peripheral nervous system. The evidence supporting this conclusion is derived from a range of in vitro and in vivo techniques, such as studying the trophic effects of growth factors on the survival of cultured neurons, on the regeneration of peripheral nerves following injury in vivo, and the effects of targeted deletion of specific growth-factor genes on development and function of the peripheral nervous system (reviewed by McMahon and Priestley 1995; see also Chaps. 3 and 4). The principle findings from in vivo studies, in animals with experimental nerve damage, are presented in a simplified version in Table 2. This illustrates that it is unlikely for any one single growth factor to be clinically useful in treating all of the different types of neuropathy that can affect the many or individual neuronal populations in man.

I. Mechanical Nerve Injury

A number of studies have demonstrated neuroprotective effects of growth factors following peripheral-nerve transection, especially in neonatal rats. The death of sensory neurons can be prevented by the neurotrophins nerve growth factor (NGF), brain-derived neurotrophic factor (BDNF) and neurotrophic factor-3 (NT-3) (Miyata et al. 1986; Eriksson et al. 1994). The survival of axotomized motor neurons is also reported to be transiently increased by treatment with the neurotrophins BDNF, NT-3 and neurotrophic factor-4/5 (NT-4/5), but not by NGF, and also by the neurocytokines ciliary neurotrophic factor (CNTF) and glial-derived neurotrophic factor (GDNF) (Sendtner et al. 1990, 1992a; Clatterbuck et al. 1994; Vejsada et al. 1994; Oppenheim et al. 1995; Yan et al. 1995).

Table 2. Neurotrophic effects of neuronal growth factors in animal assays

Growth factor	Neuronal population		
	Motor	Sensory	
		Large	Small
Nerve growth factor	X		X
Brain-derived neurotrophic factor	X	X	
Neurotrophic factor-3	X	X	
Neurotrophic factor-4/5	X	X	
Fibroblast growth factors	X	X	
Ciliary neurotrophic factor	X		
Glial-derived neurotrophic factor	X		
Insulin-like growth factor	X		X

In assays more relevant to the issue of whether such agents can also promote functional recovery from peripheral-nerve damage, there are a number of reports that neurocytokines can enhance the regeneration rate of sensory and motor axons following nerve crush injury. The insulin-like growth factors (IGF-I and IGF-II) have been shown to promote both motor and small sensory axon regeneration after local application to the site of nerve injury (Kanje et al. 1989; Near et al. 1992). Similarly, basic and acidic fibroblast growth factors (aFGF and bFGF) have been shown to promote the regeneration of large sensory and motor fibers after local or systemic administration (Aebischer et al. 1989; Laird et al. 1995).

II. Neurotoxins

There is evidence that NGF and NT-3 are able to alleviate deficits in sensory neuron function caused by neurotoxins. Systemic administration of NGF was reported to prevent the development of hypoalgesia and the depletion of substance P in the dorsal root ganglion, reflecting small sensory fiber damage (Apfel et al. 1991). In a subsequent study, NGF was also found to protect large sensory fibers from cisplatin-induced toxicity as indicated by the prevention of disturbances in proprioception (ability to balance on a rotating rod), nerve conduction velocity and depletion of CGRP levels in dorsal root ganglia (APFEL et al. 1992). Similarly, administration of NT-3 was reported to completely reverse the slowing in large sensory fiber conduction velocity caused by cisplatin in rats (GAO et al. 1995).

III. Diabetes

NGF and the IGFs are reported to reverse some aspects of the small sensory-fiber sensory neuropathy caused by streptozotocin-induced diabetes in rats. Thus, NGF prevented thermal hypoalgesia caused by streptozotocin, although slowing of the compound action potential was not ameliorated (APFEL et al. 1994). NGF (but not BDNF) also reversed the fall in substance P and CGRP content (and indeed increased it to supra-normal levels) in sciatic nerve and dorsal root ganglia of diabetic rats (APFEL et al. 1994; DIEMEL et al. 1994). Reversal of the diabetes-induced impairment in sensory fiber regeneration rate following nerve-crush injury has been reported after administration of IGF-I, IGF-II and IGF-III (ISHII and LUPIEN 1995). The effects of IGF are described in detail in Chap. 5.

IV. Motor Neuronopathy in Mice

Studies using mice with hereditary motor-neuron dysfunction provide further evidence that the neurotrophin BDNF and the neurocytokines CNTF, IGF-I and bFGF are trophic for motor neurons in vivo. In *wobbler* mice, subcutaneous administration of BDNF was able to retard the progressive decline in grip strength, reduced muscle atrophy, and protected against the loss of myelinated motor axons in the ventral roots (IKEDA et al. 1995a,b). The trophic effects of CNTF have been studied more extensively using three mutant-mouse models (*wobbler*, *pmn* and *Mnd*) that differ in their clinical features and time-course.

Subcutaneous administration of CNTF to *wobbler* mice improved grip strength and reduced paw position and walking abnormalities, although a reduction in body weight gain was also observed (MITSUMOTO et al. 1994a,b). In *pmn* mice, injection of CNTF-secreting cell lines was able to improve grip strength, reduced the loss of motor neurons in the phrenic and facial nerves, and prolonged survival time by 40% (SENDTNER et al. 1992b; SAGOT et al. 1995). CNTF was also reported to delay motor impairment in *Mnd* mice (HELGREN et al. 1992). Combined administration of BDNF with CNTF was subsequently found to completely arrest disease progression for 1 month in *wobbler* mice, indicating a synergistic interaction between these growth factors (MITSUMO et al. 1994a,b).

There is also evidence of a beneficial effect of IGF-I in murine motor neuronopathy. In *wobbler* mice, treatment with IGF-I improved grip strength and mean muscle-fiber diameter, although no effect on the reduction in skeletal muscle acetylcholine-transferase activity or the loss of spinal cord motor neurons was seen (HANTAI et al. 1995). Another neurocytokine, bFGF, also improved grip strength and retarded both muscle atrophy and the degeneration of spinal motor neurons in *wobbler* mice (IKEDA et al. 1995a,b). Finally, a recent report using GDNF failed to demonstrate beneficial effects of this agent either on the life span or axonal degeneration in *pmn* mice (SAGOT et al. 1996).

H. Drug-Development Issues

Modulation or direct administration of neuronal growth factors provides important new opportunities to develop interventions to repair nervous system damage. The production of large quantities of neurotrophic factors by recombinant techniques has made it possible to test their clinical efficacy, but important practical and conceptual difficulties remain. The inability of these large proteins to cross the blood–brain barrier has, so far, mostly limited clinical trials to investigations in MND and sensory neuropathies.

Optimizing the dose, route and duration of treatment of neurotrophic agents remains a major difficulty in the design of clinical trials. Unlike conventional drug–receptor interactions, neurotrophin signaling results in a change in the expression of specific genes. The uncertain duration of these induced changes in cell function may complicate dose titration and could cause unforeseen undesirable effects. Particular concerns include: (a) possible tumor-promoting or tumorigenic effects of growth factors, especially nonspecific mitogens, which may prohibit their use in cancer patients with nerve damage, and limit their use generally; and (b) immune responses to growth-factor therapy which might induce pathogenic antibodies capable of aggravating or causing neuronal damage.

If damaged neurons can be persuaded to regenerate, this will be of value only if they form functionally useful synaptic connections. Stimulation of neurite outgrowth by application of exogenous neurotrophic agents in a diseased nervous system might produce the desired functional re-innervation, but the critical issue of how this process can be controlled to prevent aberrant synaptic connectivity, whilst maintaining adequate trophic support to overcome the underlying pathologic process, has not yet been addressed.

I. Clinical Experience with Neurotrophic Factors

The studies described in preceding sections have provided a strong pre-clinical impetus to study the ability of neurotrophic factors to treat peripheral neuropathies in man. The outcome of ongoing trials examining the efficacy of NGF and of NT-3 in neuropathies caused by diabetes and cytotoxic drugs is keenly awaited. However, it has already been established that dose titration for NGF is likely to be problematic, since cutaneous injection of even minute doses (1–3 μg) caused long-lasting (several weeks) pressure allodynia and thermal hyperalgesia in normal volunteers (DYCK et al. 1997).

The majority of clinical trials reported to date have targeted MND, as this has clearly defined clinical assessment criteria and a more predictable time-course than other neuropathies; the current status of these studies is summarized in Table 3. CNTF was the first neurotrophic agent to be evaluated in patients with MND. Despite encouraging pre-clinical data, optimism regarding its clinical utility was short-lived following lack of efficacy and poor tolerability in man. A phase-III trial studying 720 patients revealed unacceptable side-effects including fever, weight loss and activation of herpes virus, with no improvement in muscle strength or mortality (ALS CNTF Treatment Study Group 1996). The lack of clinical efficacy of CNTF in MND may be attributable to its extremely short plasma half-life and, therefore, a recent attempt was made to overcome this problem by means of intrathecal delivery of CNTF; this trial, however, resulted in dose-limiting side-effects of headache and cramping pain in two of four patients (Penn et al. 1997). The clinical development of CNTF was discontinued in 1994.

Clinical findings using IGF-I (Myotrophin) in patients with MND remain inconclusive. Encouraging findings obtained in a phase-II/III trial in North America were not supported by a second trial performed in Europe. In May 1997, the Food and Drugs Administration refused to grant marketing approval for IGF-I because the evidence for clinical efficacy was not sufficiently robust. A third trial examining IGF-I in a further 180 patients is currently in progress (to be completed in 1998).

In 1995, Regeneron and Amgen announced exciting findings from a phase-I/II study showing that patients treated with BDNF had only half the rate of deterioration in breathing capacity seen in placebo-treated patients. Unfortunately, this observation was not replicated in a subsequent phase-III trial, although BDNF was well tolerated. Further clinical trials with subcutaneously administered BDNF are not planned for patients with MND, although studies examining intrathecal administration will be explored. The effects of subcutaneous BDNF will also be examined in patients with diabetic neuropathy. Finally, Amgen are reported to be considering phase-I trials with GDNF for possible treatment of MND (Scrip 1996a).

J. Conclusions and Future Directions

Despite the powerful pre-clinical rationale, the expectation that protein growth factors would be useful therapeutic agents in man has not yet borne fruit. The reasons for the poor clinical findings in MND require careful consideration if we are to make rational progress towards successful therapies for this and other neurodegenerative diseases.

The disappointing clinical findings in MND must call into question the predictive validity of the in vivo pre-clinical efficacy assays that were the driving force to target this patient population. The availability of mutant mice with hereditary motor neuronopathies, however, represent unusually good animal models, mimicking both the symptoms and neuropathology of MND,

Table 3. Status of clinical trials of neurotrophic factors in Motor Neuron Disease

Trophic factor	Company	Clinical findings	Reference	Current status
Ciliary Neurotrophic Factor	Regeneron	Phase-I trial in 57 patients revealed dose-limiting toxicity (fever, fatigue, cough). Phase-II/III trial in 730 patients showed no clinical improvement in muscle strength or mortality rate. Side-effects included anorexia, weight loss and cough.	ALS CNTF Treatment Study Group (1995) ALS CNTF Treatment Study Group (1996)	Development discontinued in 1994
Insulin-like Growth Factor-I (Myotrophin)	Cephalon/ Chiron/ Kyowa Hakko	U.S. Phase-II/III trial in 266 patients suggested slowing of disease progression and improved motor ability. European Phase-II/III trial in 183 patients was inconclusive. Third trial in 180 patients is in progress.	Scrip (1995a) Scrip (1995b)	NDA not approved (May 1997)
Brain-Derived Neurotrophic Factor	Regeneron/ Amgen	Phase-I/II results showed improvement in breathing capacity, but no effect on muscle strength. Phase-III trial failed to show efficacy in breathing capacity or survival.	Scrip (1995c) Scrip (1997)	Intrathecal route to be explored
Glial-derived Neurotrophic Factor	Amgen	Early clinical trials planned.	Scrip (1996a)	

that are lacking for other neurological diseases. Hence, the failure of neurotrophic factors in the clinic seems particularly difficult to explain. On closer inspection of the pre-clinical data, however, it is apparent that the *wobbler* mouse was the most frequently employed model, and it is notable that this has the least severe pathology and symptom progression of the available mutants. With the exception of CNTF, none of the other trophic factors was shown to retard disease progression or mortality in the more severely affected *pmn* and *Mnd* mutant mice. Thus, one possibility is that amelioration of motor deficits in *wobbler* mice alone is not a sufficiently rigorous criterion to predict clinical efficacy in MND.

Another critical issue relates to difficulty of establishing what should be the clinically effective dose range. In the case of CNTF, for which compelling pre-clinical data were obtained in *wobbler*, *pmn* and *Mnd* mice, it seems likely that clinical efficacy could not be demonstrated because of dose-limiting toxicity. The studies in *wobbler* mice indicate that weight loss may coincide with beneficial effects on motor symptoms, so that it may not be possible to safely achieve the equivalent dose range in man. Similar concerns limit interpretation of the negative or inconclusive clinical findings with BDNF and IGF-I; there is no simple way to determine whether these agents were administered at sufficiently high doses to adequately test their clinical utility.

Another important factor in interpreting the clinical findings is that MND may prove to be particularly intractable because of its severity and aggressive course; growth factors may well be more beneficial in other, less disabling, forms of neuropathy. It is also entirely possible that successful therapy of MND and other conditions would require concurrent administration of several growth factors together.

A number of approaches, such as gene therapy, are being explored as methods to improve the delivery of protein growth factors to the relevant target tissues and this may eventually provide a way to perform more conclusive clinical trials. However, the long-term pharmaceutical objective must be to develop small-molecule growth-factor mimetics as therapeutics. The first generation of interesting lead compounds are now emerging from pre-clinical studies into clinical trials. These include:

1. The Cephalon compound CEP1347, a K252a analogue that appears to stimulate the neurotrophin signaling pathway downstream of Trk receptors, which was reported to rescue sensory neurons from axotomy-induced cell death (Bhat et al. 1995).
2. The Sanofi compound SR 57746 A, whose mechanism of action is unknown, but which was claimed to promote regeneration of small sensory axons following sciatic nerve crush and alleviate chemical neuropathy in rats (Fournier et al. 1993). Interestingly, this compound was recently reported to be in phase-II trials in MND (Scrip 1996b).
3. Certain immunosuppressive agents, such as the Fujisawa compound FK506, and Guilford Pharmaceutical's immunophillin GPI-1046 are able to en-

hance functional and morphological recovery from sciatic nerve crush in animal assays (STEINER et al. 1997a,b).

Further consideration of the development of small-molecule neurotrophic agents will be found in Chap. 11.

Acknowledgements. The authors wish to thank Dr M Rigby and D Smith for providing the data shown in Figs. 1 and 2.

References

Aebischer P, Salessiotis AN, Winn SR (1989) Basic fibroblast growth factor released from synthetic guidance channels facilitates peripheral nerve regeneration across long nerve gaps. J Neurosci Res 23:282–289

ALS CNTF Treatment Study Group (1995) A phase I study of recombinant human ciliary neurotrophic factor (rHCNTF) in patients with amyotrophic lateral sclerosis. Clin Neuropharmacol 18:515–532

ALS CNTF Treatment Study Group (1996) A double-blind placebo-controlled clinical trial of subcutaneous recombinant human ciliary neurotrophic factor (rhCNTF) in amyotrophic lateral sclerosis. Neurology 46:1244–1249

Apfel SC, Lipson L, Arezzo JC, Kessler JA (1991) Nerve growth factor prevents toxic neuropathy in mice. Ann Neurol 29:87–89

Apfel SC, Arezzo JC, Lipson L, Kessler JA (1992) Nerve growth factor prevents experimental cisplatin neuropathy. Ann Neurol 31:76–80

Apfel SC, Arezzo JC, Brownlee M, Federoff H, Kessler JA (1994) Nerve growth factor administration protects against experimental diabetic sensory neuropathy. Brain Res 634:7–12

Arnér S, Meyerson B (1988) Lack of analgesic effect of opioids on neuropathic and idiopathic forms of pain. Pain 33:11–23

Bennett GJ (1993) Neuropathic pain. In: Wall PD, Melzack R (eds) Textbook of pain. Churchill Livingstone, London, p 38

Bensinon G, Lacomblez L, Meininger V, ALS/Riluzole Study Group (1994) A controlled trial of riluzole in amyotrophic lateral sclerosis. N Engl J Med 330:585–591

Bhat RV, Miller M, Murakata C, Contreras PC (1995) CEP-1347 rescues DRG neurons from axotomy-induced cell death. Soc Neurosci Abstr 21:308

Bisby MA, Chen S (1990) Delayed Wallerian degeneration in sciatic nerves of C57BL/Ola mice is associated with impaired regeneration of sensory axons. Brain Res 530:117–120

Boyce S, Webb JK, Carlson E, Rupniak NMJ, Hill RG, Martin J (1998) Quantitative analysis of the onset and progression of motor deficits and effects of the glycine/NMDA receptor antagonist L-701,324 and the MAO inhibitor deprenyl in the motor neurone degeneration (Mnd) mutant mouse. Exp Neurol (in press)

Brewster WJ, Fernyhough P, Diemel LT, Tomlinson DR (1994) Diabetic neuropathy, nerve growth factor and other neurotrophic factors. Trends Neurosci 17:321–325

Callahan LM, Wylen EL, Messer A, Mazurkiewicz JE (1991) Neurofilament distribution is altered in the mnd (motor neurone degeneration) mouse. J Neuropathol Exp Neurol 50:491–504

Cervero F, Meyer RA, Campbell JN (1994) A psychophysical study of secondary hyperalgesia: evidence for increased pain to input from nociceptors. Pain 58:21–28

Chabal C, Jacobson L, Russell LC, Burchiel KJ (1992) Pain response to perineuromal injection of normal saline, epinephrine and lidocaine in humans. Pain 49:9–12

Chen L, Seaber AV, Glisson RR, Davies H, Murrell GAC, Anthony DC, Urbaniak JR (1992) The functional recovery of peripheral nerves following defined acute crush injuries. J Orthop Res 10:657–664

Clatterbuck RE, Price DL, Koliatsos VE (1994) Further characterisation of the effects of brain-derived neurotrophic factor and ciliary neurotrophic factor on axotomized neonatal and adult mammalian motor neurons. J Comp Neurol 342:45–56

Contreras PC, Sterrfler C, Vaught JL (1993) rhIGF-I enhances functional recovery from sciatic crush. Time-course and dose-response study. Ann NY Acad Sci USA 27:314–316

Corteix C, Eschalier A, Lavarenne A (1993) Streptozotocin-induced diabetic rats: behavioural evidence for a model of chronic pain. Pain 53:81–88

Cuevas P, Prieto R, de Tejada IS, Gimenez-Gallego G (1996) Analgesic effects of fibroblast growth factor in the rat. Neurosci Letts 207:175–178

de Medinaceli L, Freed WJ, Wyatt RJ (1982) An index of the functional condition of rat sciatic nerve based on measurements made from walking tracks. Exp Neurol 77:634–643

Devor M (1994) Pathophysiology of damaged nerve. In: Wall PD, Melzack R (eds) Textbook of Pain. Churchill Livingstone, London, p 89

Di Stefano PS, Friedman B, Radziejewski C, Alexander C, Boland P, Schick CM, Lindsay RM, Wiegand SJ (1992) The neurotrophins BDNF, NT-3, and NGF display distinct patterns of retrograde axonal transport in peripheral and central neurons. Neuron 8:983–993

Diemel LT, Brewster WJ, Fernyhough P, Tomlinson DR (1994) Expression of neuropeptides in experimental diabetes: effects of treatment with nerve growth factor or brain-derived neurotrophic factor. Mol Brain Res 21:171–175

Donnerer J, Amann R, Schuligoi R, Skofitsch G (1996) Complete recovery by nerve growth factor of neuropeptide content and function in capsaicin-impaired sensory neurones. Brain Res 741:103–108

Duchen LW, Strich SJ (1968) An hereditary motor neurone disease with progressive denervation of muscle in the mouse: the mutant ‘wobbler’. J Neurol Neurosurg Psychiat 31:535–542

Dyck PJ, Peroutka S, Rask C, Burton E, Baker MK, Lehman KA, Gillen DA, Hokanson JL, O’Brien PC (1997) Intradermal recombinant human nerve growth factor induces pressure allodynia and lowered heat-pain threshold in humans. Neurology 48:501–505

Engelhardt JI, Appel SH (1990) IgG reactivity in the spinal cord and motor cortex in amyotrophic lateral sclerosis. Arch Neurol 47:1210–1216

Eriksson NP, Lindsay RM, Aldskogius H (1994) BDNF and NT-3 rescue sensory but not motor neurones following axotomy in the neonate. Neuroreport 5:1445–1448

Fournier J, Steinberg R, Gauthier T, Keane PE, Guzzi U, Coude FX, Bougault I, Maffrand JP, Soubrie P, Le Fur G (1993) Protective effects of SR 57746 A in central and peripheral models of neurodegenerative disorders in rodents and primates. Neuroscience 55:629–641

Fugleholm K, Schmalbruch H, Krarup C (1994) Early peripheral nerve regeneration after crushing, sectioning and freeze studied by implanted electrodes in the cat. J Neurosci 14:2659–2673

Gao W-Q, Dybdal N, Shinsky N, Murnane A, Schmelzer C, Siegel M, Keller G, Hefti F, Phillips HS, Winslow JW (1995) Neurotrophin-3 reverses experimental cisplatin-induced peripheral sensory neuropathy. Ann Neurol 38:30–37

Garruto RM, Shankar SK, Yanagihara R (1989) Low-calcium, high-aluminium diet-induced motor neuron pathology in cynomolgus monkeys. Acta Neuropathol 78:210–219

Hantai D, Akaaboune M, Lagord C, Murawsky M, Houenou LJ, Festoff BW, Vaught JL, Rieger F, Blondet B (1995) Beneficial effects of insulin-like growth factor-I on wobbler mouse motoneuron disease. J Neurol Sci 129:122–126

Helgren ME, Friedman B, Kennedy M, Lindsay RM (1992) Ciliary neurotrophic factor (CNTF) delays motor impairments in the Mnd mouse. A genetic model for motor neuron disease. Soc Neurosci Abstr 18:618

Hill RG (1994) Pharmacological considerations in the use of opioids in the management of pain associated with non-terminal disease states. Pain Rev 1:47–64

Hugon J, Tabaraud F, Rigaud M, Vallat JM, Dumas M (1989) Glutamate dehydrogenase and aspartate aminotransferase in leukocytes of patients with motor neuron disease. Neurology 39:956–958

Ikeda K, Iwasaki Y, Tagaya N, Shiojima T, Kobayashi T, Kinoshita M (1995a) Neuroprotective effect of basic fibroblast growth factor on wobbler mouse motor neuron disease. Neurol Res 17:445–448

Ikeda K, Klinkosz B, Greene T, Cedarbaum JM, Wong V, Lindsay RM, Mutsomo H (1995b) Effects of brain-derived neurotrophic factor in wobbler mouse motor neuron disease. Ann Neurol 37:505–511

Ishii DN, Lupien SB (1995) Insulin-like growth factors protect against diabetic neuropathy. Effects on sensory nerve regeneration in rats. J Neurosci Res 40:138–144

Kanje M, Skottner A, Sjoberg J, Lundborg G (1989) Insulin-like growth factor-I (IGF-I) stimulates regeneration of the rat sciatic nerve. Brain Res 486:396–398

Lacomblez L, Bensimon G, Leigh PN, Guillet P, Powe L, Durrelman S, Delumeau JC, Meiniinger V, ALS/Riluzole Study Group (1996) A confirmatory dose-ranging study of riluzole in ALS. Neurology 47:S242–S250

Laird JMA, Bennett GJ.(1993) An electrophysiological study of dorsal horn neurons in the spinal cord of rats with an experimental peripheral neuropathy. J Neurophysiol 69:2072–2085

Laird JMA, Mason GS, Thomas KA, Hargreaves RJ Hill RG (1995) Acidic fibroblast growth factor (aFGF) stimulates rat sciatic nerve regeneration after a crush injury. Neuroscience 65:209–216

Lewin GR, Mendell LM (1993) Nerve growth factor and nociception. Trends Neurosci 16:353–359

Longo FM, Powell HC, Le Beau JM, Gerrero MR, Heckman HM, Myers RR (1986) Delayed nerve regeneration in streptozotocin diabetic rats. Muscle Nerve 9:385–393

Madison R, Da Silva CF, Dikkes P (1985) Entubulation repair with protein additives increases the maximum nerve gap distance successfully bridged with tubular prostheses. Brain Res 447:325–334

Max MB, Kishore-Kumar R, Schafer SC, Meister B, Gracely RH, Smoller B, Dubner R (1991) Efficacy of desipramine in a painful diabetic neuropathy: a placebo-controlled trial. Pain 45:3–9

McLachlan EM, Janig W, Devor M, Michaelis M (1993) Peripheral nerve injury triggers noradrenergic sprouting within dorsal root ganglia. Nature 363:543–546

McMahon SB, Priestley JV (1995) Peripheral neuropathies and neurotrophic factors: animal models and clinical perspectives. Curr Opin Neurobiol 5:616–624

McQuay HJ, Tramer M, Nye BA, Carroll D, Wiffen PJ, Moore RA (1996) Systematic review of antidepressants in neuropathic pain. Pain 68:217–227

Meininger V, Duarte F, Binet S (1990) Serum monoclonal immunoglobulin in amyotrophic lateral sclerosis: a quantitative analysis using a new Western blot technique. Neurology 40:183

Mitsumoto H, Ikeda K, Holmlund T, Greene T, Cedarbaum JM, Wong V, Lindsay RM (1994a) The effects of ciliary neurotrophic factor on motor dysfunction in wobbler mouse motor neuron disease. Ann Neurol 36:142–148

Mitsumoto H, Ikeda K, Klinkosz B, Cedarbaum JM, Wong V, Lindsay RM (1994b) Arrest of motor neuron disease in wobbler mice cotreated with CNTF and BDNF. Science 265:1107–1110

Miyata Y, Kashihara Y, Homma S, Kuno M (1986) Effects of nerve growth factor on the survival and synaptic function of 1a sensory neurons axotomized in neonatal rats. J Neurosci 6:2012–2018

Mulder DW, Howard FM (1976) Patient resistance and prognosis in amyotrophic lateral sclerosis. Mayo Clin Proc 51:537–541

Near SL, Whalen LR, Miller JA, Ishii DN (1992) Insulin-like growth factor-II stimulates motor nerve regeneration. Proc Natl Acad Sci USA 89:11716–11720

Nystrom B, Hagbarth K-E (1981) Microelectrode recordings from transected nerves in amputees with phantom limb pain. Neurosci Letts 27:211–216

Oppenheim RW, Houenou LJ, Johnson JE, Lin LF, Li L, Lo AC, Newsome AL, Prevette DM, Wang S (1995) Developing motor neurons rescued from programmed and axotomy-induced cell death by GDNF. Nature 373:344–346

Plaitakis A (1990) Glutamate dysfunction and selective motor neuron degeneration in amyotrophic lateral sclerosis: a hypothesis. Ann Neurol 28:3–8

Portenoy RK, Foley KM, Inturrisi CE (1990) The nature of opioid responsiveness and its implications for neuropathic pain: new hypotheses derived from studies of opioid infusions. Pain 43:273–286

Raja SN, Treede R-D, Davis KD, Campbell JN (1991) Systemic alpha-adrenergic blockade with phentolamine: a diagnostic test for sympathetically maintained pain. Anesthesiology 74:691–698

Rothstein JD, Bristol LA, Hosler B, Brown RH, Kuncl RW (1994) Chronic inhibition of superoxide dismutase produces apototic death of spinal neurones. Proc Natl Acad Sci USA 91:4155–4158

Sagot Y, Tan SA, Baetge E, Schmalbruch H, Kato AC, Aebischer P (1995) Polymer encapsulated cell lines genetically engineered to release ciliary neurotrophic factor can slow down progressive motor neuronopathy in the mouse. Eur J Neurosci 7:1313–1322

Sagot Y, Tan SA, Hammang JP, Aebischer P, Kato AC (1996) GDNF slows loss of motoneurons but not axonal degeneration or premature death of pmn/pmn mice. J Neurosci 16:2335–2341

Sato J, Perl ER (1991) Adrenergic excitation of cutaneous pain receptors induced by peripheral nerve injury. Science 251:1608–1610

Scrip (1995a) Myotrophin slows amyotrophic lateral sclerosis (ALS) progression. Scrip 2035:21

Scrip (1995b) More modafinil rights for Cephalon. Scrip 2066:12

Scrip (1995c) Regeneron Pharmaceuticals broadens research focus. Scrip 2039:8

Scrip (1996a) U.S. biotechnology company third-quarter results. Scrip 2179:9

Scrip (1996b) Decisive year for Sanofi's research and development (R&D). Scrip 2158:11

Scrip (1997) Regeneron's s.c. brain-derived neurotrophic factor (BDNF) fails in amyotrophic lateral sclerosis (ALS). Scrip 2198:21

Sendtner M, Kreutzberg GW, Thoenen H (1990) Ciliary neurotrophic factor prevents the degeneration of motor neurons after axotomy. Nature 345:440–441

Sendtner M, Holtmann B, Kolbeck R, Thoenen H, Barde Y-A (1992a) Brain-derived neurotrophic factor prevents the death of motoneurons in newborn rats after nerve section. Nature 360:757–759

Sendtner M, Schmalbruch H, Stockli KA, Carrol P, Kreutzbery GW, Thoenen H (1992b) Ciliary neurotrophic factor prevents degeneration of motoneurons in mouse mutant progressive motoneuronopathy. Nature 358:502–504

Spencer PS, Ludolph AC, Divivedi MP (1986) Lathyrism: evidence for a role of the neuroexcitatory amino acid BOAA. Lancet ii:1066–1067

Steiner JP, Connolly MA, Valentine HL, Hamilton GS, Dawson T, Hester L, Snyder SH (1997a) Neurotrophic actions of nonimmunosuppressive analogues of immunosuppressive drugs FK506, rapamycin and cyclosporin A. Nat Med 3:421–428

Steiner JP, Hamilton GS, Ross DT, Valentine HL, Guo H, Connolly MA, Liang S, Ramsey C, Li J, Huang W, Howorth P, Soni R, Fuller M, Sauer H, Nowotnik AC, Suzdak PD (1997) Neurotrophic immunophillin ligands stimulate structural and functional recovery in neurodegenerative animal models. Proc Natl Acad Sci USA 94:2019–2024

Strong MJ, Garruto RM, Wolff AV (1990) N-Butylbenzene sulphonamide, a novel neurotoxic plasticising agent. Lancet 330:640

Tanelian DL, Brose WG (1991) Neuropathic pain can be relieved by drugs that are use-dependent sodium channel blockers: lidocaine, carbamazepine and mexiletine. Anesthesiology 74:949–951

Torebjork HE, Lundberg LER, La Motte RH (1992) Central changes in processing of mechanoreceptive input in capsaicin-induced secondary hyperalgesia in humans. J Physiol 448:765–780

Troy CM, Shelanski ML (1994) Down-regulation of copper/zinc superoxide dismutase causes apoptotic death in PC12 neuronal cells. Proc Natl Acad Sci USA 91:6384–6387

Vejsada R, Sagot Y, Kato AC (1994) BDNF-mediated rescue of axotomized motor neurones decreases with increasing dose. Neuroreport 5:1889–1892

Vergara J, Medina L, Maulen J, Inestrosa NC, Alvarez J (1993) Nerve regeneration is improved by insulin-like growth factor I (IGF-I) and basic fibroblast growth factor (bFGF). Restor Neurol Neurosci 5:181–189

Yan Q, Matheson C, Lopez OT (1995) In vivo neurotrophic effects of GDNF on neonatal and adult facial motor neurons. Nature 373:341–344

CHAPTER 7

Nerve Growth Factor Treatment for Alzheimer's Disease: The Experience of the First Attempt at Intracerebral Neurotrophic Factor Therapy

F. HEFTI

A. Introduction

The understanding of Alzheimer's disease (AD) pathology has made enormous progress during the past two decades (KOSIK 1992; SELKOE 1996; HARDY 1997). Its hallmarks are the formation of neuritic plaques, neurofibrillary tangles and neuron loss in the brain. The discovery of amyloid precursor protein (APP), the genetic analysis of familial forms of AD, and observations on transgenic animals have produced a widely accepted hypothesis which ascribes the central role in the generation of plaques to the APP fragment, Aβ. Since Aβ is neurotoxic, at least in vitro, the hypothesis includes the view that neuron loss is secondary to the initial nucleation of neuritic plaques caused by Aβ.

Neurotrophic factors have been considered from a therapeutic point of view as agents possibly able to counteract the neuron loss in AD. The approach was initially driven by the discovery that cholinergic neurons of the basal forebrain are particularly vulnerable in AD, and that these neurons respond to nerve growth factor (NGF), the protein that provided the conceptual basis for the field of neurotrophic factors. For several years, a large number of investigators provided detailed information on the nature of the trophic role of NGF in cholinergic neuron development and function. NGF was shown to be able to counteract cholinergic atrophy and cell death in a number of in vivo animal models replicating the cholinergic deficit of AD. Based on a wealth of evidence, NGF was proposed as a therapeutic agent for the disease, and initial steps towards clinical use were taken. Delivery of the protein to the target cells became an issue of particular significance because of its inability to cross the blood–brain barrier.

A small number of patients were treated with NGF infused into the lateral ventricles by a mechanical infusion device. Modest behavioral improvement was seen; however, detailed animal studies also showed hyperplasia of various nervous system cells around the spinal cord. These findings made it unlikely that intraventricular administration of NGF would represent a viable strategy for the treatment of AD, thus making this chapter the description of a probably aborted attempt to bring a conceptually new treatment to AD. However, the concept remains viable and many investigators pursue the possible use of growth factors other than NGF in AD, and attempts are underway to overcome the delivery problems by using special devices or by replacing them with small-molecule mimetics.

B. Nerve Growth Factor as a Therapeutic Agent to Counteract Cholinergic Neuron Degeneration

I. Cholinergic Neuron Atrophy in Alzheimer's Disease (AD)

AD is associated with region-specific loss of neuronal populations, particularly in areas connected to the hippocampus (Price 1986; Kosik 1992). Hippocampal inputs strongly affected include entorhinal cortex afferents, cholinergic afferents from the basal forebrain and noradrenergic afferents originating in the locus coeruleus. The cholinergic deficit has received particular attention, given the wealth of evidence linking these systems to cognitive processes. Cholinergic neuron atrophy and cell loss were established by the demonstration of reductions in the activity of choline acetyltransferase, high-affinity choline uptake, the number of nicotinic receptors and a loss of cholinergic cell bodies in the septum and nucleus basalis (Bowen et al. 1976; Davies and Maloney 1976; Whitehouse et al. 1982; DeKosky et al. 1992; Kuhl et al. 1996; Cullen et al. 1997).

A prominent role of cholinergic systems in memory processes is supported by animal studies and clinical observations. In animals, lesions of the cholinergic neurons innervating the hippocampus and cortex result in pronounced deficits in memory and cognitive functions which are reversed by drugs enhancing cholinergic function (e.g., Tilson et al. 1988; Miyamoto et al. 1989; Voytko et al. 1994; Leanza et al. 1995; Steckler et al. 1995; Wenk et al. 1994). Postmortem analysis of AD brains revealed that the extent of the cholinergic deficit correlates with the degree of memory impairment (DeKosky et al. 1992; Lehericy et al. 1993). The loss of cholinergic function was reported to be one of the earliest changes in the disease (Francis et al. 1985).

Enhancement of cholinergic function by acetyl-cholinesterase inhibitors in Alzheimer patients produce modest, but significant ameliorations (Eagger et al. 1991; Davis et al. 1992; Farlow et al. 1992). While the clinical experience provides clinical confirmation that enhancement of cholinergic function is beneficial for cognitive processing, it also points to the limits of this approach. None of the cholinesterase inhibitors tested was able to fully reverse the massive behavioral deficits of AD. It remains possible that direct cholinergic receptor agonists would be more efficacious than acetyl-cholinesterase inhibitors and that NGF treatment, by gradually stimulating regeneration and sprouting of cholinergic terminals, might produce yet more significant improvements. However, the limited efficacy of the cholinergic approach is not surprising in light of the fact that many other neuronal systems are affected in AD besides the cholinergic ones.

II. Role of NGF in Cholinergic Neuron Development and Adult Function

Contributions by many research groups during the 1980s established that NGF is a potent neurotrophic factor for forebrain cholinergic neurons during development. These studies, which have been reviewed extensively (e.g., THOENEN et al. 1987; HEFTI et al. 1989), revealed that NGF is necessary for survival, neurite extension and target innervation of the septo-hippocampal and basalo-cortical cholinergic neurons. The neurons express both the selective tyrosine kinase TrkA NGF receptor and the less selective p75 NGF receptor, whereas NGF is synthesized predominantly in the hippocampus and cortex, thus supporting the view that NGF acts as a target-derived survival and differentiation factor for these neurons. Conclusions reached from the earlier observations on cell cultures and animals injected with anti-NGF antibodies received elegant confirmation from the more-recent observations on animals with deletions of either the NGF or the TrkA receptor genes.

In NGF or TrkA knockout mice, the number of basal forebrain cholinergic cell bodies gradually decreases during development, and the innervation of the target tissue does not take place (PHILLIPS et al. 1990; SMEYNEY et al. 1994). Mice with deletion of a single NGF gene exhibit atrophy of basal forebrain cholinergic neurons as well as specific memory deficits in the Morris water-maze task (CHEN et al. 1997). The role of the p75 receptor, which can mediate apoptosis when not co-localized with TrkA (BREDESEN and RABIZADEH 1997), in cholinergic neuron function is less clear. However, reports have appeared that the number of cholinergic cell bodies is slightly reduced in mice with deletion of the corresponding gene (VANDERZEE et al. 1996).

In the adult brain, basal forebrain cholinergic neurons rather selectively express TrkA NGF and p75 NGF receptors (KORDOWER et al. 1988; HEFTI and MASH 1989; VAZQUEZ and EBENDAL 1991; HOLTZMAN et al. 1992; HECKERS et al. 1994; VENERO et al. 1995; SALEHI et al. 1996). Earlier findings that separation of the cholinergic neurons from their targets resulted in shrinkage and cell loss supported the view that NGF supports the cholinergic cell bodies as a retrogradely acting maintenance factor. More recent findings suggest a more dynamic role of neurotrophins, including NGF, as modifiers of synaptic function at much more narrow time spans and, thus, as regulating synaptic plasticity. For NGF, the work of Maffei and collaborators (CELLERINO and MAFFEI 1996) appears particularly interesting. These authors have generated a large body of evidence to support the view that NGF regulates plasticity of the visual cortex.

III. Pharmacological Effects of NGF in Animals with Experimental Cholinergic Deficits

Intracerebroventricular administration of NGF prevents cholinergic neuron atrophy caused by experimental injury or associated with normal aging in rodents and monkeys (HEFTI et al. 1984; HEFTI 1986; KOLIATSOS et al. 1991;

Haroutunian et al. 1989; Dekker et al. 1992; Garofalo et al. 1992; Tuszynski et al. 1991). The NGF treatment also corrects the behavioral deficits that accompany cholinergic neuron atrophy (Will and Hefti 1985; Fischer et al. 1987, 1991). Data of these publications and other earlier reports were summarized by Hefti and Lapchak (1993). More recently, the findings were extended and confirmed using alternative administration methodologies for NGF and more precisely defined behavioral tasks (e.g. Kordower et al. 1994; Markowska et al. 1994, 1996; Martinez-Serrano et al. 1996).

The unequivocal demonstration that NGF prevents cholinergic neuron atrophy in the adult brain was taken to suggest that NGF administration to the brain may counteract cholinergic neuron atrophy in Alzheimer's disease. The animal studies indicate that NGF administration should counteract cholinergic atrophy, irrespective of the actual cause. Thus, administration of NGF to Alzheimer patients was proposed as a pharmacological attempt to induce hypertrophy of cholinergic neurons surviving in the Alzheimer brain. NGF-induced hypertrophy in animal models manifests itself in increases in the expression of structural and transmitter-specific proteins, in a reversal of age-related degenerative changes and increased resistance to experimental insults, and in increased ability to influence postsynaptic cells. As a consequence, NGF administration to Alzheimer patients was anticipated to attenuate the rate of degeneration of cholinergic neurons and improve the functional performance of the survivors, resulting in attenuation or, perhaps, even improvement of those symptomatic behavioral changes that are a consequence of the cholinergic deficit (Hefti and Schneider 1989).

While NGF therapy of AD was not conceived as replacement therapy, considerable work went into understanding the status of NGF and neurotrophin mechanisms in AD; NGF and NGF mRNA levels remain constant or are elevated (Goedert et al. 1989; Phillips et al. 1991; Scott et al. 1995; Narisawa et al. 1996). The p75 NGF receptors remain expressed by the basal forebrain cholinergic neurons in the AD brain; however, there are conflicting reports about changes in the levels (Hefti and Mash 1989; Higgins and Mufson 1989; Loy et al. 1990; Treanor et al. 1991). The expression of TrkA NGF receptors seems to be reduced in the AD brain (Mufson et al. 1997), and evidence for reduced retrograde transport of NGF in the basalocortical cholinergic system has been reported (Mufson et al. 1995). Knowledge of the other members of the neurotrophin family is scarce, except for repeated reports of a decline in BDNF mRNA levels (Phillips et al. 1991; Murray et al. 1994; Narisawa et al. 1996), indicating that BDNF and NGF mechanisms respond in distinct ways to the events of AD pathophysiology.

IV. Human Studies with NGF: Efficacy and Possible Adverse Effects

The pre-clinical findings prompted the initiation of single patient studies. A subcutaneous infusion pump was implanted in each of the patients; via this pump, NGF was chronically infused to one of the lateral ventricles of the brain (OLSON et al. 1992; SEIGER et al. 1993). One of the patients was infused with 6.6 mg of purified mouse salivary-gland NGF over 3 months. The infusion was associated with an increase in the uptake and binding of [^{11}C]nicotine in cortical areas and an increase in cortical blood flow. Verbal episodic memory was slightly improved, whereas other cognitive measures remained unaffected (SEIGER et al. 1993).

The small improvements seen in the clinical studies were in line with the predictions from pre-clinical studies. They confirmed the view that the selectivity of NGF's action for cholinergic neurons will represent the major limitation of this therapeutic approach. Behavioral improvements produced were marginal and of similar magnitude as those obtained with inhibitors of acetyl cholinesterase. It cannot be excluded that more-extensive studies with a larger number of patients, or with patients at an earlier stage of the disease, could have produced a more significant outcome.

A second major limitation of intracerebroventricular NGF therapy of AD is given by the possible adverse effects. Besides the risk of surgery associated with implantation of the pump and the penetration of the brain tissue, other possible detrimental effects of intraventricular NGF treatment need to be considered. They include induction of aberrant cholinergic sprouting, as observed in lesioned rodents (WILLIAMS et al. 1986). Evidence that NGF may stimulate the formation or release of amyloid precursor protein mRNA gives reason for concern (MOBLEY et al. 1988; CLARRIS et al 1994; LAHIRI and NALL 1995). However, this induction was found to be limited to a mRNA species more abundant in juvenile brains and the available evidence is conflicting (OHYAGI and TABIRA 1993; FORLONI et al 1993). NGF treatment could induce the proliferation of NGF-responsive non-neuronal cells (e.g., NAKAGAWARA et al. 1993; YAAR et al. 1994; PINCELLI et al. 1994; LEVI-MONTALCINI et al. 1996). NGF infusions may act on intracerebral sympathetic neurons to produce changes in local blood flow (ISAACSON et al. 1990) or on TrkA expressing sensory afferents to the CNS, thus, changing sensory perception. Migration of Schwann cells could be stimulated by NGF treatment (ANTON et al. 1994). Finally, hypophagia was consistently observed in animals given intraventricular NGF and may occur as an adverse effect of intraventricular NGF treatment (WILLIAMS 1991).

A detailed rat study on the long-term effects of intraventricular NGF administration focused the concerns regarding adverse effects on two specific issues. WINKLER et al. (1997) found that NGF infusion over a 7-week period resulted in Schwann cell hyperplasia and sensory neuron and sympathetic neurite sprouting in the subpial region of the medulla oblongata and the spinal cord. These hyperplasic responses were reversible and disappeared after termination of the NGF treatment. While being reversible and perhaps even functionally irrelevant, the hyperplasic responses of sympathetic and sensory systems have to be considered significant undesired effects. They suggest that pharmacokinetic issues, besides the selectivity for cholinergic neurons in the brain, represent the second key limitation of the putative NGF therapy for AD.

Intracerebroventricular administration of NGF is based on the assumption that NGF infused by this route will penetrate the brain parenchyma and reach the cholinergic cell bodies or terminals at sufficient quantities to produce a trophic response. However, very few studies have addressed this problem. It was shown in rats that NGF penetration of brain parenchyma from the ventricular fluid is very limited, although sufficient to reach cholinergic neurons (Lapchak et al. 1993; Krewson et al. 1995). However, intraparenchymal injections of NGF were far more efficacious than intraventricular infusions (Venero et al. 1996). In addition, the rat may be a poor predictor of what occurs in the human brain, which has much larger diffusion distances from the ventricles to the cell body or terminal areas. The effects of NGF transported with the cerebrospinal fluid (CSF) flow have not been properly considered. The study by Winkler et al. (1997) strongly suggests that a significant portion of the infused NGF is transported to the fourth ventricle and the central canal of the spinal cord, diffusion from which will influence NGF-responsive sympathetic and sensory neurons.

V. Alternative Administration Strategies and Small-Molecule Mimetics

The problems associated with long-term intracerebroventricular administration of NGF are likely to prevent further clinical development of this protein for AD. The pharmacokinetic problems identified for NGF may provide a general limitation to the approach of using intracerebroventricular infusion of neurotrophic factors. These limitations could be overcome by methods that deliver growth factors locally, or by the use of small-molecule mimetics. Local administration by slow-releasing implants containing the neurotrophic factor in a biodegradable polymer matrix, by implanted engineered cells releasing the proteins or by synthesis from transgenes represent feasible avenues. Small organic molecules mimicking the action of a neurotrophic factor and able to penetrate freely into the brain parenchyma could be suitable for oral administration. These approaches are discussed in detail in other chapters of this volume.

C. Neurotrophic Factors for Non-Cholinergic Neurons Affected by the Disease

One of the limitations of the NGF approach could be overcome by the use of neurotrophic factors with a broader selectivity, able to affect neurons other than the cholinergic cells. BDNF and its trkB receptor are widely expressed in the brain. Neurotrophin-3 (NT-3) expression is largely confined to the hippocampus; however, its trkC receptor is as widely expressed as trkB. In contrast to the situation in the peripheral nervous system, where the presence of neurotrophins is essential for survival of sensory and sympathetic neurons, cortical and hippocampal neurons do not seem to require neurotrophins for survival during early development.

In culture, BDNF and NT-3 only marginally promote survival of developing neurons and there is no evidence of a reduction of cortical or hippocampal neurons in mice with null mutations of BDNF, NT-3, trkB or trkC genes (SNIDER 1994). However, it has been known for several years that addition of neurotrophins to cortical and hippocampal cultures stimulates their morphological and transmitter-specific molecular differentiation (COLLAZO et al. 1992; IP et al. 1993; WIDMER et al. 1993; BERNINGER et al. 1993; CROLL et al. 1994). These findings are compatible with a role of neurotrophins in development as regulators of synaptic growth and plasticity (COHEN-CORY and FRASER 1995; THOENEN 1995). In support of these concepts, hippocampal long-term potentiation has been found to change the expression of BDNF and NT-3, and long-term potentiation is impaired in BDNF knock-out mutant mice (CASTREN et al. 1993; KORTE et al. 1995). In aged animals, NGF, NT-3, and NT-4/5 were found to have beneficial effects on the behavioral impairment, whereas BDNF was ineffective (FISCHER et al. 1994). Additional studies will hopefully clarify the role of BDNF and other neurotrophins as protective agents for cortical and hippocampal neurons.

In addition to the neurotrophins, many families of growth factors fulfill a functional definition of neurotrophic factor in that they stimulate survival or differentiation of neurons in culture or in vivo. These protein families include fibroblast growth factors (FGF); epidermal growth factor-related proteins; the super family of transforming growth factor-β (TGFβ), which includes glial cell line-derived neurotrophic factor (GDNF); and insulin-like growth factors. Information on their role in cortical and hippocampal neuron function is sparse.

Basic FGF (bFGF) and its receptors are widely expressed in the brain and the factor stimulates survival and differentiation of many populations of neurons outside of the cortex (Baird 1994). Similar to NGF, bFGF prevents the loss of septal cholinergic neurons following fimbria-fornix transections. bFGF protects thalamic neurons from degeneration following ablation of the somatosensory cortex in rats (KOHMURA et al. 1994) and, of particular importance in the context of AD, intraventricular infusions of bFGF attenuated the loss of neurons in the entorhinal cortex following transection of the perforant path in adult rats (CUMMINGS et al. 1992). These findings indicate that rescue of cortical neurons can be achieved with appropriate trophic factors.

D. Relationship to Alzheimer's Disease Pathology

One of the problems of the neurotrophic factor approach to AD therapy is the absence of a clear link to the formation of plaques and tangles which provide the neuropathological definition of the disease. Indeed, neurotrophic factors are often seen as contributing to the pathology rather than being protective. Ramón and Cajal (1928) have already suggested that plaques contain a trophic substance that stimulates aberrant neurite extension into the plaques. In support of this concept, bFGF was found to be accumulated within plaques (Cummings et al. 1993). It seems possible that the protein agglomerates forming plaques may act as a sink for many soluble proteins, including neurotrophic factors, which then redirect dendrite and axon growth.

An alternative possibility is that neurotrophic factors participate in the regulation of proteins involved in the production of components of plaques and tangles. Initial evidence in support of such concepts, from studies in which the effects of NGF on APP processing was analyzed, was mentioned above as part of the discussion of possible adverse effects of NGF therapy.

The recent discovery of mutations in the presenilin family as causative factors in familial AD have opened new vistas towards the exploration of a connection between neurotrophic factors and classical pathological hallmarks. Mutations in these proteins cause the formation of plaques by inducing differential processing of APP and increased formation of the $A\beta_{1-42}$ peptide, which is believed to initiate the cascade to plaque formation. However, presenilins have also been linked to apoptotic mechanisms. A fragment of presenilin-2 was found to rescue T-cell hybridomas from *fas*-induced apoptosis (Vito et al. 1996). While the general nature of this finding has not been established, it offers a starting point for interesting speculations. There is a clear link between apoptosis and growth factors, in that growth factor deprivation leads to apoptotic death (Yamatsuji et al. 1996; Bredesen 1995). The new findings thus suggest the possibility that changes in STM2 or related proteins may change the degree of vulnerability of cells to lack of neurotrophic factor support.

E. Conclusions

The therapeutic use of NGF for AD was proposed based on a wealth of evidence for a robust trophic effect of NGF on basal forebrain cholinergic neurons and for the degeneration of these neurons in the AD brain. Limited clinical studies revealed modest beneficial effects, in line with the view that the cholinergic deficit represents one among many neuronal deficits in AD. In addition, animal studies revealed that long-term infusion of NGF in the cerebral ventricles induces hyperplasia of sympathetic and sensory neurons around the spinal cord, in line with the view that a large portion of NGF, given intracerebroventricularly, is transported with the CSF flow and is possibly able to exert adverse effects in the brain stem and spinal cord. The early experiences with NGF, thus, emphasize the need for neurotrophic factors that act on additional neuronal populations rather than on the cholinergic neurons, and for alternative administration strategies such as local delivery or small-molecule mimetics.

References

Anton ES, Weskamp G, Reichardt LF, Matthew WD (1994) Nerve growth factor and its low-affinity receptor promote Schwann cell migration. Proc Natl Acad Sci USA 91:2795–2799

Berninger B, Garcia DE, Inagaki N, Hahnel C, Lindholm D (1993) BDNF and NT-3 induce intracellular Ca^{2+} elevation in hippocampal neurones. Neuroreport 4:1303–1306

Bowen DM, Smith CB, White P et al. (1976) Neurotransmitter-related enzymes and indices of hypoxia in senile dementia and other abiotrophies. Brain 99:459–496

Bredesen DE (1995) Neural Apoptosis. Ann Neurol 38:839–851

Bredesen DE, Rabizadeh S (1997) $p75^{NTR}$ and apoptosis: Trk-dependent and Trk-independent effects. TINS 20:287–290

Castren E, Pitkanen M, Sirvio J, Parsdanian A, Lindholm D, Thoenen H, Riekkinen PJ (1993) The induction of LTP increases BDNF and NGF mRNA but decreases NT-3 mRNA in the dentate gyrus. Neuroreport 47:895–898

Cellerino A, Maffei L (1996) The action of neurotrophins in the development and plasticity of the visual cortex. Prog Neurobiol 49:53–71

Chen KS, Nishimura MC, Armanini MP, Crowley C, Spencer SD, Phillips HS (1997) Disruption of a single allele of the nerve growth factor gene results in atrophy of basal forebrain cholinergic neurons and memory deficits. J Neuroscience 17:7288–7296

Clarris HJ, Nurcombe V, Small DH, Beyreuther K, Masters CL (1994) Secretion of nerve growth factor from septum stimulates neurite outgrowth and release of the amyloid protein precursor of Alzheimer's disease from hippocampal explants. J Neurosci Res 38:248–258

Cohen-Cory S, Fraser SE (1995) Effects of brain-derived neurotrophic factor on optic axon branching and remodelling in vivo. Letters to Nature 378:192–196

Collazo D, Takahashi H, McKay RD (1992) Cellular targets and trophic functions of neurotrophin-3 in the developing rat hippocampus. Neuron 9:643–656

Croll SD, Wiegand SJ, Anderson KD, Lindsay RM, Nawa H (1994) Regulation of neuropeptides in adult rat forebrain by the neurotrophins BDNF and NGF. Eur J Neurosci 6:1343–1353

Cullen KM, Halliday GM, Double KL, Brooks WS, Creasey H, Broe G A (1997) Cell loss in the nucleus basalis is related to regional cortical atrophy in Alzheimer's Disease. Neuroscience 78:641–652

Cummings BJ, Yee GJ, Cotman CW (1992) bFGF promotes the survival of entorhinal layer II neurons after perforant path axotomy. Brain Res 591:271–276

Cummings BJ, Su JH, Cotman CW (1993) Neuritic involvement within bFGF immunopositive plaques of Alzheimer's disease. Exp Neurol 124:315–325

Davies P, Maloney AJF (1976) Selective loss of central cholinergic neurons in Alzheimer's Disease. Lancet II:1043

Davis KL, Thal LJ, Gamzu ER, Davis CS, Woolson RF, Gracon SI et al. (1992) A double-blind, placebo-controlled multicenter study of tacrine for Alzheimer's disease. The Tacrine Collaborative Study Group. N Engl J Med 327:1253–1259

Dekker AJ, Gage FH, Thal LJ (1992) Delayed treatment with nerve growth factor improves acquisition of a spatial task in rats with lesions of the nucleus basalis magnocellularis: evaluation of the involvement of different neurotransmitter systems. Neuroscience 48:111–119

DeKosky ST, Harbaugh RE, Schmitt FA, Bakay RAE, Chang Chui H, Knopman DS et al. (1992) Cortical biopsy in Alzheimer's Disease: diagnostic accuracy and neurochemical, neuropathological and cognitive correlations. Ann Neurol 32: 625–632

Eagger SA, Levy R, Sahakian BJ (1991) Tacrine in Alzheimer's disease. Lancet 337:989–992

Farlow M, Gracon SI, Hershey LA, Lewis KW, Sadowsky CH, Dolan Ureno J (1992) A controlled trial of tacrine in Alzheimer's disease. The Tacrine Study Group. JAMA 268:2523–2529

Fischer W, Wictorin K, Björklund A, Williams LR, Varon S, Gage FH (1987) Amelioration of cholinergic neuron atrophy and spatial memory impairment in aged rats by nerve growth factor. Nature 329:65–68

Fischer W, Björklund A, Chen K, Gage FH (1991) NGF improves spatial memory in aged rodents as a function of age. J Neurosci 11:1889–1906

Fischer W, Sirevaag A, Wiegand SJ, Lindsay RM, Björklund A (1994) Reversal of spatial memory impairments in aged rats by nerve growth factor and neurotrophins 3 and 4/5 but not by brain-derived neurotrophic factor. Proc Natl Acad Sci USA 91:8607–8611

Forloni G, Del Bo R, Angeretti N, Smiroldo S, Gabellini N, Vantini G (1993) Nerve growth factor does not influence the expression of b amyloid precursor protein mRNA in rat brain: in vivo and in vitro studies. Brain Res 620:292–296

Francis PT, Palmer AM, Sims NR et al. (1985) Neurochemical studies of early-onset Alzheimer's disease: possible influence on treatment. Lancet 4:7–11

Garofalo L, Ribeiro da Silva A, Cuello AC (1992) Nerve growth factor-induced synaptogenesis and hypertrophy of cortical cholinergic terminals. Proc Natl Acad Sci USA. 89:2639–2643

Goedert M, Fine A, Dawbarn D, Wilcock GK, Chao MV (1989) Nerve growth factor receptor mRNA distribution in human brain: normal levels in basal forebrain in Alzheimer's disease. Brain Res Mol Brain Res 5:1–7

Haroutunian V, Kanof PD, Davis KL (1989) Attenuation of nucleus basalis of Meynert lesion-induced cholinergic deficits by nerve growth factor. Brain Res 487:200–203

Heckers S, Ohtake T, Wiley RG, Lappi DA, Geula C, Mesulam M-M (1994) Complete and selective cholinergic denervation of rat neocortex and hippocampus but not amygdala by an immunotoxin against the p75 NGF receptor. J Neurosci 14:1271–1289

Hefti F (1986) Nerve growth factor promotes survival of septal cholinergic neurons after axonal injury. J Neurosci 6:2155–2162

Hefti F, Mash DC (1989) Localization of nerve growth factor receptors in the normal human brain and in Alzheimer's disease. Neurobiol Aging 10:75–87

Hefti F, Schneider LS (1989) Rationale for the planned clinical trials with nerve growth factor in Alzheimer's disease. Psychiatr Dev 7:297–315

Hefti F, Lapchak PA (1993) Pharmacology of nerve growth factor in the brain. Adv in Pharmacol 24:239–273

Hefti F, Dravid A, Hartikka J (1984) Chronic intraventricular injections of nerve growth factor elevate hippocampal choline acetyltransferase activity in adult rats with partial septo-hippocampal lesions. Brain Res 293:305–311

Hefti F, Hartikka J, Knusel B (1989) Function of neurotrophic factors in the adult and aging brain and their possible use in the treatment of neurodegenerative diseases. Neurobiol Aging 10:515–533

Higgins GA, Mufson EJ (1989) NGF receptor gene expression is decreased in the nucleus basalis in Alzheimer's disease. Exp Neurol 106:222–236

Holtzman DM, Li Y, Parada LF, Kinsman S, Chen CK, Valletta JS, Zhou J, Long BJ, Mobley WC (1992) p140trk mRNA marks NGF-responsive forebrain neurons: evidence that trk gene expression is induced by NGF. Neuron 9:465–478

Ip NY, Li Y, Yancopoulos GD, Lindsay RM (1993) Cultured hippocampal neurons show responses to BDNF, NT-3 and NT-4, but not NGF. J Neurosci 13:3394–3405

Isaacson LG, Saffran BN, Crutcher KA (1990) Intracerebral NGF infusion induces hyperinnervation of cerebral blood vessels. Neurobiol Aging 11:51–55

Kohmura E, Yuguchi T, Yamada K, Sakaguchi K, Hayakawa T (1994) Recombinant basic fibroblast growth factor spares thalamic neurons from retrograde degeneration after ablation of the somatosensory cortex in rats. Restorative Neurol Neurosci 6:309–316

Koliatsos VE, Clatterbuck RE, Nauta HJ, Knusel B, Burton LE, Hefti FF et al. (1991) Human nerve growth factor prevents degeneration of basal forebrain cholinergic neurons in primates. Ann Neurol 30:831–840

Kordower JH, Bartus RT, Bothwell M et al. (1988) Nerve growth factor immunoreactivity in the non-human primate (Cebus apella): distribution, morphology, and colocalization with cholinergic enzymes. J Comp Neurol 277:465–486

Kordower JH, Winn SR, Liu Y-T, Mufson EJ, Sladek JR, Hammang JP, Baetge EE, Emerich DF (1994) The aged monkey basal forebrain: rescue and sprouting of axotomized basal forebrain neurons after grafts of encapsulated cells secreting human nerve growth factor. Proc Natl Acad Sci USA 91:10898–10902

Korte M, Carroll P, Wolf E, Brem G, Thoenen H, Bonhoeffer T (1995) Hippocampal long-term potentiation is impaired in mice lacking brain-derived neurotrophic factor. Proc Natl Acad Sci USA 92:8856–8860

Kosik KS (1992) Alzheimer's disease: a cell biological perspective. Science 256:780–783

Krewson CE, Klarman ML, Saltzman WM (1995) Distribution of nerve growth factor following direct delivery to brain interstitium. Brain Res 680:196–206

Kuhl DE, Minoshima S, Fessler JA, Frey KA, Foster NL, Ficaro EP, Wieland DM, Koeppe RA (1996) In vivo mapping of cholinergic terminals in normal aging, Alzheimer's Disease, and Parkinson's Disease. Ann Neurol 40:399–410

Lahiri DJ, Nall C (1995) Promoter activity of the gene encoding the beta-amyloid precursor protein is up-regulated by growth factors, phorbol ester, retinoic acid and interleukin-1. Molecular Brain Res 32:233–240

Lapchak P A, Hefti F (1991) Effect of recombinant human nerve growth factor on presynaptic cholinergic function in rat hippocampal slices following partial septohippocampal lesions: measures of ACh synthesis, ACh release and choline acetyltransferase activity. Neuroscience 42:639–649

Lapchak PA, Araujo DM, Carswell S, Hefti F (1993) Distribution of [^{125}I]nerve growth factor in the rat brain following an intraventricular injection: sequestration by trkA mRNA expressing septal neurons. Neuroscience 54:445–460

Leanza G, Nilsson OG, Wiley RG, Björklund A (1995) Selective lesioning of the basal forebrain cholinergic system by intraventricular 192 IgG-saporin: behavioural, biochemical and stereological studies in the rat. Eur J Neurosci 7:329–343

Lehericy S, Hirsch EC, Cervera Pierot P, Hersh LB, Bakchine S, Piette F et al. (1993) Heterogeneity and selectivity of the degeneration of cholinergic neurons in the basal forebrain of patients with Alzheimer's disease. J Comp Neurol 330:15–31

Levi-Montalcini R, Skaper SD, Dal Toso R, Petrelli L, Leon A (1996) Nerve growth factor: from neurotrophin to neurokine. TINS 19:514–520

Loy R, Heyder D, Clagett-Dame M et al. (1990) Localization of NGF receptors in normal and Alzheimer's basal forebrain with monoclonal antibodies against the truncated form of the receptor. J Neurosci Res 27:651–664

Markowska AL, Koliatsos VE, Breckler SJ, Price DL, Olton DS (1994) Human nerve growth factor improves spatial memory in aged but not in young rats. J Neurosci 14:4815–4824

Markowska AL, Price DL, Koliatsos VE (1996) Selective effects of nerve growth factor on spatial recent memory as assessed by a delayed nonmatching-to-position task in the water maze. J Neurosci 16:3541–3548

Martinez-Serrano A, Fischer W, Söderström S, Ebendal T, Björklund A (1996) Long-term functional recovery from age-induced spatial memory impairments by nerve growth factor gene transfer to the rat basal forebrain. Proc Natl Acad Sci USA 93: 6355–6360

Miyamoto M, Narumi S, Nagaoka A, Coyle JT (1989) Effects of continuous infusion of cholinergic drugs on memory impairment in rats with basal forebrain lesions. J Pharm Exp Ther 248:825–835

Mobley WC, Neve RL, Prusiner SB, McKinley MP (1988) Nerve growth factor increases mRNA levels for the prion protein and the beta-amyloid protein precursor in developing hamster brain. Proc Natl Acad Sci USA 85:9811–9815

Mufson EJ, Conner JM, Kordower JH (1995) Nerve growth factor in Alzheimer's disease: defective retrograde transport to nucleus basalis. Neuroreport 6:1063–1066

Mufson EJ, Lavine N, Jaffar S, Kordower JH, Quirion R, Saragovi HU (1997) Reduction in p140-TrkA receptor protein within the nucleus basalis and cortex in Alzheimer's disease. Exp Neurol 146:91–103

Murray KD, Gall CM, Jones EG, Isackson PJ (1994) Differential regulation of brain-derived neurotrophic factor and type II calcium/calmodulin-dependent protein kinase messenger RNA expression in Alzheimer's disease. Neuroscience 60:37–48

Nakagawara A, Arima Nakagawara M, Skavarda NJ, Azar CG, Cantor AB, Brodeur GM (1993) Association between high levels of expression of the TRK gene and favorable outcome in human neuroblastoma. N Engl J Med 328:847–854

Narisawa SM, Wakabayashi K, Tsuji S, Takahashi H, Nawa H (1996) Regional specificity of alterations in NGF, BDNF and NT-3 levels in Alzheimer's disease. Neuroreport 7:2925–2928

Ohyagi Y, Tabira T (1993) Effect of growth factors and cytokines on expression of amyloid beta protein precursor mRNAs in cultured neural cells. Brain Res Mol Brain Res 18:127–132

Olson L, Nordberg A, von Holst H, Backman L, Ebendal T, Alafuzoff I et al. (1992) Nerve growth factor affects ^{11}C-nicotine binding, blood flow, EEG, and verbal episodic memory in an Alzheimer patient (case report). J Neural Transm Parkinson's Dis Dementia Sect 4:79–95

Phillips HS, Hains JN, Laramee GR et al. (1990) Widespread expression of BDNF but not NT3 by target areas of basal forebrain cholinergic neurons. Science 250:290–292

Phillips HS, Hains JM, Armanini M, Laramee GR, Johnson SA, Winslow JW (1991) BDNF mRNA is decreased in the hippocampus of individuals with Alzheimer's disease. Neuron 7:695–702

Pincelli C, Sevignani C, Manfredini R, Grande A, Fantini F, Bracci-Laudiero L et al. (1994) Expression and function of nerve growth factor and nerve growth factor receptor on cultured keratinocytes. J Invest Dermatol 103:13–18

Price D (1986) New perspectives on Alzheimer's disease. Ann Rev Neurosci 9:489–512.

Ramón Y, Cajal S (1928) Degeneration and regeneration of the nervous system. Hafner Publishing Company, London

Salehi A, Verhaagen J, Dijkhuizen PA, Swaab DF (1996) Co-localization of high-affinity neurotrophin receptors in nucleus basalis of Meynert neurons and their differential reduction in Alzheimer's disease. Neuroscience 75:373–387

Scott SA, Mufson EJ, Weingartner JA, Skau KA, Crutcher KA (1995) Nerve growth factor in Alzheimer's disease: increased levels throughout the brain coupled with declines in nucleus basalis. J Neuroscience 15:6213–6221

Seiger Å, Nordberg A, von Holst H, Bäckman L, Ebendal T, Alafuzoff I et al. (1993) Intracranial infusion of purified nerve growth factor to an Alzheimer patient: the first attempt of a possible future treatment strategy. Behav Brain Res 57:255–261

Smeyney RJ, Klein R, Schnapp A, Long LK, Bryant S, Lewin A, Lira SA, Barbacid M (1994) Severe sensory and sympathetic neuropathies in mice carrying a disrupted Trk/NGF receptor gene. Nature 368:246–249

Snider WD (1994) Functions of the neurotrophins during nervous system development: what the knockouts are teaching us. Cell 77:627–638

Steckler T, Keith AB, Wiley RG, Sahgal A (1995) Cholinergic lesions by 192 IgG-saporin and short-term recognition memory: role of the septohippocampal projection. Neuroscience 66:101–114

Thoenen H (1995) Neurotrophins and neuronal plasticity. Science 270:593–598

Thoenen H, Bandtlow C, Heumann R (1987) The physiological function of nerve growth factor in the central nervous system: comparison with the periphery. Rev Physiol Biochem Pharmacol 109:145–178

Tilson HA, McLamb RL, Shaw S, Rogers BC, Pediaditakis P, Cook L (1988) Radial-arm maze deficits produced by colchicine administered into the area of the nucleus basalis are ameliorated by cholinergic agents. Brain Res 438:83–94

Treanor JJS, Dawbarn D, Allen SJ et al. (1991) Low affinity nerve growth factor receptor binding in normal and Alzheimer's disease basal forebrain. Neurosci Lett 121:73–76

Tuszynski MH, Sang H, Yoshida K, Gage FH (1991) Recombinant human nerve growth factor infusions prevent cholinergic neuronal degeneration in the adult primate brain. Ann Neurol 30:625–636

Vanderzee CEEM, Ross GM, Riopelle RJ, Hagg T (1996) Survival of cholinergic forebrain neurons in developing p75(NGFR)-deficient mice. Science 274:1729–1732

Vazquez ME, Ebendal T (1991) Messenger RNAs for trk and the low-affinity NGF receptor in rat basal forebrain. Neuroreport 2:593–596

Venero JL, Hefti F, Beck KD (1995) Retrograde transport of nerve growth factor from hippocampus and amygdala to trkA mRNA expressing neurons in paraventricular and reuniens nuclei of the thalamus. Neuroscience 64:855–860

Venero JL, Hefti F, Knusel B (1996) Trophic effect of exogenous nerve growth factor on rat striatal cholinergic neurons: comparison between intraparenchymal and intraventricular administration. Mol Pharmacol 49:303–310

Vito P, Lacana E, D'Adamio L (1996) Interfering with apoptosis: Ca^{2+} binding protein ALG-2 and Alzheimer's disease gene ALG-3. Science 271:521–525

Voytko ML, Olton DS, Richardson RT, Gorman LK, Tobin JR, Price DL (1994) Basal forebrain lesions in monkeys disrupt attention but not learning and memory. J Neurosci 14:167–186

Wenk GL, Stoehr JD, Quintana G, Mobley S, Wiley R G (1994) Behavioral, biochemical, histological and electrophysiological effects of 192 IgG-saporin injections into the basal forebrain of rats. J Neuroscience 14:5986–5995

Whitehouse PJ, Price DL, Struble RG et al. (1982) Alzheimer's disease and senile dementia; loss of neurons in the basal forebrain. Science 215:1237–1239

Widmer HR, Kaplan DR, Rabin SJ, Beck KD, Hefti F, Knusel B (1993) Rapid phosphorylation of phospholipase C gamma3 by brain-derived neurotrophic factor and neurotrophin-3 in cultures of embryonic rat cortical neurons. J Neurochem 60:2111–2123

Will B, Hefti F (1985) Behavioural and neurochemical effects of chronic intraventricular injections of nerve growth factor in adult rats with fimbria lesions. Behav Brain Res 17:17–24

Williams LR, Varon S, Peterson GM, Wictorin K, Fischer W, Bjorklund A, Gage FH (1986) Continuous infusion of nerve growth factor prevents basal forebrain neuronal death after fimbria fornix transection. Proc Natl Acad Sci USA 83:9231–9235

Winkler J, Ramirez GA, Kuhn HG, Peterson DA, Day-Lollini PA, Steward GR, Tuszynski MH, Gage FH, Thal LJ (1997) Reversible Schwann cell hyperplasia and sprouting of sensory and sympathetic neurites after intraventricular administration of nerve growth factor. Ann Neurol 41:82–93

Yaar M, Eller MS, DiBenedetto P, Reenstra WR, Zhai S, McQuaid T et al. (1994) The trk family of receptors mediates nerve growth factor and neurotrophin-3 effects in melanocytes. J Clin Invest 94:1550–1562

Yamatsuji T, Okamoto T, Takeda S, Murayama Y, Tanaka N, Nishimoto I (1996) Expression of V642 APP mutant causes cellular apoptosis as Alzheimer trait-linked phenotype. EMBO J 15:498–509

CHAPTER 8

Neurotrophic Roles of GDNF and Related Factors

K. UNSICKER, C. SUTER-CRAZZOLARA, and K. KRIEGLSTEIN

A. Introduction

Neurotrophic factors constitute signals of intercellular communication and are widely employed in signaling from neuronal target cells, neurons and glia towards responsive neurons. Although their prime function is apparently to rescue neurons from death, the past decade of neurotrophic-factor research has taught us that there is probably no such thing as a neurotrophic factor. Even the classic paradigmatic neurotrophic factor, nerve growth factor (NGF), may be beneficial to neurons (LEVI-MONTALCINI 1987), disguise itself as a neuron killer (FRADE et al. 1996) or perform multiple functions on non-neural cells which seem to be unrelated to its neurotrophic potential (EHRHARD et al. 1993). Similarly, growth factors with long-established functions in growth and differentiation control have unveiled astonishing capacities in regulating the survival and differentiation of neurons. The transforming growth factor-β (TGF-β) superfamily harbors a number of examples to illustrate this point.

TGF-β was initially characterized by its ability to induce a transformed phenotype in mesenchymal cells (ROBERTS et al. 1981, 1983; see ROBERTS and SPORN 1990, for an early review of the field). TGF-β1 is the prototypic member of a still expanding superfamily of TGF-βs. Members of this family include the TGF-βs, activins, inhibins, bone morphogenetic proteins (BMPs), growth/differentiation factors (GDFs), mullerian-inhibiting substance, *Drosophila* decapentaplegic gene complex, *Xenopus* Vg-1 gene, and a growing subfamily of glial cell line-derived growth factor (GDNF) and related proteins (Fig. 1; cf. reviews by KINGSLEY 1994; KRIEGLSTEIN et al. 1995a; HOGAN 1996).

TGF-βs elicit diverse cellular responses depending on cell type, state of differentiation and experimental conditions. Biological actions include regulation of cell proliferation, early morphogenetic events, control of extracellular matrix production and degradation, stimulation of chondro- and osteogenesis, and modulation of numerous immune and inflammatory responses (BARNARD et al. 1990; MASSAGUE 1990; ROBERTS and SPORN 1990). The discovery that numerous members of the TGF-β superfamily are expressed in the nervous system, including TGF-β2 and -b3 (FLANDERS et al. 1991; UNSICKER et al. 1991), several BMPs (JORDAN et al. 1997; MEHLER et al. 1997), GDFs (KRIEGLSTEIN et

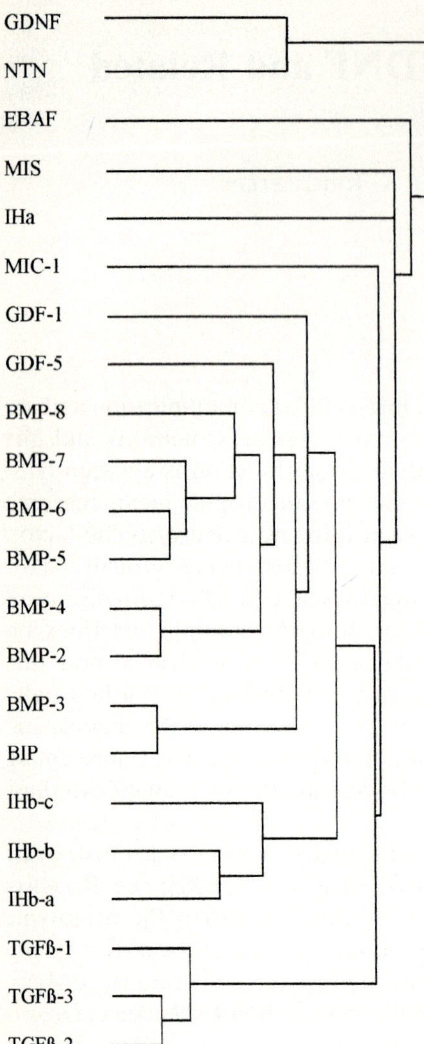

Fig. 1. GDNF and neurturin (*NTN*) are more distant members of the TGFb superfamily. For the phylogentic analysis, only peptide sequences encoding the mature proteins were applied. Analysis was carried out with the pileup program of the GCG-package

al. 1995c), and GDNF (UNSICKER 1996) prompted studies suggesting that the factors had multiple contextual activities on all types of neural cells, including trophic actions on neurons (for reviews, see KRIEGLSTEIN et al. 1995a; MEHLER et al. 1997).

This review will focus on the trophic support of developing and lesioned neurons by members of the GDNF subfamily and their receptors. The cloning and expression of GDNF, and the discovery of its survival-promoting effects on midbrain dopaminergic neurons (LIN et al. 1993) raised hopes that GDNF might become useful in the treatment of nervous system diseases. Although it seems that possible clinical applications are not within easy reach, GDNF is very likely the most promising member of the TGF-β superfamily to reach the level of applicability in the treatment of neurological diseases.

B. Molecular Structure of GDNF and Related Molecules

I. Glial Cell Line-Derived Neurotrophic Factor

GDNF was first isolated from culture supernatants of the B49 glial cell line using its ability to support the in vitro survival of embryonic midbrain neurons as a biological assay (Lin et al. 1993, 1994). GDNF binds weakly to heparin and migrates on SDS-polyacrylamide gels with an apparent molecular mass of 33–45 kDa. GDNF is heterogeneously glycosylated and behaves like a disulfide-bonded homodimer. The determined disulfide structure is highly homologous to that of TGF-β2 (Haniu et al. 1996). The apparent molecular mass of the deglycosylated monomer is about 16 kDa. The monomer has 134 amino acids. The rat, mouse and human cDNAs of GDNF have been cloned (Lin et al. 1993; N. Matsushita, unpublished data). Rat and human GDNF are 93% identical based on the amino acids, synthesized in a pre-pro form and secreted as a homodimeric glycosylated mature protein.

GDNF contains the seven conserved and typically spaced cysteine residues found in all members of the TGF-β superfamily, but shares about 20% identity with any family member (Fig. 1). As a typical TGF-β, GDNF shares a common cystine knot motif with ligands such as NGF and platelet-derived growth factor (PDGF) (Eigenbrot and Gerber 1997; McDonald and Hendrickson 1993). The human GDNF gene maps to chromosome 5p12-p13.1 (Bermingham et al. 1995; Schindelhauer et al. 1995). Transcription appears to be regulated by multiple promoters in human, mouse and rat (Suter-Crazzolara et al. 1997). The rat GDNF gene carries an intron at position 200. A similar intron at corresponding positions is also found in human and mouse (Lin et al. 1993; N. Matsushita, unpublished data).

GDNF is encoded by two mRNAs, which appear to originate from the same gene. The smaller form has a deletion of 78 bp in the pre-pro-domain encoding region and is probably the result of an alternative splicing event (Suter-Crazzolara and Unsicker 1994; Schaar et al. 1993; Springer et al. 1995). Choi-Lundberg and Bohn (1995) reported an essentially identical pattern of distribution of the two mRNA forms in all organs and tissues studied. In contrast, work from our group indicates a tissue-dependent relative abundance of these mRNA species (Suter-Crazzolara and Unsicker 1994; see also Cristina et al. 1995). As the region encoding the mature GDNF protein appears to be unaffected by the 78-bp deletion, the in vivo relevance of the mRNA forms remains to be investigated.

II. Neurturin

Neurturin, a protein structurally related to GDNF, was discovered in culture supernatants of Chinese hamster ovary (CHO) cells and purified about 400000-fold employing NGF-primed cultured sympathetic neurons as a bioassay (KOTZBAUER et al. 1996). Neurturin is thermostable, sensitive to trypsin and has a relative molecular mass of greater than 10000 in dialysis and ultrafiltration experiments. Cloning of the mouse cDNA revealed an open reading frame encoding a 195-amino acid protein, which contains a 19-amino acid signal sequence and a 76-amino acid pro-region. Mouse and human neurturin proteins are 91% identical. Neurturin shares about 42% amino acid similarity with mature GDNF and, like GDNF, its amino acid sequence similarity to other members of the TGF-β family is about 20% or less. One report suggests that neurturin, in comparison with GDNF, may be a more potent neurotrophic factor for midbrain dopaminergic neurons (LAMPE et al. 1997).

1. Persephin[1]

Existence of a third member of the GDNF subfamily has been announced in abstract form; details have not yet been published (LAMPE et al. 1997).

C. Receptors and Signal Transduction of GDNF and Neurturin

Although structural characteristics classify GDNF as a distant member of the TGF-β superfamily, the putative receptor for GDNF turned out to be unrelated to the serine/threonine receptor kinases which are employed in signal transduction by members of the TGF-β family (Fig. 2; see JOSSO and DI-CLEMENTE 1997, for a review). Striking similarities in the phenotypes of mice deficient for GDNF or the orphan tyrosine kinase receptor Ret, respectively, suggested an involvement of Ret in GDNF signal transduction. Moreover, it became apparent that Ret is just one component within a GDNF receptor complex, in which a GDNF binding protein anchored to the cell surface via a glycosyl-phosphatidylinositol (GPI) linkage has been identified as an essential component (cf. LINDSAY and YANCOPOULOS 1996; MASON 1996).

[1] After submission of this article, a full report on persephin, the third member of the GDNF family, has appeared (Neuron 20: 1–20, 1998). Like GDNF and neurturin, persephin promotes survival of embryonic and toxically impaired dopaminergic neurons in vitro and vivo. Persephin also supports the survival of motoneurons in vitro and following axotomy. In contrast to GDNF and neurturin, persephin does not support peripheral neurons in vitro. Persephin seems to signal through receptor components that are distinct from GDNF and neurturin receptors.

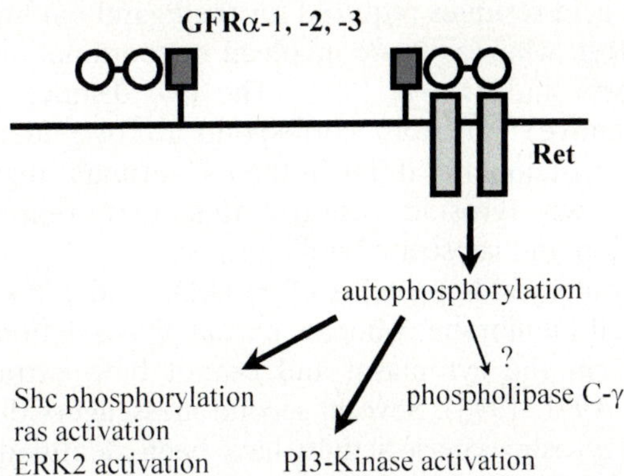

Fig. 2. Model for GDNF and NTN signaling through the Ret receptor tyrosine kinase. GDNF family members initially bind with their corresponding GFRs. Low affinity binding to other GFRs may occur. This complex interacts with Ret, which is followed by Ret autophosphorylation. Two pathways for signaling have been elucidated (VAN WEERING and BOS 1997). Whether effects of Ret are mediated by phospholipase C-γ (as has been found for several other receptor tyrosine kinases) is still not known

I. Ret

1. Molecular Structure and Signaling Pathways

The tyrosine kinase receptor Ret was discovered by transfection of NIH 3T3 mouse fibroblasts with DNA from human T-cell lymphomas (TAKAHASHI et al. 1985). Activation of the corresponding proto-oncogene was achieved by rearrangement with an unlinked DNA segment generating a new transcriptional unit encoding a fusion protein (TAKAHASHI and COOPER 1987). Since rearrangement had occurred during transfection, the proto-oncogene was named "RET" proto-oncogene (rearranged during transfection). The human RET gene is localized on chromosome 10q11.2 and contains 20 exons in a region of about 50 kb (KWOK et al. 1993; CECCHERINI et al. 1993).

Five different mRNAs (7.0, 6.0, 4.6, 4.5 and 3.9 kb) have been identified in a human neuroectodermal tumor cell line (TAHIRA et al. 1990). The 7.0, 4.5 and 3.9-kb RNAs encode an identical Ret protein of 1072 amino acids, whereas the 6.0 and 4.6-kb RNAs encode a Ret protein of 1114 amino acids. The nucleotide sequence of cDNA derived from the human RET gene (TAKAHASHI et al. 1988) predicted a protein with the typical structure of a receptor tyrosine kinase. Its tyrosine kinase domain consists of two parts separated by an "insert" and, thus, resembles the tyrosine kinase domain of the fibroblast growth factor (FGF) receptors. The extracellular portion does not resemble any other receptor tyrosine kinase extracellular domain and has a unique domain of about 110 amino acids with 30% homology to cadherins (SCHNEIDER 1992; IWAMOTO et al. 1993; KUMA et al. 1993; cf. Fig. 2). There are no indications so far, however, that Ret may act as a calcium-dependent adhesion molecule. Moreover, amino acid residues required for the ligand binding in *N*-cadherin are absent from Ret, whereas those involved in coordination of calcium are present (ROBERTSON and MASON 1997). The two distinct isoforms of Ret (see Sect. C.I.1 above) probably correspond to two identified 117-kDa and 122-kDa Ret proteins that differ in their C-terminal regions. The larger isoform includes two tyrosine residues that may represent additional autophosphorylation and substrate binding sites.

Full glycosylation yields proteins of 170 kDa and 175 kDa that can be localized to the cell membrane, whereas partial glycosylation yields proteins that are localized in the cytoplasm and cannot bind extracellular ligands (TAKAHASHI et al. 1991, 1993). Several second messengers that may serve as substrates for Ret tyrosine kinase activity have been identified (SANTORO et al. 1994). Activation of Ret in neuroblastoma cells has been shown to result in increased transcription of an Elk luciferase reporter gene, suggesting that signaling through Ret can activate the mitogen-activated protein kinase signal transduction pathway (WORBY et al. 1996; VAN WEERING and BOS 1997; cf. Fig. 2).

The recent cloning of the chick and zebrafish homologues of the ret receptor has been an important step towards the goal of understanding the full range of developmental functions of Ret, both within and outside the vertebrate nervous system (SCHUCHARDT et al. 1995; MARCOS GUTIERREZ et al. 1997).

2. Ret As a Functional Receptor for GDNF and Neurturin

Ret lost its orphan receptor identity when TRUPP et al. (1996) and DURBEC et al. (1996a) reported that Ret can serve as a functional receptor for GDNF (cf. ROBERTSON and MASON 1997, for a review). TRUPP et al. (1996) had identified a protein in a motoneuron cell line that could be cross-linked to GDNF and could be precipitated by phosphotyrosine antibodies. This protein also resembled Ret in size (about 155 kDa), occurred in the right place (motoneurons that were known to express Ret) and was, therefore, tentatively identified as a GDNF receptor. DURBEC and co-workers (1996b) noticed that GDNF was most highly expressed in gut and kidney, where the most dramatic effects were seen in Ret-deficient mice, and hypothesized that GDNF might work via Ret. In a series of experiments including a Xenopus embryo bioassay and explant cultures from wild-type and Ret-deficient mouse embryos they showed that Ret function is necessary for GDNF signaling. Activation of Ret by GDNF, as indicated by tyrosine phosphorylation of the intracellular catalytic domain, was also demonstrated by VEGA et al. (1996). These authors also reported binding of GDNF to Ret with a dissociation constant of 8 nM and coprecipitation of ^{125}I-labeled GDNF with anti-Ret antibodies.

With the discovery of a second member of the GDNF family, neurturin, it became apparent that Ret can also act as a receptor for neurturin (BALOH et al. 1997; CREEDON et al. 1997; KLEIN et al. 1997).

II. Additional Components of the Ret-Receptor Complex: α1- and α2-receptors

1. The GFR-α1 Receptor

Using expression cloning strategies (enriched populations of midbrain dopaminergic neurons, or retinal photoreceptor cells) to identify high affinity binding proteins for GDNF, two groups (JING et al. 1996; TREANOR et al. 1996) cloned identical cDNAs for a novel, GDNF binding protein. The protein, initially termed GDNFR-α (now GFR-α1; DAVIES et al. 1997) was not related to any known protein and analysis of the protein sequence suggested a GPI-anchored cell surface protein lacking an intracellular domain. In confirmation of this structure, phosphatidylinositol-specific phospholipase C (PI-PLC) treatment of cultured neurons caused them to lose responsiveness to GDNF, and re-addition of soluble GFR-α1 restored their ability to respond to GDNF.

GPI linkage and binding of GDNF with high affinity to a large complex suggested that GFR-α1 would need to interact with signaling partners. Although several lines of evidence indicated that Ret might act as a partner for GFR-α1, there was initial disagreement about the details of the receptor complex. The essential issue was whether Ret or GFR-α1 by themselves were sufficient for GDNF-mediated signaling or required co-operation with the complementary partner (cf. Fig. 2). In view of the evidence that (i) Ret-deficient embryonic tissues did not respond to GDNF, and (ii) expression of Ret in Xenopus embryos and in 3T3 fibroblasts made them responsive to GDNF (DURBEC et al. 1996a; TRUPP et al. 1996), it was assumed that Ret was sufficient for GDNF signaling. In contrast, JING et al. (1996) and TREANOR et al. (1996) had identified GFR-α1 by its capacity to bind GNDF in the absence of Ret. A possibility for reconciling these findings might be that very low levels of GFR-α1 or GDNF receptors related to GFR-α1 (see Sect. II.1 below) were present in experiments in which only Ret was assumed to be expressed. Alternatively, it is conceivable that Ret might bind GDNF in the absence of GFR-α1 at low affinity (cf. TRUPP et al. 1996), similar to ciliary neurotrophic factor (CNTF) which, at high doses, can elicit responses in the absence of the CNTFR-α and presence of its two β-receptors (DAVIS et al. 1993).

2. The Neurturin-/TrnR2-/RTL2/GFR-α2-Receptor

A novel receptor with significant sequence similarity to the GFR-α1 has recently been identified (BALOH et al. 1997; KLEIN et al. 1997; SANICOLA et al. 1997; LU et al. 1998) and termed either NTNR-a (neurturin receptor-a), TrnR2 (TGF-β-related neurotrophic factor receptor), RETL2 or GFR-α2, respectively. Like GFR-α1, GFR-α2 is a GPI-linked protein. It binds neurturin with high affinity (K_D about 10 pM; KLEIN et al. 1997); whether this receptor can also mediate GDNF signaling through Ret (BALOH et al. 1997; SANICOLA et al. 1997) is controversial (cf. KLEIN et al. 1997; BUJ-BELLO et al. 1997).

D. Distribution of GDNF, Neurturin and Their Receptors (Fig. 3)

I. GDNF and Neurturin in the Nervous System

Since GDNF had been initially identified based on its trophic functions for midbrain dopaminergic neurons (LIN et al. 1993), early expression studies focused on the nigrostriatal system. STRÖMBERG and associates (1993) demonstrated, by in situ hybridization, that expression of GDNF mRNA in the rat striatum peaked at birth, but was undetectable in the adult striatum, suggesting a retrograde messenger role in the developing nigrostriatal system. CHOI-LUNDBERG and BOHN (1995), using reverse-transcriptase polymerase chain reaction (RT-PCR) to study the distribution of GDNF mRNA, also reported the highest levels in the P0 and P10 striatum. Another study using RNase protection showed similar levels of GDNF mRNA in the striatum throughout the life span of the mouse (from 4.5 months to 24 months), even without any alterations in weaver mutants (BLUM and WEICKERT 1995). Consistent with the documented role of GDNF as a dopaminotrophic factor, TOMAC et al. (1995b) and LAPCHAK et al. (1997) provided evidence that radio-iodinated GDNF is transported from the dopaminergic target field in the striatum to the dopaminergic cell bodies in the substantia nigra. An early RT-PCR study reported that astroglial cells of the substantia nigra and neuronal cultures of embryonic substantia nigra expressed GDNF mRNA (SCHAAR et al. 1993). This contrasts with other reports that have failed to detect GDNF mRNA in cultures of embryonic midbrain neurons (KRIEGLSTEIN et al. 1995b).

Rat and human astroglial cell cultures were also reported to express GDNF mRNA (HO et al. 1995; MORETTO et al. 1996; SUTER-CRAZZOLARA and UNSICKER 1996). In cultures of striatal astrocytes, *N*-methyl-D,L-aspartic acid and kainic acid upregulate GDNF expression (HO et al. 1995). Not only the B49 glioma cells, from which GDNF was originally isolated, but also C6 glioma cells show prominent expression of GDNF mRNA. Among a large variety of compounds tested, FGF-2 and 1.25-(OH)2 D3 were among the few that caused a prominent increase of GDNF mRNA in C6 cells (SUTER-CRAZZOLARA and UNSICKER 1996; NAVEILHAN et al. 1996).

High levels of GDNF transcripts were detected in the P0 spinal cord, whereas lower levels were found in brainstem, cerebellum, diencephalon and telencephalon. While in most central nervous system (CNS) areas expression of low levels of GDNF mRNA detectable by RT-PCR persists into adulthood (CHOI-LUNDBERG and BOHN 1995; SPRINGER et al. 1994; YAMAMOTO et al. 1996), the cerebellum has a unique pattern of expression, with levels declining during early postnatal development and then increasing to adult levels after P15

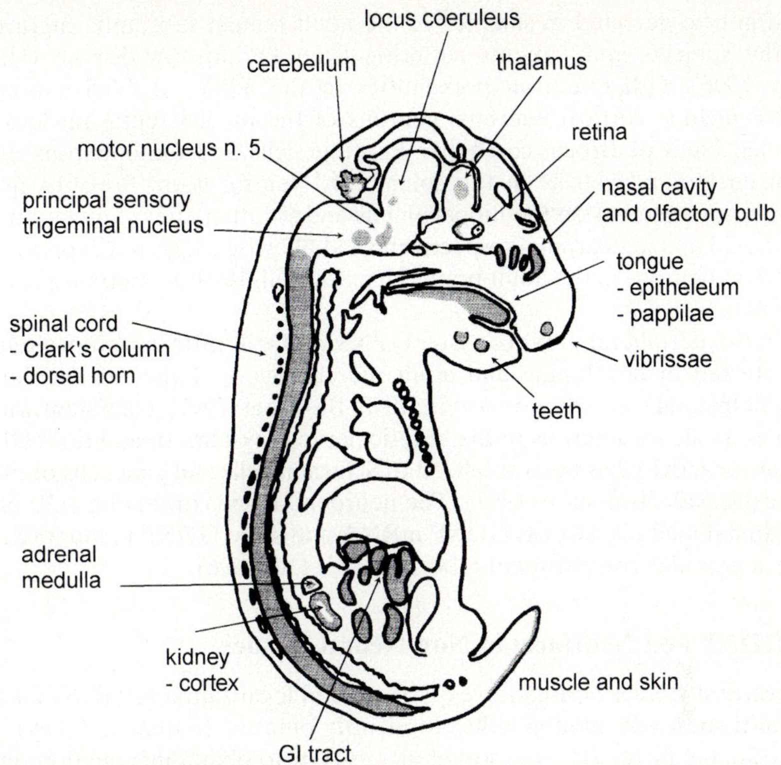

Fig. 3. Schematic diagram summarizing some of the principal regions where GDNF mRNA is expressed; sagittal section of a perinatal rat. Due to graphic limitations, some regions with GDNF expression are not included. These are striatum, hippocampus, substantia innominata, corpus pineale, inner ear, ear canal and glomus caroticum. GDNF expression in the thalamus is most likely restricted to the ventral posteromedial nucleus

(Choi-Lundberg and Bohn 1995), consistent with effects of GDNF in Purkinje cell development.

Several in situ hybridization studies have revealed more details of the regional and cellular distribution of GDNF mRNA in the embryonic and adult CNS. In addition to the embryonic striatum, Strömberg et al. (1993) and Nosrat et al. (1996) observed expression in the embryonic cerebellar anlage and spinal cord as well as in neonatal rat thalamus, cingulate cortex, pineal gland and several non-striatal dopaminergic projection areas, such as ventral pallidum, olfactory tubercle and piriform cortex. Recent studies have extended these results and shown that GDNF synthesis is maintained into adulthood and that neurons rather than glial cells are the principal sites of GDNF synthesis in the adult CNS (Pochon et al. 1997; Trupp et al. 1997).

Whether GDNF mRNA can be localized to tyrosine hydroxylase-positive dopaminergic neurons of the substantia nigra is controversial. GDNF mRNA could not be detected in samples of the adult human substantia nigra from healthy subjects and patients suffering from Parkinson's disease (HUNOT et al. 1996). Other neuron populations in the adult rat CNS expressing GDNF include cortical neurons, neurons of the medial septal nucleus and diagonal band of Broca, cerebellar Purkinje cells and motoneurons of the facial nucleus as well as in the spinal cord ventral horn. Previous in situ hybridization studies on the hippocampus and striatum after stimulation with kainic acid and pilocarpine, respectively, had likewise suggested expression of GDNF in neurons in the adult brain (HUMPEL et al. 1994; SCHMIDT-KASTNER et al. 1994).

In the peripheral nervous system (PNS), GDNF mRNA and protein can be detected in developing and adult muscle layers of the rat and human gastrointestinal tract (SUVANTO et al. 1996; BAR et al. 1997), consistent with its proposed role for neurons in the enteric nervous system. In addition, GDNF immunoreactivity has been localized to Schwann cells and glial cells of plexus in the gut wall (BAR et al. 1997). The neuroendocrine chromaffin cells of the rat adrenal medulla express GDNF mRNA and store GDNF immunoreactivity in a granular compartment (KRIEGLSTEIN et al. 1996).

II. GDNF and Neurturin in Non-Neural Tissues

The earliest studies addressing expression and localization of GDNF in non-neural tissues were aiming either to identify putative sources of GDNF as a neurotrophic factor (HENDERSON et al. 1994) or to obtain information on the relative distribution of GDNF mRNA in various tissues (SUTER-CRAZZOLARA and UNSICKER 1994; CHOI-LUNDBERG and BOHN 1995). Detection of GDNF mRNA in primary cultures of embryonic myotubes, limb buds and Schwann cells by means of RT-PCR with positive in situ hybridization signals in ventral roots, along peripheral nerves and select striated muscle (HENDERSON et al. 1994; WRIGHT and SNIDER 1996; cf. Fig. 6) suggested sites of synthesis that were different from those for the neurotrophins brain-derived neurotrophic factor (BDNF) and neurotrophin-3 (NT-3).

More detailed studies at early embryonic stages supported the view that GDNF mRNA is expressed at particularly high levels in a restricted region in proximal limb buds, where axons converge and enter the limb (WRIGHT and SNIDER 1996; Fig. 6). These studies also indicated that mesenchymal rather than Schwann cell precursors or striated muscle were the sites of GNDF synthesis at these early stages of motor and sensory axon growth. Moreover, these results suggested that GDNF in proximal limb buds may function as a transient survival factor, before motor axons reach their final targets. Highest levels of GDNF expression were detected in developing kidney, skin, teeth, whisker pad, condensing cartilages, stomach, testis and blood (SUTER-CRAZZOLARA and UNSICKER 1994; CHOI-LUNDBERG and BOHN 1995; TRUPP et al. 1995; NOSRAT et al. 1996; SUVANTO et al. 1996; LUUKKO et al. 1997; SARIOLA and SAINIO 1997).

The earliest reported developmental expression of GDNF mRNA is in the anterior neuroectoderm during early stages of mouse neurogenesis between embryonic day (E) 7.5 and E 10.5. In the E10 rat embryo, prominent signals for GDNF mRNA are found in the urogenital field and the cranial part of the gut (SUVANTO et al. 1996). At later ages (E15 and older), GDNF mRNA is particularly high in the outer metanephric kidney mesenchyme and mesenchymal/smooth muscle layers of esophagus, stomach and intestine suggesting roles for GNDF in kidney development and development of the innervation of the gastrointestinal tract (NOSRAT et al. 1996; SUVANTO et al. 1996). In the chick embryo, Northern blotting indicated that GDNF transcripts are expressed in all of the tissues that are innervated by neurons responding to GDNF (BUJ-BELLO et al. 1995).

In summary, localization of GDNF transcripts suggests multiple functions of GDNF in early morphogenesis and development of many peripheral organs, e.g., the kidney and in the nervous system. The wide expression in the adult nervous system suggests important yet enigmatic functions of GDNF on mature neurons and glial cells.

III. Expression of Ret, GFR-α1 and GFR-α2 in the Developing and Adult Nervous System

Given the large variety of neurons that are known to respond to GDNF and the fact that no other receptor tyrosine kinases that might alternatively transmit a GDNF signal have been identified (yet postulated), so far, Ret may be expected to be widely expressed on CNS and peripheral neurons. Among the earliest identified neuron populations expressing Ret were developing and adult dopaminergic neurons of the substantia nigra (TRUPP et al. 1996; NOSRAT et al. 1997), spinal motoneurons in the CNS (PACHNIS et al. 1993; TSUZUKI et al. 1995; NAKAMURA et al. 1996; NOSRAT et al. 1997; TRUPP et al. 1997), and various subpopulations of peripheral ganglionic neurons – sympathetic, nodose, enteric and some sensory (PACHNIS et al. 1993; TSUZUKI et al. 1995; NOSRAT et al. 1997).

Particularly important have been the studies that have used the demonstration of ligand and receptor expressions for resolving physiological circuits of GDNF actions (TRUPP et al. 1997). For example, GDNF expression in the adult rat striatum coincides with a complete lack of Ret and GFR-α1 mRNA expression in this location. Likewise, there is no detectable expression of Ret and GFR-α1 mRNAs in several thalamic nuclei (ventromedial, anteroventral, ventroposterolateral, ventroposteromedial) which show strong labeling for GDNF. Conversely, the reticular thalamic nucleus, zona incerta and lateral habenula display high levels of Ret and GFR-α1 mRNA labeling, but no GDNF mRNA expression. Such distributional patterns suggest functioning of GDNF as a target-derived factor.

Other GDNF-responsive neuron populations in the adult rat brain, including the noradrenergic neurons of the locus coeruleus, brain stem motoneurons and trigeminal mesencephalic sensory neurons, also show the expected pattern of co-expression of Ret and GFR-α1 mRNAs (Trupp et al. 1997). Additional populations that express both Ret and GFR-α1 are serotonergic neurons in the dorsal raphe nucleus, dorsal cochlear, lateral vestibular and several hypothalamic nuclei. An interesting segregation of Ret and GFR-α1 occurs in the basal forebrain, where Ret expression is confined to few neurons in the medial septum, whereas GFR-α mRNA is seen at high levels in neurons of the lateral septum and in peripherally located neurons of the medial septum.

In the adult rat cerebellum, Ret and GFR-α1 mRNAs are located at the external edge of the granular layer in cells that are directly adjacent to Purkinje cells. Ret mRNA expression decreases gradually towards the deeper granular layer and into the molecular layer, suggesting the existence of cells in the granular layer that express Ret but not GFR-α1. Although GDNF has been reported to have effects on Purkinje cells in mixed cultures of embryonic cerebellum, adult rat Purkinje cells do not display Ret or GFR-α1 mRNAs. GDNF itself is expressed in scattered cells of the granular layer and may act on cerebellar cortical structures with GDNF receptors, but also on GDNF receptors bearing neurons in pontine, red, cochlear and vestibular nuclei that project to the cerebellar granular layer (Trupp et al. 1997).

Segregation of Ret and GFR-α1 expressions have been found in the adult rat olfactory bulb (Trupp et al. 1997), suggesting that Ret may employ another co-receptor or recruit GFR-α1 in a soluble form from adjacent cells. Several sense organs, including the retina (Avantaggiato et al. 1994; Tsuzuki et al. 1995), the developing inner ear, olfactory epithelium and vibrissae (Nosrat et al. 1997) have been reported to display Ret and GFR-α1 mRNAs.

In a recent attempt to resolve functional circuitries for neurturin and its cognate receptor GFR-α2, Widenfalk et al. (1997) have demonstrated, using in situ hybridization, that GRF-α2 is more widely expressed than neurturin in the developing and adult CNS. They found GFR-α2 mRNA in cerebral cortex, cerebellum, thalamus, zona incerta, hypothalamus, brainstem and spinal cord, and in subpopulations of sensory neurons. Neurturin was expressed in postnatal cerebral cortex, striatum, several brainstem areas and the pineal gland. Thus, in analogy to GDNF, Ret and GFR-α1, expression patterns for neurturin and GFR-α2 are sometimes but not consistently complementary, suggesting multiple modalities of co-operativity of GDNF and neurturin in relation to their receptors.

IV. Expression of GDNF and its Receptors in the Lesioned Nervous System

Several chemical and surgical lesion paradigms of the central and peripheral nervous system have been studied with regard to the regulation of GDNF and its receptors. Kainic acid causes rapid upregulation of GDNF in the dentate gyrus that peaks at 4h (Humpel et al. 1994; Trupp et al. 1997). Transiently, there is strong GDNF expression at 12 h, apparent in all regions of the hippocampus, which remains elevated for another 12h in the CA3 and hilar regions. The GFR-α message is also elevated within the hippocampal region following kainate administration, whereas Ret mRNA is strongly expressed in only a subset of neurons.

Following transection of the adult rat sciatic nerve, GDNF and GFR-α1 mRNAs are upregulated dramatically in the distal segments, with distally increasing gradients (TRUPP et al. 1995, 1997). GDNF mRNA is also upregulated in denervated skeletal muscle (TRUPP et al. 1997). Interestingly, Ret mRNA is undetectable in the sciatic nerve, but can be demonstrated in sacrolumbar motoneurons, where both Ret and GFR-α1 mRNAS are upregulated after sciatic nerve transection (NAKAMURA et al. 1996; TRUPP et al. 1997). The functional significance of increased GFR-α1 mRNA without accompanying Ret expression in the transected sciatic nerve is enigmatic, but could indicate that GFR-α1 may be acting in Schwann cells to present GDNF to injured motor neurons.

V. Expression of Ret, GFR-α1 and GFR-α2 Outside the Nervous System: Involvement of Ret in Neuroendocrine and Gastrointestinal Disorders

Initial analysis of Ret mRNA expression indicated that mRNA levels in rat embryos, between days 9 and 11 of gestation, were 20–50 times higher than in adult tissues (brain, thymus, lung, heart, spleen, testis, small intestine) (TAHIRA et al. 1988). In situ hybridizations and immunocytochemistry showed mRNA expression and localization of the protein in the CNS and PNS, in neural crest (LO and ANDERSON 1995) and crest-derived cells (PACHNIS et al. 1993; TSUZUKI et al. 1995).

Among non-neural cells were cells at the tip of the ureteric bud (AVANTAGGIATO et al. 1994; PACHNIS et al. 1993), consistent with its role in branching morphogenesis and kidney agenesis seen in Ret-deficient mice. Sites outside the nervous system, in which GFR-α1 is expressed, include the ureteric buds of the kidney (TREANOR et al. 1996) and the dental epithelium of the developing tooth (LUUKKO et al. 1997). GFR-α2 mRNA is high in adult intestine and placenta and in fetal lung and kidney (SUVANTO et al. 1997). In the kidney, gut and adrenal gland of the E17 rat embryo, localization of GFR-α2 mRNA is distinct from that of GFR-α1 mRNA. GFR-α2 mRNA can also be detected in salivary-gland connective tissue surrounding the epithelial components and in the germ cell line. Localization of neurturin in salivary-gland epithelia and in Sertoli cells suggests co-operativities with α2-receptor bearing cells which remain to be functionally resolved (WIDENFALK et al. 1997).

Mutations in the human *RET* gene are associated with hereditary cancer syndromes, multiple endocrine neuroplasia types 2A and 2B and familial medullary thyroid carcinoma (MULLIGAN et al. 1993; CARLSON et al. 1994; EDERY et al. 1994; HOFSTRA et al. 1994; PASINI et al. 1996). In addition, mutations in the *RET* gene have been implicated in human Hirschsprung's disease, which is characterized by varying degrees of absence of parasympathetic innervation in the submucosal and myenteric plexus of the enteric nervous system. The Ret kinase null mouse (see Sect. F.II) shows similar defects in the enteric nervous system. However, mutations in the *RET* gene associated with Hirschsprung's disease are autosomal dominants, resulting in haplo-insufficiency of functional Ret (see Pasini et al. 1996, for review), whereas the ret-mutant mouse shows no defects when heterozygous for the mutant allele. Moreover, mutations in the *RET* gene only account for 50% of familial and 15%–20% of sporadic Hirschsprung's disease patients, suggesting the existence of additional gene defects as causes of Hirschsprung's disease. In 1 of 36 patients with Hirschsprung's disease, a mutation in the *GDNF* gene affecting the GDNF protein sequence has recently been reported (Ivanchuk et al. 1996).

E. Functions of GNDF and Neurturin in the Nervous System As Revealed In Vitro and In Vivo

I. Glial Cell Line-Derived Neurotrophic Factor

1. GDNF and the Nigrostriatal Dopaminergic System

a) Cultured Mesencephalic Cells

GDNF was first characterized as a survival promoting factor for cultured mesencephalic dopaminergic neurons (Lin et al. 1993). With this discovery, GDNF joined several other trophic factors and cytokines with documented survival-promoting effects on cultured dopaminergic neurons, including FGF-2 (Ferrari et al. 1989; Engele and Bohn 1991; Otto and Unsicker 1993), BDNF (Hyman et al. 1991) and the TGF-β superfamily members TGF-β1, -β2, -β3 and activin (Krieglstein and Unsicker 1994; Krieglstein et al. 1995b; Poulsen et al. 1994). Given the cellular complexity of cultures from the embryonic rat midbrain floor, a direct effect of GDNF on dopaminergic neurons is not proven, but is likely, in the light of functional GDNF receptors on dopaminergic neurons (Tomac et al. 1995a). It is also not clear whether GDNF requires co-trophic factors for eliciting its in vitro effects.

Engele and Franke (1996) have suggested that effects of GDNF on dopaminergic neurons require concurrent activation of cAMP-dependent signaling pathways. Numbers of mature glial and glial progenitor cells in mesencephalic cell cultures are not overtly increased in response to GDNF (Krieglstein et al. 1995b), suggesting but not proving that glial cells are unlikely candidates for mediating the trophic effects of GDNF. Like other neurotrophic factors, GDNF also protects cultured dopaminergic neurons from death induced by the neurotoxin 1-methyl-4-phenylpyridinium (MPP-; Hou et al. 1996).

It is now clear that the early claims of GDNF acting specifically on dopaminergic neurons in the upper brainstem cannot be maintained, since GDNF also promotes the phenotype of serotonergic (BECK et al. 1996; GALTER and UNSICKER 1998) and noradrenergic brainstem neurons (ARENAS et al. 1995).

Neurotrophic effects of GDNF and GDNF-containing fibrin glue on midbrain dopaminergic neurons have also been monitored in grafts of developing and mature mesencephalon in oculo (JOHANNSON et al. 1995; CHENG et al. 1995) and in embryonic nigral grafts (SINCLAIR et al. 1996). Similarly, fetal nigral dopaminergic grafts within the striatum also respond to GDNF by increased outgrowth of tyrosine hydroxylase-positive neurites. Moreover, animals with GDNF-treated grafts display accelerated functional recovery in models of Parkinsonism (ROSENBLAD et al. 1996; WANG et al. 1996).

In the mesencephalic dopaminergic MN9D cell line, GDNF elicits a three- to fourfold increase in the number of morphologically differentiated cells, and provides a source of monoclonal dopaminergic cells (HELLER et al. 1996).

b) Animal Models of Parkinsonism

The rescuing effect of GDNF on normal and toxin-lesioned embryonic dopaminergic neurons raised hopes that GDNF may be useful in the treatment of Parkinson's disease (see LAPCHAK et al. 1996a,b; and OLSON 1997, for reviews; see Figs. 4 and 5). Such hopes were substantiated by studies using all of the important animal models of dopaminergic nigrostriatal impairment. In the mouse 1-methyl-4-phenyl-1, 2, 3, 6-tetrahydropyridine (MPTP) model (40mg/kg s.c. MPTP on two consecutive days; TOMAC et al. 1995a; see also HOFFER et al. 1994), GDNF not only increased striatal and nigral dopamine levels, when injected 24h prior to the first MPTP injection, but even when administered into the striatum or directly above the substantia nigra 7 days after MPTP treatment, GDNF (10mg/2ml) exerted a normalizing effect on dopamine and the dopamine metabolites homovanillic acid (HVA) and dihydroxyphenylacetic acid (DOPAC). In two other classic nigrostriatal lesion paradigms, the 6-hydroxydopamine (6-OHDA) and axotomy models (Figs. 4 and 5), GDNF has also proven its protective capacity.

Following transection of the medial forebrain bundle, GDNF had an impressive protective effect on nigral dopaminergic neurons (BECK et al. 1995). Moreover, GDNF protected dopaminergic neuronal cell bodies in the substantia nigra from degeneration when applied prior, during or after setting the 6-OHDA lesion (KEARNS and GASH 1995; BOWENKAMP et al. 1995, 1996a, 1997; SAUER et al. 1995; OPACKA-JUFFRY et al. 1995; SHULTS et al. 1996). The potency of GDNF is further underscored by the observation that survival of lesioned nigral neurons persisted for at least 4 months after delayed short-term treatment in a 6-OHDA paradigm that closely mimics the slowly progressing degeneration seen in Parkinson's disease (WINKLER et al. 1996). Despite long-term rescue of nigral cells these authors did not see any significant re-innervation of the lesioned striatum or any signs of functional recovery. In contrast, pretreatment with GDNF seems to prevent 6-OHDA lesions, as evidenced by significant increases in basal and stimulated dopamine release

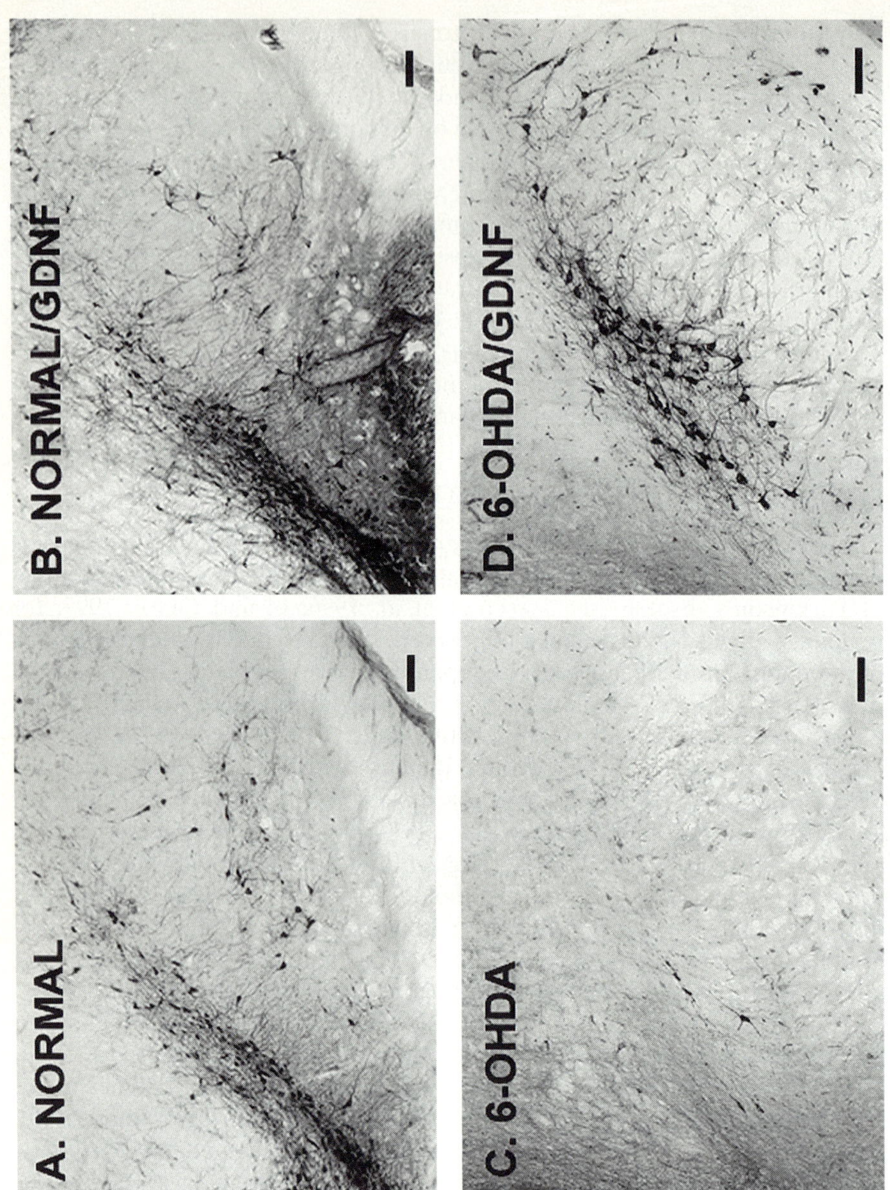
A. NORMAL
B. NORMAL/GDNF
C. 6-OHDA
D. 6-OHDA/GDNF

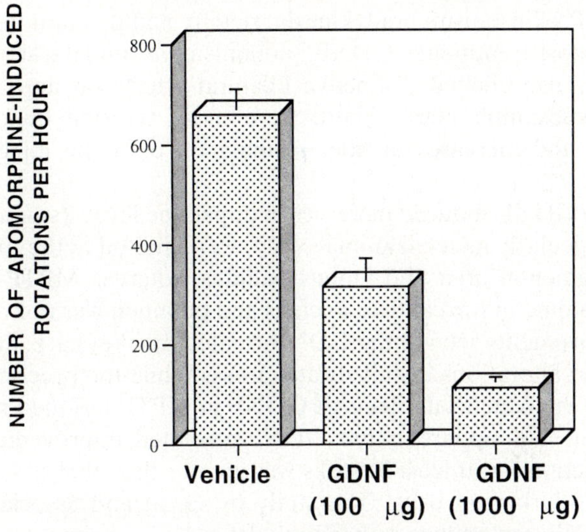

Fig. 5. Rats were lesioned with 6-OHDA and tested for dopamine receptor supersensitivity as measured by apomorphine-induced rotations (0.05 mg/kg) weekly, until a stable lesion was achieved. The rats then received intranigral injections of either vehicle or GDNF (100 μg or 1000 μg). Within 1 week of GDNF injection, a significant ($p < 0.05$) reduction in apomorphine-induced rotations was observed, suggesting a significant improvement of lesion-induced motor deficits. From: LAPCHAK et al. 1996

monitored by in vivo dialysis, and prevention of behavioral deficits (OPACKA-JUFFRY et al. 1995; SHULTS et al. 1996).

Transient reductions of behavioral deficits by GDNF in 6-OHDA-lesioned rats have also been reported in another study, in which GDNF was applied intranigrally or intracerebroventricularly (LAPCHAK et al. 1997). Behavioral improvements of intranigrally injected rats were accompanied by significant increases of nigral, but not striatal, tyrosine hydroxylase activity as well as striatal dynorphin and met-enkephalin, but not substance P levels.

GASH and co-workers (1996) extended the rodent studies to rhesus monkeys with MPTP-induced unilateral Parkinsonism. GDNF, administered by

Fig. 4. Tyrosine hydroxylase (*TH*)-positive immunostaining in normal unlesioned (**A**) and extensively 6-OHDA-lesioned (**C**) rats. 6-OHDA lesions significantly reduce the extent of TH-positive immunostaining in the substantia nigra and produce a behavioral deficit in rats. A single bolus injection of GDNF (100 μg/4 μl) into the substantia nigra upregulates TH expression in normal rats (**B**) 7 days following the injection and induces the re-expression of TH in 6-OHDA lesioned rats (**D**), also 7 days following the injection. *Bars*: 100 μm. From: LAPCHAK et al. 1996

one of the three routes: "intranigral", "intracaudate" or "intracerebroventricular", produced significant functional improvements in three of the cardinal symptoms of Parkinsonism: bradykinesia, rigidity and postural instability, within 2 weeks post-treatment. GDNF, administered unilaterally to the nigra or caudate, also elicited distinctive bilateral effects on dopaminergic neurons in the substantia nigra. There were more tyrosine hydroxylase-positive neurons and increases in fiber staining on both the injected and non-injected side.

Interestingly, GDNF-induced increases in dopamine levels (studied in the intracerebroventricularly injected animals only) were limited to the substantia nigra, ventral tegmental area and globus pallidus, whereas MPTP-induced depletion of dopamine in the caudate nucleus and putamen was not reversed. Behavioral improvements seen in the GDNF-treated monkeys are, therefore, likely to be due to alterations in sub-striatal areas. While the precise mechanisms underlying the beneficial effects of GDNF in MPTP-lesioned monkeys await clarification, it is apparent that GDNF-mediated improvement seen after a single injection for at least 3 weeks was greater than that of levodopa, the standard anti-Parkinson drug. The study by GASH and associates may suggest that GDNF can reduce behavioral deficits in a primate model of Parkinsonism by dopaminergic and non-dopaminergic mechanisms. GDNF, acting by mechanisms not involving striatal dopamine, has also been proposed in a study of rat medial forebrain transection (TSENG et al. 1997).

A recent study has shown that GDNF gene therapy may be profitably exploited to rescue 6-OHDA-lesioned nigral neurons (CHOI-LUNDBERG et al. 1997; see also OLSON 1997). A replication-defective adenoviral vector encoding human GDNF, injected near the rat substantia nigra, protected the majority of nigral neurons, retrogradely labeled from the striatum with fluorogold, that would have been destined to degenerate in control animals. Control animals were injected with an adenoviral lacZ construct or a construct encoding a biologically inactive deletion mutant GNDF. Declining transgene expression was a problem in this, as in other studies, suggesting that a rapid transfer of this method to the bedside is unlikely to occur.

Using encapsulated catecholamine- and GDNF-producing cells, LINDNER et al. (1995) were able to demonstrate protective effects in rats with unilateral dopamine depletions and Parkinsonian symptoms.

c) *Effects in Unlesioned Animals*

Putative functions of GDNF in the unlesioned nigrostriatal system have been addressed in several studies (GASH et al. 1995; MARTIN et al. 1996; LAPCHAK et al. 1996b; cf. Fig. 4). A single intracerebroventricular injection of GDNF (1–100 μg) to normal rats increased monoamine levels in the substantia nigra, striatum, ventral tegmental area, frontal cortex and hypothalamus (MARTIN et al. 1996; LAPCHAK et al. 1996b). Elevation of nigral dopamine persisted for 14 days, whereas dopamine in other areas had returned to control levels by

14 days. However, a single intranigral injection of GDNF stimulated dopamine release from striatal axon terminals at a time point when striatal dopamine levels were unaltered (HEBERT et al. 1996; HUDSON et al. 1995). A series of six intrastriatal injections of GDNF at 0.1, 1.0 or 10 μg/1.5 µl, into normal rats over a course of 2 weeks also increased the size of dopaminergic nerve cell bodies in the substantia nigra and tyrosine hydroxylase-positive axon terminals in the striatum (SHULTS et al. 1996).

When administered bilaterally to the striatum of neonatal rats, GDNF induced a transient behavioral pattern with forelimb hyperflexure, clawed toes of all limbs and a kinked tail (BECK et al. 1996). In parallel, striatal and mesencephalic dopamine and serotonin were increased up to twofold. GDNF also increased tyrosine hydroxylase activity in the mesencephalon floor, but did not alter striatal choline acetyltransferase activity and γ-aminobutyric acid (GABA) uptake. GDNF did not affect sprouting of dopaminergic neurites. Although these data provide evidence for a role of exogenously applied GDNF in the maturation of dopaminergic and serotonergic neurons early after birth, they cannot be interpreted in terms of GDNF having a physiological role in this respect.

Effects of a single injection of 150 µg human recombinant GDNF into the right substantia nigra of adult female rhesus monkeys have been analyzed by GASH and collaborators (1995). While behavioral effects over a 3-week observation period were small, in vivo electrochemical recordings in the ipsilateral caudate and putamen revealed increased potassium-evoked release of dopamine compared with vehicle-treated controls. Dopamine levels in the substantia nigra and ventral tegmental area of GDNF recipients were significantly increased after 3 weeks, suggesting that GDNF administration to the substantia nigra of normal primates clearly affects the transmitter status of the adult dopaminergic nigrostriatal system.

2. Other CNS Aminergic Neurons

Expression of GDNF in several target areas of noradrenergic and serotonergic neurons (ARENAS et al. 1995) suggested that it may also be involved in regulating survival and differentiation of non-dopaminergic neurons. In support of this notion, grafting of genetically engineered fibroblasts expressing high levels of GDNF prevented more than 80% of the 6-OHDA-induced degeneration of noradrenergic neurons in the locus coeruleus in vivo (ARENAS et al. 1995). Moreover, GDNF induced axonal sprouting, tyrosine hydroxylase levels and soma size of lesioned noradrenergic neurons. With regard to serotonergic neurons, injections of GDNF into the unlesioned striatum of neonatal rats increase levels of striatal and ventral mesencephalic serotonin (BECK et al. 1996). Comparing the protective capacity of GDNF on serotonergic and dopaminergic neurons, following methamphetamine lesions, GDNF is apparently selective in protecting dopaminergic neurons (CASS 1996). GFDN also promotes the serotonergic phenotype of neurons cultured from the embryonic rat raphe region in terms of tryptophan hydroxylase expression (GALTER and UNSICKER, unpublished observation).

3. GDNF and Intrinsic Striatal Neurons

In addition to its protective role in vitro and in vivo on dopaminergic nigrostriatal neurons, GDNF has been shown to affect intrinsic striatal parameters. Thus, GDNF can induce the phenotype of a specific subpopulation of intrinsic striatal neurons characterized by the expression of the calcium-binding protein calretinin (FARKAS et al. 1997) and enhance biosynthesis of substance P in striatal neurons in vitro (HUMPEL et al. 1996).

4. Spinal Cord and Brainstem Motoneurons

The survival of developing motoneurons depends on muscle- and CNS-derived trophic factors (OPPENHEIM 1989; HENDERSON et al. 1993). HENDERSON and co-workers were the first to find that GDNF supported the survival of purified embryonic rat motoneurons in culture and prevented losses and degeneration of axotomized facial motoneurons (HENDERSON et al. 1994). Their data were rapidly supplemented by results indicating that GDNF could also rescue developing avian motoneurons from natural programmed cell death in vivo (OPPENHEIM et al. 1995; see also HOUENOU et al. 1996). GDNF is retrogradely transported in motor axons (YAN et al. 1995). Together with its synthesis by myotubes, some striated muscle, Schwann cells (HENDERSON et al. 1994) and cells at the tips of growing motor axons (WRIGHT and SNIDER 1996; see Fig. 6), it is probably safe to conclude that GDNF has a physiological role in the early development of motoneurons. Since sites of GNDF and neurotrophin synthesis are distinct (HENDERSON et al. 1994), it is possible that the actions of GDNF and neurotrophins on developing motoneurons are different. Although GDNF turned out to be only slightly more potent than neurotrophins or CNTF in preventing programmed cell death of avian motoneurons in vivo (25% of the neurons undergoing cell death), it was significantly more potent than neurotrophins or CNTF in vitro.

Several studies suggest a potential for GDNF as a therapeutic agent in motoneuron diseases. In addition to its rescuing effects for developing and neonatal motoneurons (HENDERSON et al. 1994; YAN et al. 1995; MATHESON et al. 1997b), GDNF also partially prevented the loss of adult motoneurons following root avulsion (LI et al. 1995) as well as losses of cholinergic markers in adult axotomized motoneurons (YAN et al. 1995). The rescuing of effects of GNDF on neonatal rat facial motoneurons was also prominent, when an adenoviral vector coding for GNDF was injected into the muscular target areas (GIMENEZ et al. 1997). Studies by ZURN et al. (1994, 1996) suggest that GDNF, because of its synergistic effects with BDNF and CNTF, might be profitably combined with other trophic factors to prevent numerical and cholinergic marker losses of motoneurons. GDNF also improves other functional parameters of injured or aged motoneurons, as indicated by its positive effects

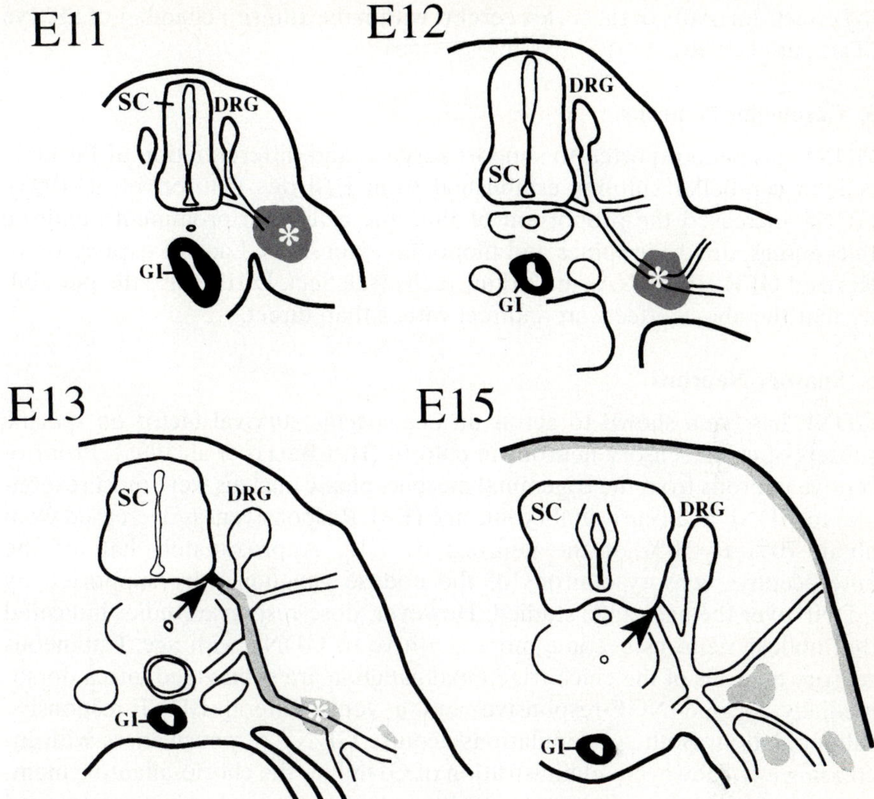

Fig. 6. Schematic diagram summarizing GDNF mRNA expression in relation to growing motor and sensory axons at the level of the forelimb. *Shaded areas* represent GDNF mRNA expression, with *darker areas* illustrating regions with higher levels of GDNF mRNA expression. The focal expression of GDNF in the limb bud (*asterisk*) is robust at E11 and remains so until E13. Sensory and motor axons are visible growing through the region expressing GDNF mRNA. GDNF is also expressed in tissues surrounding the GI tract (*GI*). Cells within the peripheral nerve that express GDNF message were most apparent at E13, particularly in the ventral roots (*arrow*) exiting the spinal cord (*SC*). At E15, GDNF mRNA is expressed in the limb, the dermis, and in a few muscles in the shoulder. DRG, dorsal root ganglion. From: WRIGHT and SNIDER 1996

on conduction velocity of transectioned tibial motor axons (MUNSON and MCMAHON 1997) and improvement of motor coordination in aged rats (BOWENKAMP et al. 1996b; EMERICH et al. 1996). In contrast to CNTF, however, encapsulated GDNF-secreting cells did not increase the life span and reduce motor axon degeneration of mutant mice with progressive motor neuropathy (*pmn*/*pmn*; SAGOT et al. 1996).

Similar to neurotrophin-4 and CNTF, GDNF has also been shown to promote the survival of corticospinal neurons cultured from neonatal rats (JUNGER and VARON 1997), but has been reported to have no survival promoting effects on grafts of rat cortex cerebri within the anterior chamber of the eye (TROK et al. 1996).

5. Cerebellar Neurons

GDNF has been reported to support survival and differentiation of Purkinje cells in cerebellar cultures established from E18 rats (MOUNT et al. 1995). GDNF increased the proportion of Purkinje cells with prominent dendritic thickenings, dendritic spines and filopodial extensions. Lack of expression of Ret and GFR-α1 mRNAs in Purkinje cells (see Sect. D.III) raise the possibility that the above effects are indirect rather than direct.

6. Sensory Neurons

GDNF has been shown to act as an age-specific survival factor on specific subsets of chick sensory neurons in culture (BUJ-BELLO et al. 1995). Proprioceptive neurons from the trigeminal mesencephalic nucleus were most responsive to GDNF at an early embryonic age (E8). Responsiveness decreased from about 70% to 50% of the neurons by E12. Approximately half of the enteroceptive sensory neurons of the nodose ganglion were supported by GDNF over the age range studied. However, dose-response studies indicated that nodose neurons become more sensitive to GDNF with age. Cutaneous sensory neurons of the chick trigeminal ganglion are subdivided into a dorsomedially located NGF-responsive and a ventro-lateral BDNF-responsive subpopulation. Both subpopulations acquire GDNF responsiveness with increasing age. However, administration of GDNF to the chorio-allantoic membrane in chick embryos augmented neither the numbers of sensory trigeminal nor nodose neurons (OPPENHEIM et al. 1995).

GDNF has also been shown to have a small survival promoting effect on dorsal root ganglionic neurons cultured from neonatal rats (MATHESON et al. 1997a). GDNF also rescued almost all dorsal root ganglionic neurons following transection of the sciatic nerve in neonatal rats. A very recent study (MOLLIVER et al. 1997) has provided evidence that a group of putatively nociceptive dorsal root ganglionic neurons in rat, characterized by binding of the plant lectin IB4 which downregulates the NGF receptor trkA after birth, initiates Ret expression between E15.5 and postnatal day 7.5 and maintains Ret expression into adulthood. These sensory neurons also express GFR-α1 and retrogradely transport ^{125}I-GNDF. In vitro, GDNF supports the survival of *Ret+/trkA*$^{-}$ neurons, suggesting that one subpopulation of rat dorsal root ganglionic neurons switches from NGF to GDNF dependence in early postnatal life.

7. Autonomic Neurons

Initial studies had reported no or only low activity of GDNF on dissociated rat sympathetic neurons (HENDERSON et al. 1994; TRUPP et al. 1995). Even so, GDNF applied to sympathetic and parasympathetic chick ganglia embedded in collagen gel produced marked neurite outgrowth (EBENDAL et al. 1995), suggesting that GDNF actions in these systems may require co-trophic factors.

Age-specific survival effects of GDNF on cultured chick sympathetic and parasympathetic neurons were reported by BUJ-BELLO et al. (1995). Both sympathetic and parasympathetic neurons become less responsive to GDNF with age. Half-maximally effective doses for ciliary ganglionic neurons increased 10-fold from 0.8 ng/ml to 8 ng/ml between E6 and E12. With sympathetic neurons, the EC50 increased approximately twofold, from 2.6 ng/ml at E10 to 5.7 ng/ml at E14. Although saturating levels of GDNF were as effective as NGF in promoting survival of sympathetic neurons, GDNF was less potent than NGF. The EC50 for E12 sympathetic neurons responding to GNDF (3.4 ng/ml) was more than two orders of magnitude greater than the EC50 for E12 sympathetic neurons (0.02 ng/ml) responding to NGF. In agreement with the observation that GDNF increases the in vitro survival of embryonic chick sympathetic neurons, administration of GDNF to the chorio-allantoic membrane of chick embryos resulted in significantly higher numbers of neurons in sympathetic ganglia than in control embryos (OPPENHEIM et al. 1995). However, no significant increases in ciliary neurons were observed in GDNF-treated embryos.

8. Neural Crest

Growth of mouse neural-crest cell cultures, in the presence of GDNF, has been shown to result in a dramatic increase in the number of tyrosine hydroxylase-positive cells with neuronal morphologies (MAXWELL et al. 1996). The effects were specific in that several BMPs and TGF-βs did not induce tyrosine hydroxylase-positive cells. However, NT-3 and FGF-2 elicited increases in the number of immunoreactive cells, similar to that seen in response to GDNF. The inductive effect of GDNF on neural crest cells generating adrenergic neurons, in vitro, may reflect a physiological function of GNDF in vivo since subpopulations of noradrenergic neurons and neuroendocrine cells are affected in GDNF- or Ret-deficient mice (see Sect. F below).

9. GDNF in CNS Lesion Models Other Than Parkinsonism

The cholinergic septohippocampal projection through the fimbria/fornix is of particular neurological interest, because cholinergic deficits are a hallmark of Alzheimer's disease and other memory dysfunctions. Unilateral knife transection of the fimbria/fornix causes a 70% loss of choline acetyltransferase-positive neurons and a reduction of p75-immunoreactive cells in the medial septum. Losses of phenotypic markers are associated with atrophy and shrinkage. GDNF, applied at 10 μg/day, completely prevented the loss of p75-positive neurons and significantly reduced the loss of choline acetyltransferase-positive neurons (WILLIAMS et al. 1996; LAPCHAK et al. 1996b). GDNF is one order of magnitude less potent than NGF, but one order of magnitude more potent than BDNF.

Upregulation of GDNF mRNA in kainate-induced excitation (HUMPEL et al. 1994) and after pilocarpine-induced status epilepticus (SCHMIDT-KASTNER et al. 1994) suggested physiological roles of GDNF in the protection against neurotoxic damage. In support of this notion, GDNF injected intracerebroventricularly suppressed kainic acid-induced seizure activity as well as the associated neuronal cell loss in hippocampal, thalamic and amygdala regions (MARTIN et al. 1995).

Both intracerebroventricular and intraparenchymal administration of GDNF protect cerebral hemispheres from damage induced by transient middle cerebral artery occlusion (WANG et al. 1997). GDNF also blocks the elevation of NO that accompanies arterial occlusion and reperfusion, and may therefore become important in the treatment of cerebrovascular occlusive disease.

II. Neurturin

The spectrum of neuron populations that respond to neurturin is only beginning to emerge. Sympathetic neurons from the rat superior cervical ganglion were used for monitoring the purification of neurturin (KOTZBAUER et al. 1996). The neurturin effect requires priming sympathetic neurons by NGF, suggesting that neurturin belongs to a category of neurotrophic factors that are not only molecularly, but conceptually distinct from neurotrophins. In addition to sympathetic neurons, neurturin has been reported to support the survival of motoneurons, nodose, dorsal root ganglionic and dopaminergic midbrain neurons (KOTZBAUER et al. 1996).

F. Developmental Roles of GDNF, Neurturin and Their Receptors As Revealed by Gene Targeting

I. Glial Cell Line-Derived Neurotrophic Factor

GDNF-deficient mice have simultaneously been generated in three laboratories (SANCHEZ et al. 1996; PICHEL et al. 1996; MOORE et al. 1996), with the following phenotypic features: GDNF−/− animals display kidney agenesis as a major deficit outside the nervous system. Surprisingly, the number of TH-immunoreactivie neurons in the substantia nigra and the density of dopaminergic nerve terminals in the striatum were identical in GDNF −/− and wild-type mice. In addition, there were no apparent nigrostriatal deficits in heterozygous GDNF knockouts examined at postnatal day 42 (MOORE et al. 1996). Maturation of the dopaminergic nigrostriatal projection both prior to and after birth, including a second wave of ontogenetic neuron death after birth are well documented (OO and BURKE 1997). Analysis of GDNF-deficient mice, therefore, suggests that GDNF is not a major survival or neurite promoting factor for prenatal dopaminergic neurons, but may be more important in postnatal maturation of the system. Neurons in the locus coeruleus which also respond to GDNF in vitro and in vivo were not altered in GDNF-deficient mice in terms of neuron number. However, their packing density was clearly decreased (GRANHOLM et al. 1997).

Whereas the number of facial motoneurons of GDNF −/− mice at birth was unaltered compared with wild-type mice, there was a small, yet significant, deficit in the number of lumbar motoneurons (−21%, MOORE et al. 1996; −31%, PICHEL et al. 1996) and trigeminal motoneurons (PICHEL et al. 1996). Numbers of trigeminal sensory neurons, nodose-petrosal (−40%) and dorsal root ganglionic neurons (−23%) were also reduced in number (PICHEL et al. 1996; MOORE et al. 1996). Superior cervical ganglionic neurons showed a numerical reduction by 35% (MOORE et al. 1996), whereas other paravertebral sympathetic neurons were apparently unaltered. Remaining neurons in the superior cervical ganglion exhibited decreased levels of TH immunoreactivity (GRANHOLM et al. 1997). Moreover, the sympathetic innervation of blood vessels and glands in the head was significantly decreased.

Consistent with the observation that GDNF mRNA is abundantly expressed in the muscle layers of the intestine during embryogenesis (HELLMICH et al. 1996), neurons in the Meissner and Auerbach plexus, at the levels of the small and large intestine, that are colonized by vagal neural-crest-derived cells were completely absent in GDNF −/− mice except for a few neurons in the stomach (MOORE et al. 1996; SANCHEZ et al. 1996; PICHEL et al. 1996). Whether these data indicate that GDNF directs commitment, migration or survival of enteric neuronal precursor cells remains to be examined.

II. Ret

Similar to GDNF-deficient mice, in the case of Ret-kinase null mice, metanephric kidneys are absent. The enteric nervous system is completely lacking from levels below the esophagus and stomach (SCHUCHARDT et al. 1994, 1996; DURBEC et al. 1996b). In contrast to the GDNF knockout, enteric precursors of Ret-deficient mice are able to survive and differentiate. The superior cervical sympathetic neurons, which are partly affected in GDNF-deficient mice, are entirely absent in mice lacking Ret, although neural crest cells migrate to the position of the ganglion to form its anlage (DURBEC et al. 1996b). Interestingly, precursors of the superior cervical ganglion can be mapped to the vagal region of the neural tube (DURBEC et al. 1996b), i.e., the same region from which the majority of enteric nervous system precursors are derived.

III. Neurturin

Neurturin-deficient mice have been generated recently, but their phenotype has only been published in abstract form (HEUCKEROTH et al. 1997). Unlike mice lacking GDNF, neurturin −/− mice have normal kidneys and an intact enteric nervous system.

G. Perspectives

I. Clinical Relevance

At present, it seems unlikely that GDNF will soon make the jump from bench to bedside. There are no reports as yet indicating that any clinical trial with GDNF, in particular its application in patients with Parkinson's disease, has been or is about to become successful. For those who have been working in the field of TGF-βs, the apparent mismatch of expectations and apparent therapeutic failure of GDNF may not come as a surprise. TGF-βs, much unlike neurotrophins (as they are commonly thought of), are not only multifunctional, but, first of all, contextually acting growth factors (Sporn and Roberts, 1990), and GDNF may not be an exception in this regard. Responses elicited by TGF-βs are significantly influenced by the simultaneous presence of other cytokines that may activate additional signaling pathways or influence receptor components. The recent discovery of Smad as a common component in the BMP and EGF signaling pathways underscores this point (KRETZSCHMAR et al. 1997).

Although GDNF has shown its efficiency in a number of animal models of Parkinsonism, underlying mechanisms have not been fully elucidated. There is sufficient evidence to suggest that both direct and indirect actions on the dopaminergic system account for the efficacy of GDNF. Even more importantly, a major discrepancy in the pathophysiology of human Parkinsonism and an animal lesion model of Parkinsonism probably resides in trauma-associated alterations in the expression of cytokines within the nigrostriatal system after an acute versus a chronic lesion. Upregulation of endogenous cytokines that may potentially synergize with exogenously applied GDNF in animal models of Parkinsonism has not been seriously considered as an explanation for the beneficial effects of GDNF in animal models. It is, therefore, safe to assume that the success of GDNF as a future therapeutic agent is likely to depend on a thorough analysis of potential co-trophic agents of GDNF.

II. Neurobiological Relevance

As with many other neurotrophic molecules, *physiological* functions of GDNF in the adult nervous system are still far from being understood. Most of the current knowledge concerns roles of GDNF in development or in lesion and cell culture paradigms as deduced from transgenic animal analyses and pharmacological effects. Conditional knockouts will provide a major step towards the goal of understanding physiological roles of GDNF in the adult animal. In addition, perturbation experiments using neutralizing antibodies and antisense constructs will help to further clarify functions of endogenous GDNF, neurturin, persephin and other GDNF family members that might emerge in the future.

References

Arenas E, Trupp M, Akerud P, Ibanez CF (1995) GDNF prevents degeneration and promotes the phenotype of brain noradrenergic neurons in vivo. Neuron 15:1465–1473

Avantaggiato V, Dathan NA, Grieco M, Fabien N, Lazzaro D, Fusco A, Simeone A, Santoro M (1994) Developmental expression of the RET protooncogene. Cell Growth Differ 5:305–311

Baloh RH, Tansey MG, Golden JP, Creedon DJ, Heuckeroth RO, Keck CL, Zimonjic DB, Popescu NC, Johnson EM, Jr., Milbrandt J (1997) TrnR2, a novel receptor that mediates neurturin and GDNF signaling through Ret. Neuron 18:793–802

Bar KJ, Facer P, Williams NS, Tam PK, Anand P (1997) Glial-derived neurotrophic factor in human adult and fetal intestine and in Hirschsprung's disease. Gastroenterology 112:1381–1385

Barnard JA, Lyons RM, Moses HL (1990) The cell biology of transforming growth factor beta. Biochim Biophys Acta 1032:79–87

Beck KD, Valverde J, Alexi T, Poulsen K, Moffat B, Vandlen RA, Rosenthal A, Hefti F (1995) Mesencephalic dopaminergic neurons protected by GDNF from axotomy-induced degeneration in the adult brain. Nature 373:339–341

Beck KD, Irwin I, Valverde J, Brennan TJ, Langston JW, Hefti F (1996) GDNF induces a dystonia-like state in neonatal rats and stimulates dopamine and serotonin synthesis. Neuron 16:665–673

Bermingham N, Hillermann R, Gilmour F, Martin JE, Fisher EM (1995) Human glial cell line-derived neurotrophic factor (GDNF) maps to chromosome 5. Hum Genet 96:671–673

Blum M, Weickert CS (1995) GDNF mRNA expression in normal postnatal development, aging, and in Weaver mutant mice. Neurobiol Aging 16:925–929

Bowenkamp KE, Hoffman AF, Gerhardt GA, Henry MA, Biddle PT, Hoffer BJ, Granholm AC (1995) Glial cell line-derived neurotrophic factor supports survival of injured midbrain dopaminergic neurons. J Comp Neurol 355:479–489

Bowenkamp KE, David D, Lapchak PL, Henry MA, Granholm AC, Hoffer BJ, Mahalik TJ (1996a) 6-hydroxydopamine induces the loss of the dopaminergic phenotype in substantia nigra neurons of the rat. A possible mechanism for restoration of the nigrostriatal circuit mediated by glial cell line-derived neurotrophic factor. Exp Brain Res 111:1–7

Bowenkamp KE, Lapchak PA, Hoffer BJ, Bickford PC (1996b) Glial cell line-derived neurotrophic factor reverses motor impairment in 16–17 month old rats. Neurosci Lett 211:81–84

Bowenkamp KE, Lapchak PA, Hoffer BJ, Miller PJ, Bickford PC (1997) Intracerebroventricular glial cell line-derived neurotrophic factor improves motor function and supports nigrostriatal dopamine neurons in bilaterally 6-hydroxydopamine lesioned rats. Exp Neurol 145:104–117

Buj-Bello A, Buchman VL, Horton A, Rosenthal A, Davies AM (1995) GDNF is an age-specific survival factor for sensory and autonomic neurons. Neuron 15:821–828

Buj-Bello A, Adu J, Pinon LG, Horton A, Thompson J, Rosenthal A, Chinchetru M, Buchman VL, Davies AM (1997) Neurturin responsiveness requires a GPI-linked receptor and the Ret receptor tyrosine kinase. Nature 387:721–724

Carlson KM, Dou S, Chi D, Scavarda N, Toshima K, Jackson CE, Wells SA, Jr., Goodfellow PJ, Donis Keller H (1994) Single missense mutation in the tyrosine kinase catalytic domain of the RET protooncogene is associated with multiple endocrine neoplasia type 2B. Proc Natl Acad Sci USA 91:1579–1583

Cass WA (1996) GDNF selectively protects dopamine neurons over serotonin neurons against the neurotoxic effects of methamphetamine. J Neurosci 16:8132–8139

Ceccherini I, Bocciardi R, Luo Y, Pasini B, Hofstra R, Takahashi M, Romeo G (1993) Exon structure and flanking intronic sequences of the human RET proto-oncogene. Biochem Biophys Res Commun 196:1288–1295

Cheng H, Hoffer B, Strömberg I, Russell D, Olson L (1995) The effect of glial cell line-derived neurotrophic factor in fibrin glue on developing dopamine neurons. Exp Brain Res 104:199–206

Choi-Lundberg DL, Bohn MC (1995) Ontogeny and distribution of glial cell line-derived neurotrophic factor (GDNF) mRNA in rat. Brain Res Dev Brain Res 85:80–88

Choi-Lundberg DL, Lin Q, Chang YN, Chiang YL, Hay CM, Mohajeri H, Davidson BL, Bohn MC (1997) Dopaminergic neurons protected from degeneration by GDNF gene therapy. Science 275:838–841

Creedon DJ, Tansey MG, Baloh RH, Osborne PA, Lampe PA, Fahrner TJ, Heuckeroth RO, Milbrandt J, Johnson EM, Jr. (1997) Neurturin shares receptors and signal transduction pathways with glial cell line-derived neurotrophic factor in sympathetic neurons. Proc Natl Acad Sci USA 94:7018–7023

Cristina N, Chatellard-Causse C, Manier M, Feuerstein C (1995) GDNF: existance of a second transcript in the brain. Brain Res Mol Brain Res 32:354–357

Davies AM, Dixon JE, Fox GM, Ibanez CF, Jing SQ, Johnson E, Milbrandt J, Phillips H, Rosenthal A, Saarma M, Sanicola M, Treanor J, Vega QC (1997) Nomenclature of GPI-linked receptors for the GDNF ligand family. Neuron 19:485

Davis S, Aldrich TH, Stahl N, Pan L, Taga T, Kishimoto T, Ip NY, Yancopoulos GD (1993) LIFR beta and gp130 as heterodimerizing signal transducers of the tripartite CNTF receptor. Science 260:1805–1808

Durbec P, Marcos Gutierrez CV, Kilkenny C, Grigoriou M, Wartiowaara K, Suvanto P, Smith D, Ponder B, Costantini F, Saarma M, Sariola H, Pachnis V (1996a) GDNF signalling through the Ret receptor tyrosine kinase. Nature 381:789–793

Durbec PL, Larsson Blomberg LB, Schuchardt A, Costantini F, Pachnis V (1996b) Common origin and developmental dependence on c-ret of subsets of enteric and sympathetic neuroblasts. Development 122:349–358

Ebendal T, Tomac A, Hoffer BJ, Olson L (1995) Glial cell line-derived neurotrophic factor stimulates fiber formation and survival in cultured neurons from peripheral autonomic ganglia. J Neurosci Res 40:276–284

Edery P, Pelet A, Mulligan LM, Abel L, Attie T, Dow E, Bonneau D, David A, Flintoff W, Jan D et al. (1994) Long segment and short segment familial Hirschsprung's disease: variable clinical expression at the RET locus. J Med Genet 31:602–606

Ehrhard PB, Ganter U, Stadler A, Bauer J, Otten U (1993) Expression of functional trk protooncogene in human monocytes. Proc Natl Acad Sci USA 90:5423–5427

Eigenbrot C, Gerber N (1997) X-ray structure of glial cell-derived neurotrophic factor at 1.9 A resolution and implications for receptor binding. Nat Struct Biol 4:435–438

Emerich DF, Plone M, Francis J, Frydel BR, Winn SR, Lindner MD (1996) Alleviation of behavioral deficits in aged rodents following implantation of encapsulated GDNF-producing fibroblasts. Brain Res 736:99–110

Engele J, Bohn MC (1991) The neurotrophic effects of fibroblast growth factors on dopaminergic neurons in vitro are mediated by mesencephalic glia. J Neurosci 11:3070–3078

Engele J, Franke B (1996) Effects of glial cell line-derived neurotrophic factor (GDNF) on dopaminergic neurons require concurrent activation of cAMP-dependent signaling pathways. Cell Tissue Res 286:235–240

Farkas LM, Suter-Crazzolara C, Unsicker K (1997) GDNF induces the calretinin phenotype in cultures of embryonic striatal neurons. J Neurosci Res 50:361–372

Ferrari G, Minozzi M-C, Toffano G, Leon A, Skaper AD (1989) Basic fibroblast growth factor promotes the survival and development of mesencephalic neurons in culture. Dev Biol 133:140–147

Flanders KC, Lüdecke G, Engels S, Cissel DS, Roberts AB, Kondaiah P, Lafyatis R, Sporn MB, Unsicker K (1991) Immunhistochemical localization of transforming growth factor-βs in the nervous system of the mouse embryo. Development 113:183–191

Frade JM, Rodriguez-Tebar A, Barde YA (1996) Induction of cell death by endogenous nerve growth factor through its p75 receptor. Nature 383:166–168

Gash DM, Zhang Z, Cass WA, Ovadia A, Simmerman L, Martin D, Russell D, Collins F, Hoffer BJ, Gerhardt GA (1995) Morphological and functional effects of intranigrally administered GDNF in normal rhesus monkeys. J Comp Neurol 363:345–358

Gash DM, Zhang Z, Ovadia A, Cass WA, Yi A, Simmerman L, Russell D, Martin D, Lapchak PA, Collins F, Hoffer BJ, Gerhardt GA (1996) Functional recovery in parkinsonian monkeys treated with GDNF. Nature 380:252–255

Gimenez Y, Revah F, Pradier L, Loquet I, Mallet J, Privat A (1997) Prevention of motoneuron death by adenovirus-mediated neurotrophic factors. J Neurosci Res 48:281–285

Granholm AC, Srivastava N, Mott JL, Henry S, Henry M, Westphal H, Pichel JG, Shen L, Hoffer BJ (1997) Morphological alterations in the peripheral and central nervous systems of mice lacking glial cell line-derived neurotrophic factor (GDNF): immunohistochemical studies. J Neurosci 17:1168–1178

Haniu M, Hui J, Young Y, Le J, Katta V, Lee R, Shimamoto G, Rohde MF (1996) Glial cell line-derived neurotrophic factor: selective reduction of the intermolecular disulfide linkage and characterization of its disulfide structure. Biochemistry 35:16799–16805

Hebert MA, Van Horne CG, Hoffer BJ, Gerhardt GA (1996) Functional effects of GDNF in normal rat striatum: presynaptic studies using in vivo electrochemistry and microdialysis. J Pharmacol Exp Ther 279:1181–1190

Heller A, Price S, Won L (1996) Glial-derived neurotrophic factor (GDNF) induced morphological differentiation of an immortalized monoclonal hybrid dopaminergic cell line of mesencephalic neuronal origin. Brain Res 725:132–136

Hellmich HL, Kos L, Cho ES, Mahon KA, Zimmer A (1996) Embryonic expression of glial cell-line derived neurotrophic factor (GDNF) suggests multiple developmental roles in neural differentiation and epithelial-mesenchymal interactions. Mech Dev 54:95–105

Henderson CE, Bloch-Gallego E, Camu W, Gouin A, Mettling C (1993) Restorative Neurol Neurosci 5:15

Henderson CE, Phillips HS, Pollock RA, Davies AM, Lemeulle C, Armanini M, Simmons L, Moffet B, Vandlen RA, Simpson LC, Moffet B, Vandlen RA, Koliatsos VE, Rosenthal A (1994) GDNF: a potent survival factor for motoneurons present in peripheral nerve and muscle. Science 266:1062–1064

Heuckeroth RO, Tourtellotte L, Gavrilina G, Johnson E, Milbrandt J (1997) Characterization of the neurturin knockout mouse. Soc Neurosci Abstr 23:1704

Ho A, Gore AC, Weickert CS, Blum M (1995) Glutamate regulation of GDNF gene expression in the striatum and primary striatal astrocytes. Neuroreport 6:1454–1458

Hoffer BJ, Hoffman A, Bowenkamp K, Huettl P, Hudson J, Martin D, Lin LF, Gerhardt GA (1994) Glial cell line-derived neurotrophic factor reverses toxin-induced injury to midbrain dopaminergic neurons in vivo. Neurosci Lett 182:107–111

Hofstra RM, Landsvater RM, Ceccherini I, Stulp RP, Stelwagen T, Luo Y, Pasini B, Hoppener JW, van Amstel HK, Romeo G et al. (1994) A mutation in the RET proto-oncogene associated with multiple endocrine neoplasia type 2B and sporadic medullary thyroid carcinoma. Nature 367:375–376

Hogan BL (1996) Bone morphogenetic proteins: multifunctional regulators of vertebrate development. Genes Dev 10:1580–1594

Hou JG, Lin LF, Mytilineou C (1996) Glial cell line-derived neurotrophic factor exerts neurotrophic effects on dopaminergic neurons in vitro and promotes their survival and regrowth after damage by 1-methyl-4-phenylpyridinium. J Neurochem 66:74–82

Houenou LJ, Oppenheim RW, Li L, Lo AC, Prevette D (1996) Regulation of spinal motoneuron survival by GDNF during development and following injury. Cell Tissue Res 286:219–223

Hudson J, Granholm AC, Gerhardt GA, Henry MA, Hoffman A, Biddle P, Leela NS, Mackerlova L, Lile JD, Collins F, Hoffer BJ (1995) Glial cell line-derived neurotrophic factor augments midbrain dopaminergic circuits in vivo. Brain Res Bull 36:425–432

Humpel C, Hoffer B, Strömberg I, Bektesh S, Collins F, Olson L (1994) Neurons of the hippocampal formation express glial cell line-derived neurotrophic factor messenger RNA in response to kainate-induced excitation. Neuroscience 59:791–795

Humpel C, Marksteiner J, Saria A (1996) Glial-cell-line-derived neurotrophic factor enhances biosynthesis of substance P in striatal neurons in vitro. Cell Tissue Res 286:249–255

Hunot S, Bernard V, Faucheux B, Boissiere F, Leguern E, Brana C, Gautris PP, Guerin J, Bloch B, Agid Y, Hirsch EC (1996) Glial cell line-derived neurotrophic factor (GDNF) gene expression in the human brain: a post mortem in situ hybridization study with special reference to Parkinson's disease. J Neural Transm 103:1043–1052

Hyman C, Hofer M, Barde Y-A, Juhasz M, Yancopoulos GD, Squinto SP, Lindsay RM (1991) BDNF is a neurotrophic factor for dopaminergic neurons of the substantia nigra. Nature 350:230–232

Ivanchuk SM, Myers SM, Eng C, Mulligan LM (1996) De novo mutation of GDNF, ligand for the RET/GDNFR-alpha receptor complex, in Hirschsprung's disease. Hum Mol Genet 5:2023–2026

Iwamoto T, Taniguchi M, Asai N, Ohkusu K, Nakashima I, Takahashi M (1993) cDNA cloning of mouse ret proto-oncogene and its sequence similarity to the cadherin superfamily. Oncogene 8:1087–1091

Jing S, Wen D, Yu Y, Holst PL, Luo Y, Fang M, Tamir R, Antonio L, Hu Z, Cupples R, Louis JC, Hu S, Altrock BW, Fox GM (1996) GDNF-induced activation of the ret protein tyrosine kinase is mediated by GDNFR-alpha, a novel receptor for GDNF. Cell 85:1113–1124

Johansson M, Friedemann M, Hoffer B, Strömberg I (1995) Effects of glial cell line-derived neurotrophic factor on developing and mature ventral mesencephalic grafts in oculo. Exp Neurol 134:25–34

Jordan J, Böttner J, M, Schluesener H, Unsicker K, Krieglstein K (1997) Bone Morphogenetic Proteins: Neurotrophic roles for midbrain dopaminergic neurons and implications of astroglial cells. Eur J Neurosci 9:1699–1710

Josso N, di Clemente N (1997) Serine/threonine kinase receptors and ligands. Curr Opin Genet Dev 7:371–377

Junger H, Varon S (1997) Neurotrophin-4 (NT-4) and glial cell line-derived neurotrophic factor (GDNF) promote the survival of corticospinal motor neurons of neonatal rats in vitro. Brain Res 762:56–60

Kearns CM, Gash DM (1995) GDNF protects nigral dopamine neurons against 6-hydroxydopamine in vivo. Brain Res 672:104–111

Kingsley DM (1994) The TGF-β superfamily: new members, new receptors, and new genetic tests of function in different organisms. Genes Dev 8:133–146

Klein RD, Sherman D, Ho WH, Stone D, Bennett GL, Moffat B, Vandlen R, Simmons L, Gu Q, Hongo JA, Devaux B, Poulsen K, Armanini M, Nozaki C, Asai N, Goddard A, Phillips H, Henderson CE, Takahashi M, Rosenthal A (1997) A GPI-linked protein that interacts with Ret to form a candidate neurturin receptor. Nature 387:717–721

Kotzbauer PT, Lampe PA, Heuckeroth RO, Golden JP, Creedon DJ, Johnson EM, Jr., Milbrandt J (1996) Neurturin, a relative of glial-cell-line-derived neurotrophic factor. Nature 384:467–470

Kretzschmar M, Doody J, Massague J (1997) Opposing BMP and EGF signalling pathways converge on the TGF-β family mediator Smad1. Nature 389:618–622

Krieglstein K, Unsicker K (1994) Transforming growth factor-β promotes survival of midbrain dopaminergic neurons and protects them against N-methyl-4-phenylpyridinium ion toxicity. Neuroscience 63:1189–1196

Krieglstein K, Rufer M, Suter-Crazzolara C, Unsicker K (1995a) Neural functions of the transforming growth factor b. Int J Dev Neurosci 13:301–315

Krieglstein K, Suter Crazzolara C, Fischer WH, Unsicker K (1995b) TGF-beta superfamily members promote survival of midbrain dopaminergic neurons and protect them against MPP+ toxicity. EMBO J 14:736–742

Krieglstein K, Suter Crazzolara C, Hotten G, Pohl J, Unsicker K (1995c) Trophic and protective effects of growth/differentiation factor 5, a member of the transforming growth factor-beta superfamily, on midbrain dopaminergic neurons. J Neurosci Res 42:724–732

Krieglstein K, Deimling F, Suter Crazzolara C, Unsicker K (1996) Expression and localization of GDNF in developing and adult adrenal chromaffin cells. Cell Tissue Res 286:263–268

Kuma K, Iwabe N, Miyata T (1993) Motifs of cadherin- and fibronectin type III-related sequences and evolution of the receptor-type-protein tyrosine kinases: sequence similarity between proto-oncogene ret and cadherin family. Mol Biol Evol 10:539–551

Kwok JB, Gardner E, Warner JP, Ponder BA, Mulligan LM (1993) Structural analysis of the human ret proto-oncogene using exon trapping. Oncogene 8:2575–2582

Lampe PA, Leitner ML, Golden JP, Milbrandt JD, Johnson EM Jr (1997) Members of TRN (TGF-β related neurotrophic factors) family promote survival of mesencephalic neurons. Soc Neurosci Abstr 23:625

Lapchak PA, Jiao S, Miller PJ, Williams LR, Cummins V, Inouye G, Matheson CR, Yan Q (1996a) Pharmacological characterization of glial cell line-derived neurotrophic factor (GDNF): implications for GDNF as a therapeutic molecule for treating neurodegenerative diseases. Cell Tissue Res 286:179–189

Lapchak PA, Miller PJ, Jiao S, Araujo DM, Hilt D, Collins F (1996b) Biology of glial cell line-derived neurotrophic factor (GDNF): implications for the use of GDNF to treat Parkinson's disease. Neurodegeneration 5:197–205

Lapchak PA, Jiao S, Collins F, Miller PJ (1997) Glial cell line-derived neurotrophic factor: distribution and pharmacology in the rat following a bolus intraventricular injection. Brain Res 747:92–102

Levi-Montalcini R (1987) The nerve growth factor 35 years later. Science 237:1154–1162

Li L, Wu W, Lin LF, Lei M, Oppenheim RW, Houenou LJ (1995) Rescue of adult mouse motoneurons from injury-induced cell death by glial cell line-derived neurotrophic factor. Proc Natl Acad Sci USA 92:9771–9775

Lin LF, Doherty DH, Lile JD, Bektesh S, Collins F (1993) GDNF: a glial cell line-derived neurotrophic factor for midbrain dopaminergic neurons. Science 260:1130–1132

Lin LF, Zhang TJ, Collins F, Armes LG (1994) Purification and initial characterization of rat B49 glial cell line-derived neurotrophic factor. J Neurochem 63:758–768

Lindner MD, Winn SR, Baetge EE, Hammang JP, Gentile FT, Doherty E, McDermott PE, Frydel B, Ullman MD, Schallert T et al. (1995) Implantation of encapsulated catecholamin and GDNF-producing cells in rats with unilateral dopamine depletions and parkinsonian symptomms. Exp Neurol 132:62–76

Lindsay RM, Yancopoulos GD (1996) GDNF in a bind with known orphan: accessory implicated in new twist. Neuron 17:571–574

Lo L, Anderson DJ (1995) Postmigratory neural crest cells expressing c-RET display restricted developmental and proliferative capacities. Neuron 15:527–539

Lu B, Ni J, Jiang H, Hsu TA, Dugich-Djordjevic M, Feng L, Zhang M, Mei L, Gentz R (1998) Cloning and characterization of glial cell line-derived neurotrophic factor receptor-B: a novel receptor for members of glial cell line-derived neurotrophic factor family of neurotrophic factors Neurosci 83:7–14

Luukko K, Suvanto P, Saarma M, Thesleff I (1997) Expression of GDNF and its receptors in developing tooth is developmentally regulated and suggests multiple roles in innervation and organogenesis. Dev Dyn 210:463–471

Marcos Gutierrez CV, Wilson SW, Holder N, Pachnis V (1997) The zebrafish homologue of the ret receptor and its pattern of expression during embryogenesis. Oncogene 14:879–889

Martin D, Miller G, Rosendahl M, Russell DA (1995) Potent inhibitory effects of glial derived neurotrophic factor against kainic acid mediated seizures in the rat. Brain Res 683:172–178

Martin D, Miller G, Cullen T, Fischer N, Dix D, Russell D (1996) Intranigral or intrastriatal injections of GDNF: effects on monoamine levels and behavior in rats. Eur J Pharmacol 317:247–256

Mason I (1996) The GDNF receptor: recent progress and unanswered questions. Mol Cell Neurosci 8:112–119

Massague J (1990) The transforming growth factor-beta family. Annu Rev Cell Biol 6:597–641

Matheson CR, Carnahan J, Urich JL, Bocangel D, Zhang TJ, Yan Q (1997a) Glial cell line-derived neurotrophic factor (GDNF) is a neurotrophic factor for sensory neurons: comparison with the effects of the neurotrophins. J Neurobiol 32:22–32

Matheson CR, Wang J, Collins FD, Yan Q (1997b) Long-term survival effects of GDNF on neonatal rat facial motoneurons after axotomy. Neuroreport 8:1739–1742

Maxwell GD, Reid K, Elefanty A, Bartlett PF, Murphy M (1996) Glial cell line-derived neurotrophic factor promotes the development of adrenergic neurons in mouse neural crest cultures. Proc Natl Acad Sci USA 93:13274–13279

McDonald NQ, Hendrickson WA (1993) A structural superfamily of growth factors containing a cystine knot motif. Cell 73:421–424

Mehler MF, Mabie PC, Zhang D, Kessler JA (1997) Bone morphogenetic proteins in the nervous system. Trends Neurosci 20:309–317

Molliver DC, Wright DE, Leitner ML, Parsadanian AS, Doster K, Wen D, Yan Q, Snider WD (1997) IB4-binding DRG neurons switch from NGF to GDNF dependence in early postnatal life. Neuron 19:849–861

Moore MW, Klein RD, Farinas I, Sauer H, Armanini M, Phillips H, Reichardt LF, Ryan AM, Carver Moore K, Rosenthal A (1996) Renal and neuronal abnormalities in mice lacking GDNF. Nature 382:76–79

Moretto G, Walker DG, Lanteri P, Taioli F, Zaffagnini S, Xu RY, Rizzuto N (1996) Expression and regulation of glial-cell-line-derived neurotrophic factor (GDNF) mRNA in human astrocytes in vitro. Cell Tissue Res 286:257–262

Mount HT, Dean DO, Alberch J, Dreyfus CF, Black IB (1995) Glial cell line-derived neurotrophic factor promotes the survival and morphologic differentiation of Purkinje cells. Proc Natl Acad Sci USA 92:9092–9096

Mulligan LM, Kwok JB, Healey CS, Elsdon MJ, Eng C, Gardner E, Love DR, Cole SE, Moore JK, Papi L, et al. (1993) Germ-line mutations of the RET proto-oncogene in multiple endocrine neoplasia type 2 A. Nature 363:458–460

Munson JB, McMahon SB (1997) Effects of GDNF on axotomized sensory and motor neurons in adult rats. Eur J Neurosci 9:1126–1129

Nakamura M, Ohta K, Hirokawa K, Fukushima M, Uchino M, Ando M, Tanaka H (1996) Developmental and denervation changes in c-ret proto-oncogene expression in chick motoneurons. Brain Res Mol Brain Res 39:1–11

Naveilhan P, Neveu I, Wion D, Brachet P (1996) 1,25-Dihydroxyvitamin D3, an inducer of glial cell line-derived neurotrophic factor. Neuroreport 7:2171–2175

Nosrat CA, Tomac A, Lindqvist E, Lindskog S, Humpel C, Strömberg I, Ebendal T, Hoffer BJ, Olson L (1996) Cellular expression of GDNF mRNA suggests multiple functions inside and outside the nervous system. Cell Tissue Res 286:191–207

Nosrat CA, Tomac A, Hoffer BJ, Olson L (1997) Cellular and developmental patterns of expression of Ret and glial cell line-derived neurotrophic factor receptor alpha mRNAs. Exp Brain Res 115:410–422.

Olson L (1997) The coming age of the GDNF family and its receptors: gene delivery in a rat Parkinson model may have clinical implications. Trends Neurosci 20:277–279

Oo TF, Burke RE (1997) The time course of developmental cell death in phenotypically defined dopaminergic neurons of the substantia nigra. Brain Res Dev Brain Res 98:191–196

Opacka Juffry J, Ashworth S, Hume SP, Martin D, Brooks DJ, Blunt SB (1995) GDNF protects against 6-OHDA nigrostriatal lesion: in vivo study with microdialysis and PET. Neuroreport 7:348–352

Oppenheim RW (1989) The neurotrophic theory and naturally occurring motoneuron death. Trends Neurosci 12:252–255

Oppenheim RW, Houenou LJ, Johnson JE, Lin LF, Li L, Lo AC, Newsome AL, Prevette DM, Wang S (1995) Developing motor neurons rescued from programmed and axotomy-induced cell death by GDNF. Nature 373:344–346

Otto D, Unsicker K (1993) FGF-2 mediated protection of cultured mesencephalic dopaminergic neurons against MPTP and MPP+ – specificity and impact of culture condition, non-dopaminergic neurons, and astroglial cells. J Neurosci Res 34:382–393

Pachnis V, Mankoo B, Costantini F (1993) Expression of the c-ret proto-oncogene during mouse embryogenesis. Development 119:1005–1017

Pasini B, Ceccherini I, Romeo G (1996) RET mutations in human disease. Trends Genet 12:138–144

Pichel JG, Shen L, Sheng HZ, Granholm AC, Drago J, Grinberg A, Lee EJ, Huang SP, Saarma M, Hoffer BJ, Sariola H, Westphal H (1996) Defects in enteric innervation and kidney development in mice lacking GDNF. Nature 382:73–76

Pochon NA, Menoud A, Tseng JL, Zurn AD, Aebischer P (1997) Neuronal GDNF expression in the adult rat nervous system identified by in situ hybridization. Eur J Neurosci 9:463–471

Poulsen KT, Armanini MP, Klein RD, Hynes MA, Phillips HS, Rosenthal A (1994) TGF beta 2 and TGF beta 3 are potent survival factors for midbrain dopaminergic neurons. Neuron 13:1245–1252

Roberts AB, Sporn MB (1990) The transforming growth factors-bs. In: Sporn MB, Roberts AB (eds) Peptide growth factors and their receptors. Springer, Berlin Heidelberg New York, pp 419–472 (Handbook of Experimental Pharmacology, Vol. 95)

Roberts AB, Anzano MA, Lamb LC, Smith JM, Sporn MB (1981) New class of transforming growth factors potentiated by epidermal growth factor. Proc Natl Acad Sci USA 78:5339–5343

Roberts AB, Anzano MA, Meyers CA, Wideman J, Blacher R, Pan Y-C, Stein S, Lehrman SR, Smith JM, Lamb LC, Sporn MB (1983) Purification and properties of a type beta transforming growth factor from bovine kidney. Biochemistry 22:5692–5698

Robertson K, Mason I (1997) The GDNF-RET signalling partnership. Trends Genet 13:1–3

Rosenblad C, Martinez-Serrano A, Björklund A (1996) Glial cell line-derived neurotrophic factor increases survival growth and function of intrastriatal fetal nigral dopaminergic grafts. Neuroscience 75:979–985

Sagot Y, Tan SA, Hammang JP, Aebischer P, Kato AC (1996) GDNF slows loss of motoneurons but not axonal degeneration or premature death of pmn/pmn mice. J Neurosci 16:2335–2341

Sanchez MP, Silos Santiago I, Frisen J, He B, Lira SA, Barbacid M (1996) Renal agenesis and the absence of enteric neurons in mice lacking GDNF. Nature 382:70–73

Sanicola M, Hession C, Worley D, Carmillo P, Ehrenfels C, Walus L, Robinson S, Jaworski G, Wei H, Tizard R, Whitty A, Pepinsky RB, Cate RL (1997) Glial cell line-derived neurotrophic factor-dependent RET activation can be mediated by two different cell-surface accessory proteins. Proc Natl Acad Sci USA 94:6238–6243

Santoro M, Wong WT, Aroca P, Santos E, Matoskova B, Grieco M, Fusco A, di Fiore PP (1994) An epidermal growth factor receptor/ret chimera generates mitogenic and transforming signals: evidence for a ret-specific signaling pathway. Mol Cell Biol 14:663–675

Sariola H, Sainio K (1997) The tip-top branching ureter. Curr Opin Cell Biol 9:877–884

Sauer H, Rosenblad C, Bjorklund A (1995) Glial cell line-derived neurotrophic factor but not transforming growth factor beta 3 prevents delayed degeneration of nigral dopaminergic neurons following striatal 6-hydroxydopamine lesion. Proc Natl Acad Sci USA 92:8935–8939

Schaar DG, Sieber BA, Dreyfus CF, Black IB (1993) Regional and cell-specific expression of GDNF in rat brain. Exp Neurol 124:368–371

Schindelhauer D, Schuffenhauer S, Gasser T, Steinkasserer A, Meitinger T (1995) The gene coding for glial cell line derived neurotrophic factor (GDNF) maps to chromosome 5p12-p13.1. Genomics 28:605–607

Schmidt Kastner R, Tomac A, Hoffer B, Bektesh S, Rosenzweig B, Olson L (1994) Glial cell-line derived neurotrophic factor (GDNF) mRNA upregulation in striatum and cortical areas after pilocarpine-induced status epilepticus in rats. Brain Res Mol Brain Res 26:325–330

Schneider R (1992) The human proto-oncogene ret: a communicative cadherin? Trends Biochem Sci 17:468–469

Schuchardt A, D'Agati V, Larsson Blomberg L, Costantini F, Pachnis V (1994) Defects in the kidney and enteric nervous system of mice lacking the tyrosine kinase receptor Ret. Nature 367:380–383

Schuchardt A, Srinivas S, Pachnis V, Costantini F (1995) Isolation and characterization of a chicken homolog of the c-ret proto-oncogene. Oncogene 10:641–649

Schuchardt A, D'Agati V, Pachnis V, Costantini F (1996) Renal agenesis and hypodysplasia in ret-k- mutant mice result from defects in ureteric bud development. Development 122:1919–1929

Shults CW, Kimber T, Martin D (1996) Intrastriatal injection of GDNF attenuates the effects of 6-hydroxydopamine. Neuroreport 7:627–631

Sinclair SR, Svendsen CN, Torres EM, Martin D, Fawcett JW, Dunnett SB (1996) GDNF enhances dopaminergic cell survival and fibre outgrowth in embryonic nigral grafts. Neuroreport 7:2547–2552

Springer JE, Mu X, Bergmann LW, Trojanowski JQ (1994) Expression of GDNF mRNA in rat and human nervous tissue. Exp Neurol 127:167–170

Springer JE, Seeburger JL, He J, Gabrea A, Blankenhorn EP, Bergman LW (1995) cDNA sequence and differential mRNA regulation of two forms of glial cell line-derived neurotrophic factor in Schwann cells and rat skeletal muscle. Exp Neurol 131:47–52

Strömberg I, Bjorklund L, Johansson M, Tomac A, Collins F, Olson L, Hoffer B, Humpel C (1993) Glial cell line-derived neurotrophic factor is expressed in the developing but not adult striatum and stimulates developing dopamine neurons in vivo. Exp Neurol 124:401–412

Suter-Crazzolara C, Unsicker K (1994) GDNF is expressed in two forms in many tissues outside the CNS. Neuroreport 5:2486–2488

Suter-Crazzolara C, Unsicker K (1996) GDNF mRNA levels are induced by FGF-2 in rat C6 glioblastoma cells. Brain Res Mol Brain Res 41:175–182

Suter-Crazzolara C, Baeker PA, Johnson RM, Unsicker K (1997) Characterization of a human GDNF gene promotor. Soc Neurosci Abstr. 23, 90

Suvanto P, Hiltunen JO, Arumae U, Moshnyakov M, Sariola H, Sainio K, Saarma M (1996) Localization of glial cell line-derived neurotrophic factor (GDNF) mRNA in embryonic rat by in situ hybridization. Eur J Neurosci 8:816–822

Suvanto P, Wartiovaara, Lindahl M, Arumäe U, Moshnyakov M, Horelli-Kuitunen N, Airaksinen MS, Palotie A, Sariola H, Saarma M (1997) Cloning, mRNA distribution and chromosomal localisation of the gene or glial cell line-derived neurotrophic factor receptor b, a homologue to GDNFR-α. Hum Mol Genetics 6:1267–1273

Tahira T, Ishizaka Y, Sugimura T, Nagao M (1988) Expression of proto-ret mRNA in embryonic and adult rat tissues. Biochem Biophys Res Commun 153:1290–1295

Tahira T, Ishizaka Y, Itoh F, Sugimura T, Nagao M (1990) Characterization of ret proto-oncogene mRNAs encoding two isoforms of the protein product in a human neuroblastoma cell line. Oncogene 5:97–102

Takahashi M, Cooper GM (1987) ret transforming gene encodes a fusion protein homologous to tyrosine kinases. Mol Cell Biol 7:1378–1385

Takahashi M, Buma Y, Iwamoto T, Inaguma Y, Ikeda H, Hiai H (1988) Cloning and expression of the ret proto-oncogene encoding a tyrosine kinase with two potential transmembrane domains. Oncogene 3:571–578

Takahashi M, Buma Y, Taniguchi M (1991) Identification of the ret proto-oncogene products in neuroblastoma and leukemia cells. Oncogene 6:297–301

Takahashi M, Asai N, Iwashita T, Isomura T, Miyazaki K, Matsuyama M (1993) Characterization of the ret proto-oncogene products expressed in mouse L cells. Oncogene 8:2925–2929

Takahashi M, Ritz J, Cooper GM (1985) Activation of a novel human transforming gene, ret, by DNA rearrangement. Cell 42:581–588

Tomac A, Lindqvist E, Lin LF, Ogren SO, Young D, Hoffer BJ, Olson L (1995a) Protection and repair of the nigrostriatal dopaminergic system by GDNF in vivo [see comments]. Nature 373:335–339

Tomac A, Widenfalk J, Lin LF, Kohno T, Ebendal T, Hoffer BJ, Olson L (1995b) Retrograde axonal transport of glial cell line-derived neurotrophic factor in the adult nigrostriatal system suggests a trophic role in the adult. Proc Natl Acad Sci USA 92:8274–8278

Treanor JJ, Goodman L, de Sauvage F, Stone DM, Poulsen KT, Beck CD, Gray C, Armanini MP, Pollock RA, Hefti F, Phillips HS, Goddard A, Moore MW, Buj Bello A, Davies AM, Asai N, Takahashi M, Vandlen R, Henderson CE, Rosenthal A (1996) Characterization of a multicomponent receptor for GDNF [see comments]. Nature 382:80–83

Trok K, Almstrom S, Olson L (1996) A comparison of the effects of glial cell line-derived neurotrophic factor on spinal cord and cortex cerebri grafts. J Pharmacol Exp Ther 278:941–949

Trupp M, Ryden M, Jornvall H, Funakoshi H, Timmusk T, Arenas E, Ibanez CF (1995) Peripheral expression and biological activities of GDNF, a new neurotrophic factor for avian and mammalian peripheral neurons. J Cell Biol 130:137–148

Trupp M, Arenas E, Fainzilber M, Nilsson AS, Sieber BA, Grigoriou M, Kilkenny C, Salazar Grueso E, Pachnis V, Arumäe U, Sariola H, Saarma M, Ibanez CF (1996) Functional receptor for GDNF encoded by the c-ret proto-oncogene. Nature 381:785–788

Trupp M, Belluardo N, Funakoshi H, Ibanez CF (1997) Complementary and overlapping expression of glial cell line-derived neurotrophic factor (GDNF), c-ret proto-oncogene, and GDNF receptor-alpha indicates multiple mechanisms of trophic actions in the adult rat CNS. J Neurosci 17:3554–3567

Tseng JL, Baetge EE, Zurn AD, Aebischer P (1997) GDNF reduces drug-induced rotational behavior after medial forebrain bundle transection by a mechanism not involving striatal dopamine. J Neurosci 17:325–333

Tsuzuki T, Takahashi M, Asai N, Iwashita T, Matsuyama M, Asai J (1995) Spatial and temporal expression of the ret proto-oncogene product in embryonic, infant and adult rat tissues. Oncogene 10:191–198

Unsicker K (1996) GDNF: a cytokine at the interface of TGF-betas and neurotrophins. Cell Tissue Res 286:175–178

Unsicker K, Flanders KC, Cissel DS, Lafyatis R, Sporn MB (1991) Transforming growth factor beta isoforms in the adult rat central and peripheral nervous system. Neuroscience 44:613–625

van Weering DH, Bos JL (1997) Glial cell line-derived neurotrophic factor induces Ret-mediated lamellipodia formation. J Biol Chem 272:249–254

Vega QC, Worby CA, Lechner MS, Dixon JE, Dressler GR (1996) Glial cell line-derived neurotrophic factor activates the receptor tyrosine kinase RET and promotes kidney morphogenesis. Proc Natl Acad Sci USA 93:10657–10661

Wang Y, Tien LT, Lapchak PA, Hoffer BJ (1996) GDNF triggers fiber outgrowth of fetal ventral mesencephalic grafts from nigra to striatum in 6-OHDA-lesioned rats. Cell Tissue Res 286:225–233

Wang Y, Lin SZ, Chiou AL, Williams LR, Hoffer BJ (1997) Glial cell line-derived neurotrophic factor protects against ischemia-induced injury in the cerebral cortex. J Neurosci 17:4341–4348

Widenfalk J, Nosrat C, Tomac A, Westphal H, Hoffer B, Olson L (1997) Neurturin and glial cell line-derived neurotrophic factor receptor-b (GDNFR-b), novel proteins related to GDNF and GDNFR-α with specific cellular patterns of expression suggesting roles in the developing and adult nervous system and in peripheral organs. J Neurosci 17:8506–8519

Williams LR, Inouye G, Cummins V, Pelleymounter MA (1996) Glial cell line-derived neurotrophic factor sustains axotomized basal forebrain cholinergic neurons in vivo: dose-response comparison to nerve growth factor and brain-derived neurotrophic factor. J Pharmacol Exp Ther 277:1140–1151

Winkler C, Sauer H, Lee CS, Bjorklund A (1996) Short-term GDNF treatment provides long-term rescue of lesioned nigral dopaminergic neurons in a rat model of Parkinson's disease. J Neurosci 16:7206–7215

Worby CA, Vega QC, Zhao Y, Chao HHJ, Seasholtz AF, Dixon JE (1996) Glial cell line-derived neurotrophic factor signals through the RET receptor and activates mitogen-activated protein kinase. J Biol Chem 271:23619–23622

Wright DE, Snider WD (1996) Focal expression of glial cell line-derived neurotrophic factor in developing mouse limb bud. Cell Tissue Res 286:209–217

Yamamoto M, Sobue G, Yamamoto K, Terao S, Mitsuma T (1996) Expression of mRNAs for neurotrophic factors (NGF, BDNF, NT-3, and GDNF) and their receptors (p75NGFR, trkA, trkB, and trkC) in the adult human peripheral nervous system and non-neural tissues. Neurochem Res 21:929–938

Yan Q, Matheson C, Lopez OT (1995) In vivo neurotrophic effects of GDNF on neonatal and adult facial motor neurons [see comments]. Nature 373:341–344

Zurn AD, Baetge EE, Hammang JP, Tan SA, Aebischer P (1994) Glial cell line-derived neurotrophic factor (GDNF), a new neurotrophic factor for motoneurones. Neuroreport 6:113–118

Zurn AD, Winkel L, Menoud A, Djabali K, Aebischer P (1996) Combined effects of GDNF, BDNF, and CNTF on motoneuron differentiation in vitro. J Neurosci Res 44:133–141

CHAPTER 9

Role of Neurotrophic Factors in Cerebral Ischemia

K. Nikolics

A. Neurotrophic Factors, Their Receptors and Their Expression in the Central Nervous System (CNS)

I. Neurotrophic Factors Support Survival and Functionality of Neurons

A growing number of studies suggest that neurotrophic factors may be beneficial in protecting neurons from cell death or in delaying neuronal cell death in in vitro and in vivo models of hypoxic-ischemic CNS injury. Protection from neuronal cell death also leads to a better retention and recovery of neurological and behavioral functions. In this chapter, we review the potential role and utility of neurotrophic factors in the ischemically injured brain.

Neurotrophic factors and neuronal growth factors and cytokines control the proliferation and phenotypic differentiation of neuronal precursor cells and the survival, phenotype, neurite outgrowth and synaptic function of specific neuronal populations in the embryonic and postnatal nervous system. The expression of neurotrophic factors in the developing and normal adult CNS and peripheral nervous system (PNS) is regulated by afferent neuronal activity, suggesting that they play functional roles in neuronal plasticity, survival and maintenance of synaptic connectivity and structural integrity (Barde 1989; Korsching 1993; Snider 1994; Davies 1996). In the adult CNS, the expression of neurotrophic factors is also dynamically regulated by various types of injury, suggesting that they play specific roles in acute and slow neurodegenerative response mechanisms and in synaptic rearrangements following injury (Lindvall et al. 1994; Isackson 1995).

Animal models of different types of human-brain insults, such as global and focal hypoxic-ischemic injuries, mechanical lesions, and chemically and electrically induced seizures, have been found to cause changes in neurotrophic factor expression by neuronal and glial cells. Acute nervous-system injury and chronic neurodegenerative diseases cause structural damage, induce reactive plasticity and it is likely that neurotrophic factors play protective and regenerative functions in responses to injury. Neurotrophic factors, thus, may offer a therapeutic opportunity by reversing the atrophy of the nerve cell body and its synapses and, perhaps, by stimulating the re-establishment of lost synaptic connections. Neurotrophic factors have been extensively studied in various animal models of acute nervous-system injury and neurodegenerative diseases and, based on such results, some have subsequently moved into clinical evaluation (Hefti 1994, 1997).

II. Neurotrophic-Factor Families

1. Neurotrophins

The protein family called "neurotrophins" (Barde 1989; Snider 1994) includes nerve growth factor (NGF), brain-derived neurotrophic factor (BDNF), neurotrophin-3 (NT-3) and neurotrophin-4/5 (NT-4/5). Studies with NGF led to the formulation of the neurotrophic hypothesis according to which innervated target cells provide trophic signals for innervating neurons by a mechanism involving the retrograde axonal transport of the neurotrophic factor. The neurotrophins bind to and stimulate protein kinase receptors of the Trk family and they bind to and activate a lower affinity receptor, referred to as $p75^{NTR}$ or $p75^{NGFR}$ (Kaplan and Stephens 1994; Chao and Hempstead 1995; Barbacid 1995). The interaction between the neurotrophins and their cognate Trk receptors leads to a stimulation of autophosphorylation of the kinase domain of the receptor which, in turn, triggers a series of intracellular kinases.

NGF is the ligand of the Trk protein, BDNF and NT-4/5 are the ligands of the TrkB protein. NT-3 binds with high affinity to the TrkC protein, but it is also able to bind to the TrkB and Trk proteins at higher concentrations. $p75^{NTR}$ is a member of the Fas/tumor necrosis factor-receptor family of proteins which activates intracellular processes via Trk-independent mechanisms. With the exception of NGF, the other neurotrophins stimulate the phosphorylation of TrkB and TrkC receptors in cultured hippocampal cells (Ip et al. 1993). In rat hippocampal slice cultures, which retain some of the characteristic cytoarchitecture and connectivity between the hippocampal layers, BDNF and NT-3 have been reported to stimulate synaptic transmission at the Schaffer collateral-CA1 synapses (Kang and Schuman 1995).

2. Glial-Derived Neurotrophic Factor (GDNF) and Transforming Growth Factors (TGFs)

GDNF was originally purified as a differentiation factor for mesencephalic dopaminergic neurons which raised the possibility that it may provide a therapeutic basis for the treatment of Parkinson's disease (Lin et al. 1993). GDNF is a distant member of the TGF-b family of proteins. GDNF is expressed in target areas of dopaminergic neurons of the substantia nigra and it acts as a dopaminergic neurotrophic factor both in vitro and in vivo (Beck et al. 1995; Sauer et al. 1995; Tomac et al. 1995). GDNF acts both as a differentiation factor for mesencephalic dopaminergic neurons and as a protective agent against neurotoxic damage. In addition to its effect on dopaminergic neurons, GDNF also acts as a potent trophic factor for motoneurons, cerebellar Purkinje cells and peripheral sympathetic and ciliary ganglionic neurons.

TGF-β2 and -β3 and activin, which is also a member of the TGF-β growth factor family, act as very potent trophic factors for central dopaminergic neurons, spinal motoneurons and retinal ganglionic neurons (SCHUBERT et al. 1990; POULSEN et al. 1994). Another member of the TGF-β family, bone morphogenetic protein-6 (BMP-6) has been found to show a neuronal expression pattern and has trophic activities (TOMIZAWA MATSUI et al. 1995). TGF-β family members appear to be broad-spectrum factors regulating morphogenetic, trophic, inflammatory and wound responses in various tissues.

3. Ciliary Neurotrophic factor (CNTF), Fibroblast Growth Factors (FGFs), Insulin-Like Growth Factors (IGFs) and Other Factors

CNTF was originally purified from the eye as a trophic factor for parasympathetic neurons of ciliary ganglia (LIN et al. 1989). Later it was found that CNTF can support the survival of several other neuronal populations, including peripheral and central cholinergic neurons and spinal motoneurons (ARAKAWA et al. 1990; HAGG et al. 1992).

Acidic and basic FGFs (aFGF, bFGF) and FGF-2 and -5 act as neurotrophic factors for several central and peripheral neuronal cell types (WALICKE et al. 1986; GOMEZ-PINILLA et al. 1992). The IGF-1 and IGF-2 have potent neurotrophic effects on several central and peripheral neuronal types, including central cholinergic, spinal motoneurons and peripheral sensory neurons (RECIO-PINTO et al. 1986).

Midkine and heparin-binding growth associated molecule (HB-GAM) (also known as pleiotrophin or heparin-binding neurotrophic factor), two related novel proteins, were purified based on their ability to promote neurite outgrowth of embryonic brain cells (LI et al. 1990; MERENMIES and RAUVALA 1990; YASUHARA et al. 1993). Based on their biological activities in cell culture studies or their expression patterns in the brain hepatocyte growth factor (HGF), interleukins (IL)-1, -2, -3 and -6, erythropoietin, and granulocyte-macrophage colony stimulating factor have been tentatively identified as neurotrophic factors (HONDA et al. 1995; KAMEGAI et al. 1990; HAMA et al. 1991; KONISHI et al. 1993). The effects of all of these factors, where identified, are mediated through receptor protein kinases, either tyrosine kinases or serine/threonine kinases which, in turn, stimulate intracellular pathways involving the phosphorylation of a cascade of mediator proteins.

Growth factors acting as regulatory agents for glial cells have also been identified. Among others, glia maturation factor-b (GMF-b; LIM et al. 1989), Platelet-Derived Growth Factors (NOBLE et al. 1989; YEH et al. 1991), various isoforms of heregulin/ARIA/glial growth factor (HOLMES et al. 1992; MARCHIONNI et al. 1993; FALLS et al. 1993) and others have been found to act as growth factors regulating glial cell functions. Progress has also been made towards understanding vascular growth factors (LEUNG et al. 1989; BREIER et al. 1997; Maisonpierre et al. 1997) which may be able to protect endothelial cells from death in hypoxic-ischemic brain injury. Although in this review we will focus our attention on neuronal trophic factors, based on recent work, it appears that similar trophic mechanisms are likely to apply to glial and vascular cells, as well.

III. Afferent Activity Regulates Neurotrophic Factor Expression

Neurotrophins are synthesized in the brain at very different levels in different cell types and regions. NGF is produced at the highest levels by GABAergic interneurons in the hippocampus (Lauterborn et al. 1993). TrkA, the high affinity NGF receptor, is not expressed in the hippocampus, but in cholinergic nuclei (Merlio et al. 1992). mRNAs for BDNF and NT-3 are found in excitatory neurons of the dentate gyrus and in the CA1–3 pyramidal cell layer; their receptors, TrkB and TrkC, are also expressed by neurons of the dentate gyrus and the pyramidal cell layer (Merlio et al. 1993).

The recognition that neuronal activity can cause changes in the expression of the neurotrophins is very recent. The first of such observations was made in studies using epileptogenic seizures which increase neurotrophin and TrkB mRNA expression in cortical and hippocampal neurons (Gall and Isackson 1989; Isackson et al. 1991; Ernfors et al. 1991; Rocamora et al. 1992; Merlio et al. 1993). Seizures induced by a dentate hilar lesion (Rocamora et al. 1992), kindling (Bengzon et al. 1992, 1993) or injection of kainate (Gall et al. 1991; Dugich-Djordjevic et al. 1992; Lowenstein et al. 1993; Suzuki et al. 1995) have been found to increase NGF, BDNF, and trk and trkB mRNA, and to decrease NT-3 mRNA in cortical and hippocampal neurons.

Since increased sprouting and synaptic reorganization follow epileptic seizures, these findings raised the possibility that increased neurotrophin gene expression following epileptic seizures might be responsible for the increased sprouting and synaptic rearrangements. Kainate-induced seizures also markedly increased GDNF mRNA levels in neurons of the dentate gyrus as early as 3 h after kainate injection, peaking at about 6 h and returning to normal basal levels by 24 h (Humpel et al. 1994). GDNF mRNA was also highly elevated in the striatum, hippocampus and cortex following pilocarpine-induced epileptic seizures (Schmidt-Kastner et al. 1994). Seizures were found to induce the expression of FGF-5 and FGF-2, as well as the FGF receptor (Gomez-Pinilla et al. 1995).

Physiological levels of afferent activity can induce changes in the expression of neurotrophins: NGF, BDNF and NT-3 were found to be induced by long-term potentiation (LTP) (Lindefors et al. 1992; Patterson et al. 1992; Castrén et al. 1993; Dragunow et al. 1993). BDNF mRNA was found to be significantly increased in the rat visual cortex upon retinal light exposure (Castrén et al. 1992). Physical exercise increases cortical and hippocampal BDNF levels (Neeper et al. 1996). Spreading depression was found to induce a rapid and transient increase of BDNF and TrkB mRNA levels in the cortex

(Kokaia et al. 1993). *N*-Methyl-D-aspartate (NMDA)-receptor activation (Gwag et al. 1993) led to elevated levels of hippocampal and cortical neurotrophin expression. Cholinergic deafferentation by fimbrial transection caused a decrease in BDNF mRNA in the hippocampus (Lapchak et al. 1993).

B. Hypoxic-Ischemic Injury Regulates the Expression of Neurotrophic Factors and Their Receptors in the Central Nervous System

Earlier studies suggested that the synthesis of neurotrophic activity increased after different types of brain injury (Ebendal et al. 1980; Nieto-Sampedro et al. 1982). Using an assay responsive to most known polypeptide growth factors, based on the stimulation of proliferation of a fibroblast cell line, it was shown that growth-factor activity was increased in hypoxic-ischemic brain tissue (Finklestein et al. 1990). A neurotrophic activity induced by hypoxic-ischemic injury was partially purified from rat brain (Yamada et al. 1992). More recently, it was observed that the degree of tyrosine phosphorylation increased in the injured brain after transient ischemia, suggesting the activation of receptor protein kinases (Hu and Wieloch 1993). Using more specific methods, many known growth factors have been reported to be induced or inhibited in the injured brain.

I. Global Hypoxic-Ischemic Injury

Studies, primarily in rodents, have established that permanent neuronal damage is caused by global forebrain hypoxia-ischemia lasting longer than 3–4 min. Interestingly, shorter sub-lethal periods of hypoxia-ischemia (2–3 min) provide protection from subsequent longer hypoxic-ischemic periods, a phenomenon referred to as ischemic tolerance or preconditioning (Kirino 1982; Kirino et al. 1996). In the adult rat or gerbil, delayed cell death occurs in the CA1 area of the hippocampus following 5–12 min of transient forebrain ischemia. CA1 pyramidal cells are selectively vulnerable to ischemia and die 1–3 days after such transient ischemia. Longer periods of hypoxia-ischemia (20–60 min) cause cortical and striatal damage beyond the hippocampal cell death. Hypoxic-ischemic injury can also be studied in vitro. Cortical neurons in culture can be subjected to brief or prolonged oxygen and glucose deprivation mimicking the in vivo hypoxia-ischemia. Brief exposures have been found to be protective, whereas longer exposures cause cell death (Goldberg and Choi 1993; Sakaki et al. 1995). Both in vivo and in vitro systems have been widely used for analyzing the expression of neurotrophic factors, as well as for testing potential protective effects of various agents.

Hypoxic-ischemic brain injury and other types of insults, such as hypoglycemic, excitotoxic, epileptic and mechanical brain injuries, induce significant changes in the expression of neurotrophic factor and neurotrophic factor-receptor genes. It is possible that these changes represent an intrinsic neuroprotective response, and/or sprouting and synaptic rearrangement which follows such insults. However, elevated levels of neurotrophic factors could also increase synaptic transmission during the early post-ischemic phase which may contribute to the initiation and propagation of epileptogenesis.

1. Neurotrophins

The expression of members of the neurotrophin family has been found to be regulated after CNS injury (reviewed by Lindvall et al. 1994; Isackson 1995). Different types of CNS injury cause different patterns of neurotrophin mRNA expression. In general, a biphasic or multiphasic pattern of neurotrophin expression has been observed with a rapid first phase (from 15 min to several hours following the injury) and a longer-lasting second or third phase (days, up to weeks following the injury).

Short periods of transient global forebrain ischemia that do not cause neuronal cell death were found to increase NGF, BDNF and TrkB mRNA levels in dentate granule cells (Ballarin et al. 1991; Shozuhara et al. 1992; Lindvall et al. 1992; Takeda et al. 1993). NT-3 mRNA was reduced under these conditions. By one day following the challenge, all mRNA levels returned to baseline values. Under severe, damaging ischemic conditions (20 min global forebrain ischemia), the early transient changes were similar to the mild insult; however, the increase in NGF and BDNF mRNA was more delayed than in the mild insult, and BDNF mRNA also increased in the CA3 region. The early induction of BDNF expression parallels several known immediate early genes (Dragunow et al. 1994).

The rat BDNF gene consists of four short 5′ exons linked to separate promoters and one 3′ exon encoding the mature BDNF protein. Kindling-induced seizures and cerebral ischemia were found to increase BDNF mRNA levels by specific usage of three of the promoters of the BDNF gene (Lindvall et al. 1992; Kokaia et al. 1994). Both brief (2 min) and longer (10 min) periods of global forebrain ischemia induced significant and major increases only of exon-III mRNA in the dentate gyrus. Single and multiple hippocampal seizures highly induced the expression of exon-I, -II and -III mRNAs in dentate granule cells. Multiple seizures induced both exon-I and -III mRNAs in the CA3 region, amygdala, piriform cortex and neocortex; however, in the hippocampal CA1 region, an increase was detected only for exon-III mRNA. Neither of the insults had any effect on exon-IV mRNA in the brain.

In a recent study, Kokaia et al. (1996) measured levels of BDNF mRNA and protein simultaneously. BDNF protein was highest in the dentate gyrus, while the levels in CA3, CA1 and parietal cortex were significant, but lower. A 10 min period of global forebrain ischemia caused a transient increase in BDNF protein in the dentate 6 h after the insult and in the CA3 region 1 week after the insult. In the CA1 region and parietal cortex, BDNF protein decreased after 24 h. In contrast, BDNF mRNA in dentate granule cells and in the CA3 pyramidal layer was elevated 2 h after the same insult, whereas no change was detected in CA1 or the neocortex. Thus, BDNF protein and mRNA levels partially correlate with regional differences in cellular resistance to ischemic damage. These results are consistent with the hypothesis of a neuroprotective role of BDNF.

TrkB mRNA was found to be transiently increased in the dentate gyrus following transient cerebral ischemia, whereas trk and trkC mRNAs did not change (Merlio et al. 1993). Hippocampal CA1 neurons immunoreactive for the calcium-binding protein parvalbumin are resistant to short transient forebrain ischemia. Ferrer et al. (1997) found that BDNF immunoreactivity was localized in all neurons of the CA1 area in gerbils, whereas only a fraction of CA1 neurons were TrkB immunoreactive. The number of BDNF-immunoreactive cells in the ischemic CA1 region was dramatically reduced 24 h after ischemia, whereas the number of TrkB-immunoreactive cells in the CA1 area remained stable. BDNF and TrkB were found to be co-localized in about 95% of CA1 neurons surviving the ischemic insult. Almost all of these BDNF- and TrkB-immunoreactive cells in ischemic gerbils co-localized with parvalbumin. These data would suggest that a subpopulation of CA1 hippocampal neurons in the gerbil hippocampus may utilize a BDNF/TrkB autocrine or paracrine system that increases cell survival and stimulates synaptic remodeling following transient forebrain ischemia.

2. Basic Fibroblast Growth Factor

In CA1 pyramidal cells exposed to a short period of 10 min of transient forebrain ischemia, bFGF mRNA was found to be induced within 6h, with a maximal level within 24 h of ischemia (Endoh et al. 1994). In the same study, mRNA for the FGF receptor, flg, was present in the pyramidal cell layer, and decreased almost completely in parallel with neuronal death. In the granule cell layer of the dentate gyrus, the expression of bFGF mRNA increased more rapidly. It peaked at 6h and returned to basal level within 3 days. In the hilus of the dentate gyrus, bFGF expression was maximal at 24h and returned to control levels within 3 days. In contrast, there was no significant change of bFGF immunoreactivity in either the CA1 pyramidal cell layer or in the granule cell layer of dentate gyrus within 3 days of ischemia. Predominantly in reactive glial cells, bFGF and FGFR mRNA and bFGF immunoreactivity increased dramatically in the CA1 area from 7 days until 30 days after ischemia.

In a culture model of hypoxic injury, cortical neurons were exposed to short (4-h) and long (24-h) periods of hypoxia (Sakaki et al. 1995). The long treatment caused significant neuronal death, whereas the short treatment protected against subsequent hypoxic damage. The brief hypoxia caused an increase in bFGF mRNA and protein levels 1 day after the treatment. The longer, damaging hypoxia caused an increase in the expression of bFGF mRNA after 2 days, but no increase in protein levels until 3 days after the treatment. When the cells were subjected to prolonged hypoxia, 2 days after the protective brief hypoxia, no increase in bFGF mRNA was observed, while bFGF protein levels remained elevated.

3. IGFs, TGF-b and Other Factors

mRNAs encoding the insulin-like growth factors IGF-I and IGF-II were found to be significantly elevated following carotid-artery occlusion combined with hypoxia in young rats, primarily in cortical regions and in the dentate gyrus on the ipsilateral side (Gluckman et al. 1992; Beilharz et al. 1995a). This increase was very high within 3 days of the lesion. By 5 days, subcortical areas, including the thalamus and the striatum, also showed elevated IGF-I mRNA levels. The predominant site of IGF-I expression, which is very low in the uninjured brain, was astrocytic. In a similar model of hypoxic-ischemic insult, IGF-I and the type-I receptor were found to be induced rapidly and widely in the contralateral hemisphere and within 24 h in the hippocampus and the thalamus (Lee et al. 1992). In 21-day-old rats subjected to carotid-artery occlusion for 60 min, IGF-II was found to be significantly increased in the infarcted cortex 5–7 days following the insult (Beilharz et al. 1995a). A demyelinating lesion was found to cause a substantial elevation of IGF-1 mRNA expression in astrocytes (Komoly et al. 1992).

The expression of TGF-β was significantly elevated in the infant rat brain following global hypoxia (Klempt et al. 1992). The levels of TGF-β were highest in the infarcted cortex and hippocampus, and reached maximal levels by three days following the initial insult. Hippocampal and striatal deafferentation, as well as kainate-induced limbic seizures caused a significant increase in TGF-β mRNA (Morgan et al. 1993; Pasinetti et al. 1993). In all of these studies, TGF-β was expressed predominantly in astrocytes, microglial cells or macrophages. In most areas, the resting levels of TGF-b expression were practically undetectable, and the increases in expression were several-fold.

HGF, the ligand of the c-Met proto-oncogene product, prolonged the survival of embryonic hippocampal neurons in primary culture at a potency similar to NGF (Honda et al. 1995). HGF mRNA and protein were present in cerebral cortex, hippocampus and amygdala, and the expression of both HGF and c-Met/HGF receptor mRNAs was markedly induced in response to ischemic brain injury.

Astrocytes exposed to hypoxia/reoxygenation (H/R) expressed increased levels of mRNA and released increased amounts of IL-6, whereas levels of tumor necrosis factor and IL-1 remained undetectable (Maeda et al. 1994). Conditioned medium from H/R astrocytes increased the survival of PC12 cells exposed to H/R, an effect blocked by neutralizing anti-IL-6 antibody. In a gerbil model of global forebrain ischemia, IL-6 activity was lower in the hippocampus. IL-6 protein was increased in astrocytes from ischemic regions of gerbil brain.

II. Focal Hypoxic-Ischemic Injury

1. Neurotrophins

NGF immunoreactivity was found to increase following focal ischemic brain injury in the rat hippocampus and striatum and to a lesser degree in the cortex (Lorez et al. 1989). However, at the time of this study, other neurotrophins were not known and, therefore, the specificity of the antibody used was not tested against other neurotrophins. Thus, it is not impossible that some of the NGF immunoreactivity was caused by other neurotrophins.

Photochemical stroke caused a rapid increase in BDNF and its receptor, TrkB, mRNA in the hippocampus and cortex ipsilateral to the lesion (Comelli et al. 1992, 1993). This effect paralleled the pattern of expression of several immediate early-inducible genes, and it could be inhibited by NMDA antagonist treatment, suggesting the involvement of excitatory amino acid neurotransmission.

In a transient middle cerebral artery-occlusion (MCAO) model, elevated levels of NGF and BDNF mRNA were recorded in a biphasic pattern, along with a number of immediate early genes involved in transcriptional regulation (Hsu et al. 1993). Transient MCAO was found to regulate the expression of the neurotrophins and their receptors in a biphasic pattern. Short-term (15 min) MCAO, which does not cause neuronal death, induced BDNF expression in the ipsilateral frontal and cingulate cortices outside the ischemic area. Longer (2 h), transient MCAO which leads to cortical infarction, induced more elevated BDNF mRNA levels bilaterally in dentate granule cells and CA1 and CA3 pyramidal neurons. BDNF expression peaked after 2 h of reperfusion and, within 24 h, BDNF mRNA expression returned to normal. This and other types of brain injury appear to stimulate BDNF expression using different transcriptional controls. MCAO induced a marked increase of exon-III mRNA, but only small increases of exon-I and -II mRNAs in cortex and hippocampus. The longer MCAO also induced transient, bilateral increases of NGF and TrkB mRNA levels and a decrease of NT-3 mRNA expression in the dentate gyrus. In general, the expression of BDNF and NGF appears to increase following transient ischemia, whereas the expression of NT-3 remains stable or decreases.

Kokaia et al. (1995) measured mRNAs for c-fos, NGF, BDNF, NT-3, TrkB, and TrkC using in situ hybridization in the rat brain at different reperfusion times after unilateral MCAO. Short-term (15 min) MCAO, which does not cause neuronal death, induced elevated BDNF mRNA expression in the ipsilateral frontal and cingulate cortices outside the ischemic area. With a 2 h MCAO, which causes cortical infarction, the increase was more marked, and elevated BDNF mRNA levels were also detected bilaterally in dentate granule cells and CA1 and CA3 pyramidal neurons. Maximum expression was found after 2 h of reperfusion.

At 24h, BDNF mRNA expression had returned to control values. In the ischemic core of the parietal cortex, only scattered neurons were expressing high levels of BDNF mRNA after 15 min and 2 h of MCAO. Analysis of different BDNF transcripts showed that MCAO induced a marked increase of exon-III mRNA, but only small increases of exon-I and -II mRNAs in cortex and hippocampus. Two hours of MCAO also induced transient, bilateral increases of NGF and TrkB mRNA levels and a decrease of NT-3 mRNA expression in dentate granule cells. Similar results were obtained by Arai et al. (1996) who found elevated BDNF and trkB mRNA levels in a widespread region of the ipsilateral cortex outside the infarct, 4 h after MCAO. They were also highly induced in the bilateral hippocampus outside of the ischemic MCA region. These results are consistent with the hypothesis that changes in neurotrophin and neurotrophin-receptor gene expression may reflect a protective response in the areas outside the infarct that are injured, but can recover following the injury. In contrast to transient MCAO, permanent MCAO caused a decrease in TrkB mRNA 1 day, 4 days, and 7 days after the occlusion (Chan et al. 1996).

2. Basic Fibroblast Growth Factor

The levels of bFGF protein were greatly stimulated in adult rat brain 7 days after focal ischemic brain injury (Finklestein et al. 1988). Permanent MCAO in adult rats was followed by an increase in bFGF protein levels, 7–14 days after the occlusion (Kumon et al. 1993). Astrocytic cells appeared to be the predominant source of bFGF, although neuronal cells also contained increased bFGF immunoreactivity.

Focal cerebral ischemia induced by Rose bengal resulted in a global upregulation of bFGF gene expression after 24 h (Lippoldt et al. 1993). This upregulation in bFGF gene expression was largely due to an upregulation in glial bFGF expression in most of the areas, as assessed by in situ hybridization. However, in the piriform cortex, neuronal upregulation of bFGF could also be detected. There were substantial increases in bFGF mRNA expression in the cingulate cortex and in the neostriatum. No changes in bFGF gene expression were seen in the CA1 region of the hippocampus on the lesioned side and in the dentate gyrus. Significant changes in bFGF upregulation in the caudate putamen, the piriform cortex and the amygdaloid region and the frontoparietal cortex were found.

Speliotes et al. (1996) studied bFGF expression in permanent MCAO in the rat and found a fourfold increase in bFGF mRNA in tissue surrounding focal infarcts at 1 day after ischemia. Astrocytic cells in several cortical regions, including the frontoparietal, temporal and cingulate cortex, and in caudoputamen, globus pallidus, septal nuclei, nucleus accumbens and olfactory tubercle in the ipsilateral hemisphere showed significant increases in bFGF mRNA. Double immunostaining identified bFGF-IR cells as astroglia in these structures; however, in the piriform cortex, both increased bFGF mRNA levels and increased bFGF-IR were found in neurons 1 day after ischemia. The peak of increased bFGF expression preceded the peak in expression of the astroglial marker GFAP within the ipsilateral hemisphere.

The expression of four members of the FGF receptor family was analyzed in rats subjected to temporal middle cerebral-artery occlusion by MASUMURA et al. (1996). FGFR-1 mRNA was highly expressed in neurons in the cerebral cortex, whereas mRNAs of FGFR-2, -3 and -4 were not expressed. After temporal MCAO, expression of FGFR-1 mRNA in cortical neurons markedly increased in association with the progression of neuronal death, lasting for about 5 days after the focal ischemia.

3. Other Factors

Focal cerebral ischemia caused a prolonged (up to 2 weeks) increase in the levels of TGF-β mRNA that correlated with the increase in monocyte/macrophage accumulation and with the formation of extracellular matrix in the area of the infarct (WANG et al. 1995). TGF-β mRNA and protein were significantly elevated in the penumbra region of human cortex obtained from post-stroke tissue samples (KRUPINSKI et al. 1996). The mRNA encoding the receptor PDGF-R β (was found to be highly induced following focal ischemia in the rat, in cortical areas surrounding the infarct (IIHARA 1996). PDGF-A and PDGF-B mRNAs were also found mainly in neurons in penumbra, but also in astrocytes in post-stroke human tissues (KRUPINSKI 1997). PDGF-R a and PDGF-R β were found mainly on neurons, and PDGF-R b on some endothelial cells. Midkine was found to be present in the surrounding ischemic zone of the infarct, but not in the necrotic lesion between the fourth and the fourteenth days following focal hypoxic-ischemic injury (YOSHIDA et al. 1995).

C. Specific Growth Factors Can Attenuate Morphological and Functional Damage Caused by Hypoxic-Ischemic Brain Injury

The recognition that specific neurotrophic factors are expressed at highly increased levels in the acutely injured brain, rapidly following injury, some of them responding along with immediate early genes, suggested that this phenomenon may represent a protective response by the injured neurons or glia, or by those indirectly affected by the injury. Recent studies with several growth factors using different models of hypoxic ischemic and other types of brain injury are suggestive that some neurotrophic factors in specific models of ischemia can reduce neuronal damage. This may present a pharmacological opportunity in applying growth factors for the treatment of hypoxic-ischemic brain injury.

A growing number of studies have accumulated over the past years that suggest that some growth factors may increase neuronal survival in vitro and in vivo and may enhance recovery after brain injury. It is somewhat difficult to compare the various reports, due to the use of biochemically very different factors applied in various different injury models. Nevertheless, some of the neurotrophic factors, tested so far, appear to show beneficial effects in reducing neuronal damage in various paradigms. However, a recent study cautions against this generalized view as, in a specific system, a trophic factor contributed to increased necrotic cell death.

I. Global Ischemic Injury

Models of neonatal and adult global hypoxic-ischemic brain injury have been developed in various species, including rodents and sheep (GUNN et al. 1990; JOHNSTON et al. 1996). The degree of neuronal damage can be controlled by the length of the hypoxic-ischemic conditions. Short exposure leads to selective hippocampal neuronal cell death, whereas long exposure also causes cortical and striatal damage.

1. Neurotrophins

A single intracerebroventricular (ICV) application of NGF was found to be protective against delayed cell death in a model of forebrain ischemia, in rats, produced by transient bilateral occlusion of the common carotid arteries and lowering blood pressure for 8min (TANAKA et al. 1994). Cell death in the hippocampal CA1 region was assessed 7 days after ischemia. NGF reduced cell death from about 87% in controls to about 14%. Intraventricular injection of NGF, either before or after 5min of forebrain ischemia in the gerbil, significantly reduced the occurrence of delayed hippocampal cell death (SHIGENO et al. 1991). A large amount of NGF in transient global ischemia in the gerbil was delivered with the atelo-collagen mini-pellet system. NGF, when given continuously at such high concentrations, prevented pyramidal cell damage (YAMAMOTO et al. 1992). In dissociated hippocampal cell cultures subjected to hypoglycemia or excitotoxic conditions, NGF was found to be a relatively potent protective agent, whereas BDNF and NT-3 only had weak protective effects (CHENG and MATTSON 1991, 1994).

A continuous ICV infusion of BDNF for 7 days starting immediately before the onset of transient forebrain ischemia in the rat significantly decreased cell death in the CA1 region of the hippocampus (BECK et al. 1994). Increased trkB hybridization in the CA1 area was observed during the postischemic phase. A single ICV injection of BDNF prior to global forebrain ischemia was found to be highly protective for hippocampal CA1 neurons (TSUKAHARA et al. 1994). Oxygen and glucose deprivation-induced ischemia in organotypic hippocampal cultures causes cell death similar to that observed in vivo in global ischemia. Pre- but not post-ischemic addition of BDNF produced a concentration-dependent reduction in neuronal damage in this system (PRINGLE et al. 1996) whereas neurotrophin-3 did not have an effect on hippocampal cell death under the same conditions. A single ICV injection of BDNF resulted in rapid and robust phosphorylation of trk receptors in multiple brain regions in the postnatal day (PD) 7 rat brain (Cheng et al. 1997). BDNF also markedly protected against hypoxic-ischemic brain injury at PD7. It protected against 90% of tissue loss due to hypoxic-ischemia when given just prior to the insult and against 50% of tissue loss when given after the insult. In contrast, ICV injection of BDNF in PD21 and adult rats resulted in little trk phosphorylation and less dramatic protection against unilateral hypoxic-ischemic injury at PD21.

2. Basic Fibroblast Growth Factor

In 7-day rat pups, bFGF when injected intraperitoneally 30 min prior to a combined carotid artery ligation and hypoxia followed by striatal NMDA injections, reduced the rate and size of cortical and striatal damage (Nozaki et al. 1993a,b). In a similar study, using the same model, bFGFs protective effect could be extended up to 1 h after the injury (Nozaki et al. 1993b). Acidic fibroblast factor, when applied prior to ischemia, protected hippocampal CA1 neurons (Sasaki et al. 1992). Gerbil hippocampal CA1 neurons could be protected by continuos ICV bFGF infusion (Nakata et al. 1993).

bFGF can also protect neurons in cell culture. Various central neuronal populations are protected by bFGF from excitotoxicity and other toxic agents in vitro (Freese et al. 1992; Fernandez-Sanchez and Novelli 1993; Zhang et al. 1993). bFGF in combination with the N-methyl-D-aspartate (NMDA) receptor antagonist MK-801 was found to be protective in organotypic hippocampal slice cultures that were exposed to combined oxygen and glucose deprivation. bFGF alone reduced neuronal cell death, although not as effectively as MK-801. However, the two compounds together provided a high degree of protection that was synergistic (Barth et al. 1996). Sakaki et al. (1995) found bFGF added to cultured cortical neurons exposed to hypoxia for 24 h significantly reduced neuronal injury. bFGF mRNA and protein were strongly induced in these cultures upon exposure to a brief period of tolerizing hypoxia. Basic FGF may have contributed to the protection in this model. Transgenic mice expressing bovine basic fibroblast growth factor were exposed to right carotid artery ligation, hyperglycemia, and 20 min of 1% carbon monoxide (MacMillan et al. 1993). The number of surviving CA1 neurons in the right hippocampus was almost two-fold in hypoxic-ischemic transgenic mice compared with nontransgenic controls.

3. TGF-b, IGF-I and Other Factors

In a rat model using transient (10 min) bilateral carotid artery occlusion combined with hypoxia, TGF-b in a single dose of 10 ng injected intracerebroventricularly 2 h following hypoxia, reduced infarction in the cortex, striatum, thalamus, and dentate gyrus, and improved neurobehavioral performance (McNeill et al. 1994). In a similar model of transient forebrain ischemia induced by bilateral occlusion of the carotid arteries combined with systemic hypotension for 10 min, 4 ng TGF-beta 1 was found to be protective when injected intracerebroventricularly or intrahippocampally 1 h before ischemia. However, lower or higher amounts (0.5, 50 ng) were ineffective (Henrich-Noack et al. 1996). In vitro, a 24-h pretreatment of cultured hippocampal neurons with TGF-beta 1 (0.1 to 10 ng/mL) significantly inhibited nitric oxide and staurosporine induced neurotoxicity. Posttreatment with TGF-beta 1 (10 ng/mL) also inhibited staurosporine neurotoxicity but potentiated nitric oxide-induced neuronal injury (Henrich-Noack et al. 1996).

In a rat model of carotid artery occlusion combined with hypoxia, a single intraventricular injection of IGF-I caused a significant reduction of cerebral infarct size, particularly in the cortex and the dentate gyrus, whereas insulin had no significant effect (Gluckman et al. 1992; Guan et al. 1993). The protective effects of IGF-I were most significant in the cortex, striatum, and the dentate gyrus, with a marginal effect in the CA 1–4 regions of the hippocampus. An equivalent amount of insulin, or des(1–3) IGF-I had no significant effects. In a similar model of global ischemia, however in fetal sheep, the administration of very small doses of IGF-I proved to be highly protective for cortical, hippocampal, and striatal neurons (Johnston et al. 1996). In the rat model, the administration of IGF-I 30 min before the hypoxic ischemic insult did not seem to have any beneficial effects (Bergstedt and Wieloch 1993). Similarly, IGF-I was ineffective in decreasing hippocampal neuronal loss when applied 30 min before or 30 min after a hypoxia model using a 2-vessel occlusion in rats (Bergstedt and Wieloch 1993). Insulin was found to be more potent than IGF-I in decreasing the number of cortical and striatal necrotic neurons when applied as a constant ventricular infusion over a one-week period after a mild transient forebrain ischemia in rats (Voll and Auer 1991; Zhu and Auer 1994). IGF-I and -II protected cultured hippocampal and septal neurons from hypoglycemic neuronal cell death (Cheng and Mattson 1992).

CNTF infused continuously for 1 week ICV into gerbils starting 2 h before a brief transient forebrain ischemia. This treatment prevented ischemia-induced learning disability in a dose-dependent manner as analyzed in a step-down passive avoidance task. Light and electron microscopic examination showed that pyramidal neurons in the CA1 region of the hippocampus as well as synapses within the molecular layer were highly preserved in gerbils infused with CNTF than in controls (Wen et al. 1995b). However, CNTF was found to be ineffective in a model of rat transient forebrain ischemia (Ogata et al. 1996). In this experiment, CNTF was infused continuously starting 1 week before the induction of ischemia and continued until 1 week after the ischemia which was induced by 7 min of bilateral carotid occlusion with hypotension. Neuronal cell death in the hippocampal CA1 area was evaluated 1 week after the ischemia. Although cell death was slightly lower in the CNTF-treated group as compared with controls, this was statistically not different. Prosaposin, saposin C, and a18-mer saposin fragment promoted survival and neurite outgrowth of cultured rat hippocampal neurons in a dose-dependent manner. Infusion of the 18-mer peptide into the lateral ventricle of gerbils, starting either 2h before or immediately after 3min of forebrain ischemia lasting for 7 days, protected ischemia-induced learning disability and hippocampal CA1 neuronal loss (KOTANI et al. 1996).

II. Focal Ischemic Injury

1. Neuroprotective Effects of Neurotrophins

NGF and to a lesser extent BDNF produced by the hippocampus act as trophic factors for innervating cholinergic neurons (HEFTI 1986; KNÜSEL et al. 1992). BDNF also acts as a survival factor for cortical neurons in culture (GHOSH et al. 1992). BDNF attenuated apoptotic cell death caused by serum-deprivation of cortical neurons in vitro (KOH et al. 1995). Based on a large number of studies, neurotrophins may act as target-derived trophic factors, as well as autocrine or local paracrine factors in the hippocampus, for innervating neuronal populations, and for cortical neurons.

After transient MCAO, upregulation of BDNF mRNA in cortical neurons suggests that BDNF potentially plays a neuroprotective role in focal cerebral ischemia. SCHABITZ et al. (1997) analyzed the effect of ICV infusion of BDNF (2.1 micrograms/day for 8 days), beginning 1 day before the permanent MCAO in rats. Neurological deficit assessed daily, improved in BDNF-treated animals as compared with controls. Mean total infarct volume in BDNF-treated animals was about 40% lower than in controls whereas cortical infarct volume in BDNF-treated animals was about 70% lower than in controls.

In an in vitro study, however, instead of acting as protectant, BDNF potentiated the necrotic cell death of cortical neurons induced by oxygen-glucose deprivation or by NMDA (CHOI 1995). BDNF pretreatment of cortical cultures increased Ca2+ uptake induced by oxygen-glucose deprivation. The NMDA-antagonist MK-801 inhibited this increase in Ca2+ influx, as well as neuronal death but the kainate-antagonist NBQX did not have any influence. It appears that BDNF pretreatment may have made cortical neurons more vulnerable to the subsequent insult rather than making them more resistant as would have been expected from previous work. Thus, the protective effects of neurotrophic factors cannot be generalized and it is possible that the two types of cell death (apoptosis vs necrosis) involve different mechanisms differently influenced by the same neurotrophic agents.

As TrkB was highly induced following transient MCAO in the cortex, the only other member of the neurotrophin family acting via this receptor, neurotrophin-4/5 (NT-4/5) was evaluated for its possible effect in permanent focal cerebral ischemia in the rat (CHAN et al. 1996). Permanent focal cerebral ischemia in rats was produced by right side MCAO. NT-4/5 was administered ICV one day before and immediately following occlusion. NT-4/5 treatment reduced infarction volume by 34% when compared to control rats one day after the permanent MCAO. Infarction volume was unaltered by the neurotrophin treatment 4 to 7 days after occlusion. In contrast to transient MCAO, the permanent MCAO used in this study led to a significant reduction in levels of mRNAs coding for catalytic and truncated TrkB receptors which remained unaffected by NT-4/5 treatment.

Unoki and LaVail (1994) studied the effects of BDNF in a model of retinal ischemia in rats that can be established by increasing intraocular pressure. This treatment causes a thinning and a decrease in cell numbers in the inner retinal layers, but not in the photoreceptor nuclear layer. BDNF reduced this damage when injected intravitreally 2 days before ischemia. At 7 days postischemia, the inner retinal layers were far less damaged, and more ganglion cells were present. If a second injection of BDNF was made 5 days after the ischemic insult, then the inner retinal layers were more preserved than controls at 14 days postischemia, but the survival of ganglion cells was not enhanced. A single injection of BDNF at either 1 or 3 days postischemia reduced the degree of inner retinal damage and increased the number of surviving ganglion cells over controls.

2. Neuroprotective Effects of bFGF

bFGF in different models has, in most cases, significant neuroprotective effects. In an adult rat permanent MCAO model, intracisternally administered bFGF significantly reduced thalamic cell death (Yamada et al. 1991). bFGF was first given one day after the lesion, and then repeatedly once a week for up to four weeks.

In a mouse MCAO model, bFGF administered intravenously for 2–6 days starting 15 min postischemia, reduced the number of astrocytes and macrophages analyzed 7 days later (Brown et al. 1993). In a permanent MCAO model in the rat, Koketsu et al. (1994) found that continuous ICV infusion of basic FGF (1.2 micrograms/day; with or without heparin) for 3 days before focal ischemic infarcts protected from ischemic damage. The occlusion was made in the right lateral cerebral cortex by permanent distal MCAO and temporary (45 min) bilateral carotid occlusion. There was a 25% reduction in infarct volume in basic fibroblast growth factor- versus vehicle-treated animals which was not influenced by the addition of heparin.

These studies have shown that bFGF, administered ICV or intravenously, before or within several hours after ischemia, reduces infarct size and neurological deficits in permanent focal cerebral ischemia in the rat. In separate studies, using the same model, Fisher et al. (1995) found that delayed administration of bFGF after MCAO improved morphological recovery. Kawamata et al. (1996) tested the hypothesis that bFGF, also administered at later time points after ischemia, might improve behavioral recovery, even without affecting the size of infarction. Rats were injected intracisternally with bFGF twice weekly for 4 weeks, starting 1 day after permanent MCAO. Within 4 weeks after ischemia, there was no difference in infarct volume between bFGF- and vehicle-treated animals. However, there was a clear enhancement in the rate and degree of behavioral recovery among bFGF-treated animals, suggesting that trophic-factor treatment may be beneficial beyond improving morphological measurements.

bFGF was also found to be protective in a model of transient MCAO (Jiang et al. 1996). After 2h of occlusion, bFGF was infused intravenously for 3h. There was a 40% reduction in infarct volume in bFGF-treated compared with the vehicle-treated rats. This was associated with improved neurological outcome and regained body weight in bFGF-treated animals.

Ren and Finklestein (1997) reported that the time dependence of bFGF infusion on infarct reduction was an important factor in clinically evaluating bFGF. They reported a significant reduction in infarct volume when the bFGF infusion (50 μg/kg per hour for 3h) was begun up to 3h, but not 4h after the onset of ischemia. The infarct-reducing effects of bFGF were not altered by co-infusion of heparin.

In one study, a lack of neuroprotection with bFGF, when applied following MCAO, was reported (Tenjin et al. 1995). The number of live neurons in the peri-infarction cortex was significantly decreased compared with the contralateral control cortex 1 week after MCAO. The chronic administration of bFGF, starting 2 days after MCAO, did not result in either a significant increase in neovascularization or a higher number of live neurons in the peri-infarction cortex.

3. Neuroprotective Effects of IGF-I, TGF-β and Other Growth Factors

Cerebral ischemia induces delayed neuronal death in stroke-prone spontaneously hypertensive rats (SP-SHR). Cultured cortical neurons from SP-SHR were more vulnerable than neurons from Wistar rats when treated with nitric oxide and NMDA (Tagami et al. 1997). IGF-1 protected neurons prepared from SP-SHR against NO- and NMDA-mediated neurotoxicity. Wortmannin, a phosphatidyl inositol (PI)-3-kinase inhibitor, lowered the protective effects of IGF-1 against NO-mediated toxicity.

In a rabbit model of thrombo-embolic stroke, a single intracarotid injection of 10 μg TGF-b, applied at the time of embolization, reduced infarct size by about 45% compared with controls (Gross et al. 1993). TGF-b also protected cortical neurons in culture from glutamate toxicity in a concentration-dependent manner in the low ng/ml range (Prehn et al. 1993; Henrich-Noack et al. 1994). The effect of TGF-β at low concentrations was protective against glutamate-induced excitotoxic neuronal cell death, whereas at high concentrations it potentiated cell death (Prehn and Krieglstein 1994). In a mouse model of permanent MCAO, ICV-applied TGFb-1 significantly reduced the size of the infarcted cortical area (Henrich-Noack et al. 1994).

ICV and intraparenchymal administration of GDNF greatly protected from cortical infarction induced by transient MCAO. In addition, the increase in nitric oxide that accompanies MCAO and subsequent reperfusion is blocked almost completely by GDNF (Wang et al. 1997).

CNTF was infused continuously, ICV, for 4 weeks, starting just after permanent occlusion of the left middle cerebral artery (MCA) in SP-SHRs (Kumon et al. 1996). CNTF infusion prevented ischemia-induced learning disability in a dose-dependent manner in rats subjected to the Morris water-maze test (Wen et al. 1995a,b). Cortical infarction and retrograde degeneration of ipsilateral thalamic neurons in ischemic rats infused with CNTF were significantly less severe than in controls.

4. Protection Via Neurotrophic-Factor Induction

Several small molecules have been described that induce the expression of neurotrophic factors in the brain. Several of these compounds have been tested in models of cerebral ischemia. L-Threo-3,4-dihydroxyphenylserine (DOPS) increased nerve growth factor (NGF) synthesis in cultured mouse L-M fibroblast and astroglial cells. Lee et al. (1994) found that DOPS protected hippocampal CA1 from cell death in a dose-dependent manner after transient forebrain ischemia in gerbils.

Clenbuterol, a $\beta 2$-adrenergic receptor agonist, enhances NGF synthesis in the adult rat brain. Exposure of mixed neuronal/glial hippocampal cultures to clenbuterol led to elevated NGF secretion (Semkova et al. 1996a). When cultures were exposed to 1 mM L-glutamate for 1 h in serum-free medium, NGF protected hippocampal neurons from excitotoxic damage, when added to the medium 4 h before induction of the injury and continued until 18 h after. Clenbuterol was similarly as protective as NGF under the same experimental conditions. The neuroprotective activity of clenbuterol against glutamate-induced damage in hippocampal cultures was blocked by anti-NGF monoclonal antibodies added to the medium during the clenbuterol exposure, demonstrating that the neuronal rescue is mediated by NGF.

Propranolol, a β-adrenergic receptor antagonist, added 20 min before and kept in the medium during exposure of the cultures to clenbuterol, reversed the neuroprotective activity, suggesting that the induction of NGF and neuroprotection caused by clenbuterol are mediated via β-adrenergic receptor activation. The capacity of clenbuterol to protect hippocampal neurons was also demonstrated in vivo in a rat model of transient forebrain ischemia. Clenbuterol (4×1 mg/kg) administered intraperitoneally (i.p.) increased the number of viable neurons in the CA1 subfield of the rat hippocampus. Furthermore, clenbuterol [0.3 mg/kg and 1 mg/kg, i.p., and 1 mg/kg, subcutaneously (s.c.)] reduced the infarct area on the mouse brain surface significantly, after occlusion of the MCA (Semkova et al. 1996a).

Selegiline, a monoamine oxidase-B (MAO-B) inhibitor, potentiates glial reaction to injury and has "trophic-like" activities which do not depend on the inhibition of MAO-B. Selegiline induced NGF mRNA levels in cultured rat cortical astrocytes, resulting in an increased NGF protein secretion into astrocyte-conditioned medium. Exposure of hippocampal cultures to selegiline enhanced the secretion of NGF after 6 h of incubation. Selegiline, when added 6h before the exposure to glutamate and continued until 18h after, protected hippocampal neurons from excitotoxic death. Furthermore, the drug enhanced the expression of the NGF message in intact rat cerebral cortex and protected rat cortical tissue from ischemic insult caused by permanent MCAO. The neuroprotective activity of selegiline was also demonstrated in a mouse model of focal cerebral ischemia (SEMKOVA et al. 1996b).

D. Therapeutic Potential of Neurotrophic Factors in Hypoxic-Ischemic Brain Injury

Hypoxic-ischemic brain injuries increase the expression of many neurotrophic factor and neurotrophic factor-receptor genes. These, produced in and around the injured area, increase the survival of specific neurons, help retain their connections and, thus, improve the retention of neural functions. In addition, neurotrophic factors can also enhance neurite outgrowth, and this may contribute to increased plasticity following the injury. Neurotrophic factors may become important components of an efficient post-ischemic treatment regimen along with thrombolytic agents and other neuroprotective compounds.

Despite all of the positive data, neurotrophic factors are not always beneficial. They enhance synaptic transmission, and this activity may contribute to the propagation of seizure activity following hypoxic-ischemic injury. In a recent study, BDNF was found to increase hypoxic-ischemic necrotic cell death. Hypoxic-ischemic brain injury in survivors of perinatal asphyxia is a frequently encountered clinical problem for which there is currently no effective therapy. NTs, IGFs and other agents can protect responsive neurons against cell death in some injury paradigms.

It appears that rapid cell death following long-term oxygen-glucose deprivation or excitotoxic insults, is necrotic and not apoptotic. This process takes place in the core of the infarct of focal ischemic brain injury. In contrast, in transient global ischemia and in the penumbral area of focal ischemia, a type of cell death has been observed which has been described as delayed neuronal cell death. This process has apoptotic characteristics according to recent studies (HERON et al. 1993; BEILHARZ et al. 1995a; NITATORI et al. 1995). In agreement with the hypothesis that neurotrophic factors protect from hypoxic-ischemic injury by inhibiting apoptosis, overexpressing positive intracellular regulators of apoptosis or inhibiting negative regulators have been found to lead to increased survival of hypoxic-ischemic brain injuries. MARTINOU et al. (1994) found that transgenic mice overexpressing the anti-apoptotic *bcl-2* gene, when subjected to hypoxic-ischemic injury, showed significantly less damage than controls.

FRIEDLANDER et al. (1997) constructed transgenic mice expressing a mutant IL-1b converting enzyme (ICE) gene that acts as a dominant negative ICE inhibitor. After permanent focal ischemia by MCAO, the mutant transgenic mice showed significantly reduced brain injury and less behavioral deficits than the wild-type controls.

In addition to their direct effects on neuronal survival and resistance, growth factors can also protect neurons indirectly, by inhibiting processes which would lead to neuronal cell death. Among these, several growth factors, including TGF-b and some ILs, have been shown to inhibit the proliferation of microglia and the infiltration of macrophages into the CNS (BARNUM and JONES 1994; HUNTER et al. 1993; SUZUMURA et al. 1993).

For practical application, it is important to consider the available time window within which a factor has beneficial physiological effects. It appears that the majority of neurotrophic factors are most potent when applied prior to or immediately following the injury.

For therapeutic utility, the route of administration of trophic factors is an important problem to be solved. In the studies reviewed above, exogenous growth factors were applied by various routes. bFGF, IGF-1, TGF-β, for example, are all effective when injected or infused ICV; there seems to be sufficient uptake of growth-factor proteins from the ventricular surface into the brain parenchyma. For potential future clinical plans, however, systemic routes of administration may be more practical. bFGF and TGF-β were also efficacious when administered intravenously or intra-arterially, respectively. In hypoxic-ischemic brain injury, the blood–brain barrier is compromised in the infarcted area which may be beneficial for the administration of exogenous factors.

In one clinical study, young children with mental retardation due to perinatal hypoxia were treated with bFGF and were found to show improvement in their mental development. Bovine bFGF was administered intramuscularly in children, aged 1–15 years, once or twice a month, over 7–12 months. Development as assessed by psychometric measurements increased significantly in treated children and their IQ rose by more than 10 points (AGUILAR et al. 1993).

Perhaps the factor studied most extensively in focal ischemic brain injury is bFGF. Based on the large amount of encouraging pharmacological data, bFGF has recently entered clinical testing for the treatment of stroke.

References

Aguilar LC, Islas A, Rosique P, Hernandez B, Portillo E, Herrera JM, Cortes R, Cruz S, Alfaro F, Martin R (1993) Psychometric analysis in children with mental retardation due to perinatal hypoxia treated with fibroblast growth factor (FGF) and showing improvement in mental development. J Intellect Disabil Res 37:507–520

Arai S, Kinouchi H, Akabane A, Owada Y, Kamii H, Kawase M, Yoshimoto T (1996) Induction of brain-derived neurotrophic factor (BDNF) and the receptor trk B mRNA following middle cerebral artery occlusion in rat. Neurosci Lett 211:57–60

Arakawa Y, Sendtner M, Thoenen H (1990) Survival effect of ciliary neurotrophic factor (CNTF) on chick embryonic motoneurons in culture: comparison with other neurotrophic factors and cytokines. J Neurosci 10:3507–3515

Ballarin M, Ernfors P, Lindefors N, Persson H (1991) Hippocampal damage and kainic acid injection induce a rapid increase in mRNA for BDNF and NGF in the rat brain. Exp Neurol 114:35–43

Barbacid M (1995) Neurotrophic factors and their receptors. Curr Opin Cell Biol 7:148–155

Barde Y-A (1989) Trophic factors and neuronal survival. Neuron 2:1525–1534

Barnum SR, Jones JL (1994) Transforming growth factor-beta 1 inhibits inflammatory cytokine-induced C3 gene expression in astrocytes. J Immunol 152:765–773

Barth A, Barth L, Morrison RS, Newell DW (1996) bFGF enhances the protective effects of MK-801 against ischemic neuronal injury in vitro. Neuroreport 7:1461–1464

Beck KD, Valverde J, Alexi T et al. (1995) Mesencephalic dopaminergic neurons protected by GDNF from axotomy-induced degeneration in the adult brain. Nature 373:339–41

Beck T, Lindholm D, Castren E, Wree A (1994) Brain-derived neurotrophic factor protects against ischemic cell damage in rat hippocampus. J Cereb Blood Flow Metab 14:689–692

Beilharz E, Williams CE, Dragunow M, Sirimanne ES, Gluckman PD (1995a) Mechanisms of delayed cell death following hypoxic-ischemic injury in the immature rat: evidence for apoptosis during selective neuronal loss. Mol Brain Res 29:1–14

Beilharz EJ, Bassett NS, Sirimanne ES, Williams CE, Gluckman PD (1995b) Insulin-like growth factor II is induced during wound repair following hypoxic-ischemic injury in the developing brain. Mol Brain Res 29:81–91

Bengzon J, Kokaia Z, Ernfors P et al. (1993) Regulation of neurotrophin and trkA, trkB and trkC tyrosine kinase receptor messenger RNA expression in kindling. Neuroscience 53:433–446

Bengzon J, Söderström S, Kokaia Z et al. (1992) Widespread increase of nerve growth factor protein in the rat forebrain after kindling-induced seizures. Brain Res 4:396–403

Bergstedt K, Wieloch T (1993) Changes in insulin-like growth factor 1 receptor density after transient cerebral ischemia in the rat. Lack of protection against ischemic brain damage following injection of insulin-like growth factor 1. J Cereb Blood Flow Metab 13:895–898

Breier G, Damert A, Plate KH, Risau W (1997) Angiogenesis in embryos and ischemic diseases. Thromb Haemost 78:678–683

Brown CM, Calder C, Emmett C, Spedding M (1993) Neuroprotective properties of bFGF in a mouse model of focal ischemia. Br J Pharmacol 109:204P

Castr+n E, Zafra F, Thoenen H, Lindholm D (1992) Light regulates expression of brain-derived neurotrophic factor mRNA in rat visual cortex. Proc Natl Acad Sci U S A 89:9444–9448

Chan KM, Lam DT, Pong K, Widmer HR, Hefti F (1996) Neurotrophin-4/5 treatment reduces infarct size in rats with middle cerebral artery occlusion. Neurochem Res 21:763–767

Chao MV, Hempstead BL (1995) p75 and Trk: a two-receptor system. Trends Neurosci 18:321–326

Cheng B, Mattson MP (1991) NGF and bFGF protect rat hippocampal and human cortical neurons against hypoglycemic damage by stabilizing calcium homeostasis. Neuron 7:1031–1041

Cheng B, Mattson MP (1992) IGF-I and IGF-II protect cultured hippocampal and septal neurons against calcium-mediated hypoglycemic damage. J Neurosci 12:1558–1566

Cheng B, Mattson MP (1944) NT-3 and BDNF protect CNS neurons against metabolic/excitotoxic insults. Brain Res 640:56–67

Cheng B, Mattson MP (1994) NT-3 and BDNF protect CNS neurons against metabolic/excitotoxic insults. Brain Res 640:56–67

Cheng Y, Gidday JM, Yan Q, Shah AR, Holtzman DM (1997) Marked age-dependent neuroprotection by brain-derived neurotrophic factor against neonatal hypoxic-ischemic brain injury. Ann Neurol 41:521–529

Comelli MC, Seren MS, Guidolin D et al. (1992) Photochemical stroke and brain derived neurotrophic factor (BDNF) mRNA expression. Neuroreport 3:473–476

Comelli MC, Guidolin D, Seren MS et al. (1993) Time course, localization and pharmacological modulation of immediate early inducible genes, brain derived neurotrophic factor and trkB messenger RNAs in the rat brain following photochemical stroke. Neuroscience 55:473–490

Davies AM (1996) The neurotrophic hypothesis: where does it stand? Philos Trans R Soc Lond B Biol Sci 351:389–394

Dragunow M, Beilharz E, Mason B, Lawlor P, Abraham W, Gluckman P (1993) Brain-derived neurotrophic factor expression after long-term potentiation. Neurosci Lett 160:232–236

Dragunow M, Beilharz E, Sirimanne E, Lawlor P, Williams C, Bravo R, Gluckman P (1994) Immediate-early gene protein expression in neurons undergoing delayed death, but not necrosis, following hypoxic-ischaemic injury to the young rat brain. Mol Brain Res 25:19–33

Dugich-Djordjevic MM, Tocco G, Willoughby DA, Najm I, Pasinetti G, Thompson RF, Baudry M, Lapchak PA, Hefti F (1992) BDNF mRNA expression in the developing brain following kainic acid-induced limbic seizure activity. Neuron 8:1127–1138

Ebendal T, Olson L, Seiger A, Hedlund K-O (1980) Nerve growth factors in the rat iris. Nature 286:461–470

Endoh M, Pulsinelli WA, Wagner JA (1994) Transient global ischemia induces dynamic changes in the expression of bFGF and the FGF receptor. Mol Brain Res 22:76–88

Ernfors P, Bengzon J, Kokaia Z, Persson H, Lindvall O (1991) Increased levels of messenger RNAs for neurotrophic factors in the brain during kindling epileptogenesis. Neuron 7:165–176

Falls DL, Rosen KM, Corfas G, Lane WS, Fischbach GD (1993) ARIA, a protein that stimulates acetylcholine receptor synthesis, is a member of the neu ligand family. Cell 72:801–815

Fernandez-Sanchez MT, Novelli A (1993) Basic fibroblast growth factor protects cerebellar neurons in primary culture from NMDA and non-NMDA receptor mediated neurotixicity. FEBS Lett 335:124–131

Ferrer I, Ballabriga J, Marti E, Pozas E, Planas AM, Blasi J (1997) BDNF and TrkB co-localize in CA1 neurons resistant to transient forebrain ischemia in the adult gerbil. J Neuropathol Exp Neurol 56:790–797

Finklestein SP, Apostolides PJ, Caday CG, Prosser J, Philips MF, Klagsbrun M (1988) Increased basic fibroblast growth factor (bFGF) immunoreactivity at the site of focal brain wounds. Brain Res 460:253–259

Finklestein SP, Caday CG, Kano M et al. (1990) Growth factor expression after stroke. Stroke 21 [Suppl III]: 122–124

Fisher M, Meadows ME, Do T, Weise J, Trubetskoy V, Charette M, Finklestein SP (1995) Delayed treatment with intravenous basic fibroblast growth factor reduces infarct size following permanent focal cerebral ischemia in rats. J Cereb Blood Flow Metab 15:953–959

Freese A, Finklestein SP, DiFiglia M (1992) Basic fibroblast growth factor protects striatal neurons in vitro from NMDA receptor mediated excitotoxicity. Brain Res 575:351–355

Friedlander RM, Gagliardini V, Hara H, Fink KB, Li W, MacDonald G, Fishman MC, Greenberg AH, Moskowitz MA, Yuan J (1997) Expression of a dominant negative mutant of interleukin-1 beta converting enzyme in transgenic mice prevents neuronal cell death induced by trophic factor withdrawal and ischemic brain injury. J Exp Med 185:933–940

Gall CM, Isackson PJ (1989) Limbic seizures increase neuronal production of mRNA for nerve growth factor. Science 245:758–761

Gall C, Murray K, Isackson PJ (1991) Kainic acid-induced seizures stimulate increased expression of nerve growth factor mRNA in rat hippocampus. Brain Res Mol Brain Res 9:113–123

Gall CM, Berschauer R, Isackson PJ (1994) Seizures increase basic fibroblast growth factor mRNA in adult rat forebrain neurons and glia. Mol Brain Res 21:190–205

Ghosh A, Carnahan J, Greenberg ME (1992) Requirement for BDNF in activity-dependent survival of cortical neurons. Science 263:1618–1623

Gluckman P, Klempt N, Guan J, et al. (1992) A role for IGF-1 in the rescue of CNS neurons following hypoxic-ischemic injury. Biochem Biophys Res Comm 182:593–599

Goldberg MP, Choi DW (1993) Combined oxygen and glucose deprivation in cortical cell culture: calcium-dependent and calcium-independent mechanisms of neuronal injury. J Neurosci 13:3510–3524

Gomez-Pinilla F, Lee JW, Cotman CW (1992) Basic FGF in adult rat brain: cellular distribution and response to entorhinal lesion and fimbria-fornix transection. J Neurosci 12:345–355

Gomez-Pinilla F, van der Wal EA, Cotman CW (1995) Possible coordinated gene expressions for FGF receptor, FGF-5 and FGF-2 following seizures. Exp Neurol 133:164–174

Gross CE, Bednar MM, Howard DB, Sporn MB (1993) Transforming growth factor-b1 reduces infarct size after experimental cerebral ischemia in a rabbit model. Stroke 24:558–562

Guan J, William CE Gunning M, Mallard EC, Gluckman PD (1993) The effects of IGF-1 treatment after hypoxic-ischemic brain injury in adult rats. J Cereb Blood Flow Metab 13:609–616

Gunn AJ, Dragunow M, Faull RL, Gluckman PD (1990) Effects of hypoxia-ischaemia and seizures on neuronal and glial-like c-fos protein levels in the infant rat. Brain Res 531:105–116

Gwag BJ, Sessler FM, Waterhouse BD, Springer JE (1993) Regulation of nerve growth factor mRNA in the hippocampal formation: effects of N-methyl-D-aspartate receptor activation. Exp Neurol 121:160–171

Hagg T, Quon D, Higaki J, Varon S (1992) Ciliary neurotrophic factor prevents neuronal degeneration and promotes low affinity NGF receptor expression in the adult rat CNS. Neuron 8:145–158

Hama T, Kushima Y, Miyamoto M, Kubota M, Takei N, Hatanaka H (1991) Interleukin-6 improves the survival of mesencephalic catecholaminergic and septal cholinergic neurons from postnatal two-week old rats in cultures. Neuroscience 40:445–452

Hefti F (1986) Nerve growth factor promotes survival of septal cholinergic neurons after fimbrial transections. J Neurosci 8:2155–2162

Hefti F (1994) Neurotrophic factor therapy for nervous system degenerative diseases. J Neurobiol 25:1418–1435

Hefti F (1997) Pharmacology of neurotrophic factors. Annu Rev Pharmacol Toxicol 37:239–267

Henrich-Noack P, Prehn JH, Krieglstein J (1994) Neuroprotective effects of TGF-beta 1. J Neural Transm Suppl 43:33–45

Henrich-Noack P, Prehn JH, Krieglstein J (1996) TGF-beta 1 protects hippocampal neurons against degeneration caused by transient global ischemia. Dose-response relationship and potential neuroprotective mechanisms. Stroke 27:1609–1614

Heron A, Pollard H, Dessi F, Moreau J, Lasbennes F, Ben-Ari Y, Charriaut-Marlangue C (1993) Regional variability in DNA fragmentation after global ischemia evidenced by combined histological and gel electrophoresis observations in the rat brain. J Neurochem 61:1973–1976

Holmes WE, Sliwkowski MX, Akita RW et al. (1992) Identification of heregulin, a specific activator of p185erbB2. Science 256:1205–1208

Honda S, Kagoshima M, Wanaka A, Tohyama M, Matsumoto K, Nakamura T (1995) Localization and functional coupling of HGF and c-Met/HGF receptor in rat brain: implication as neurotrophic factor. Brain Res Mol Brain Res 32:197–210

Hsu CY, An G, Liu JS, Xue JJ, He YY, Lin TN (1993) Expression of immediate early gene and growth factor mRNAs in a focal cerebral ischemia model in the rat. Stroke 24:178–188

Hu BR, Wieloch T (1993) Changes in tyrosine phosphorylation in neocortex following transient cerebral ischemia. Neuroreport 4:219–222

Humpel C, Hoffer B, Stromberg I, Bektesh S, Collins F, Olson L (1994) Neurons of the hippocampal formation express glial cell line-derived neurotrophic factor messenger RNA in response to kainate-induced excitation. Neuroscience 59:791–795

Hunter KE, Sporn MB, Davies AM (1993) Transforming growth factor-betas inhibit mitogen-stimulated proliferation of astrocytes. Glia 7:203–211

Iihara K (1996) Induction of platelet-derived growth factor beta-receptor in focal ischemia of rat brain. J Cereb Blood Flow Metab 16:941–949

Ip NY, Li Y, Yancopoulos GD, Lindsay RM (1993) Cultured hippocampal neurons show responses to BDNF, NT-3 and NT-4, but not NGF. J Neurosci 13:3394–3405

Isackson PJ (1995) Trophic factor response to neuronal stimuli or injury. Curr Opin Neurobiol 5:350–357

Isackson Pj, Huntsman MM, Murray KD, Gall CM (1991) BDNF mRNA expression is increased in adult rat forebrain after limbic seizures: temporal patterns of induction distinct from NGF. Neuron 6:937–948

Jiang N, Finklestein SP, Do T, Caday CG, Charette M, Chopp M (1996) Delayed intravenous administration of basic fibroblast growth factor (bFGF) reduces infarct volume in a model of focal cerebral ischemia/reperfusion in the rat. J Neurol Sci 139:173–179

Johnston BM et al. (1996) Insulin-like growth factor-1 is a potent neuronal rescue agent after hypoxic-ischemic injury in fetal lambs. J Clin Invest 97:300–308

Kamegai M, Niijima K, Kunishita T et al. (1990) Interleukin 3 as a trophic factor for central cholinergic neurons in vitro and in vivo. Neuron 2:429–436

Kang H, Schuman EM (1995) Long-lasting neurotrophin-induced enhancement of synaptic transmission in the adult hippocampus. Science 267:1658–1662

Kaplan DR, Stephens RM (1994) Neurotrophin signal transduction by the Trk receptor. J Neurobiol 25:1404–1417

Kawamata T, Alexis NE, Dietrich WD, Finklestein SP (1996) Intracisternal basic fibroblast growth factor (bFGF) enhances behavioral recovery following focal cerebral infarction in the rat. J Cereb Blood Flow Metab 16:542–547

Kirino T (1982) Delayed neuronal death in the gerbil hippocampus following ischemia. Brain Res 239:57–69

Kirino T, Nakagomi T, Kanemitsu H, Tamura A (1996) Ischemic tolerance. Adv Neurol 71:505–511

Klempt ND, Sirimanne E, Gunn AJ et al. (1992) Hypoxia-ischemia induces transforming growth factor beta 1 mRNA in the infant brain. Mol Brain Res 13:93–101

Knüsel B, Beck KD, Winslow JW et al. (1992) Brain-derived neurotrophic factor administration protects basal forebrain cholinergic but not nigral dopaminergic neurons from degenerative changes after axotomy in the adult brain. J Neurosci 12:4391–4402

Koh JY, Gwag BJ, Lobner D, Choi DW (1995) Potentiated necrosis of cultured cortical neurons by neurotrophins. Science 268:573–575

Kokaia Z, Gidö G, Ringstedt T et al. (1993) Rapid increase of BDNF mRNA levels in cortical neurons following spreading depression: regulation by glutamatergic mechanisms independent of seizure activity. Mol Brain Res 19:277–286

Kokaia Z, Metsis M, Kokaia M, Bengzon J, Elmer E, Smith ML, Timmusk T, Siesjo BK, Persson H, Lindvall O (1994) Brain insults in rats induce increased expression of the BDNF gene through differential use of multiple promoters. Eur J Neurosci 6:587–596

Kokaia Z, Zhao Q, Kokaia M, Elmer E, Metsis M, Smith ML, Siesjo BK, Lindvall O (1995) Regulation of brain-derived neurotrophic factor gene expression after transient middle cerebral artery occlusion with and without brain damage. Exp Neurol 136:73–88

Kokaia Z, Nawa H, Uchino H, Elmer E, Kokaia M, Carnahan J, Smith ML, Siesjo BK, Lindvall O (1996) Regional brain-derived neurotrophic factor mRNA and protein levels following transient forebrain ischemia in the rat. Brain Res Mol Brain Res 38:139–144

Koketsu N, Berlove DJ, Moskowitz MA, Kowall NW, Caday CG, Finklestein SP (1994) Pretreatment with intraventricular basic fibroblast growth factor decreases infarct size following focal cerebral ischemia in rats. Ann Neurol 35:451–457

Komoly S, Hudson LD, Webster HD, Bondy CA (1992) Insulin-like growth factor I gene expression is induced in astrocytes during experimental demyelination. Proc Natl Acad Sci USA 89:1894–1898

Konishi Y, Chui DH, Hirose H, Kunishita T, Tabira T (1993) Trophic effect of erythropoietin and other hemopoietic factors on central cholinergic neurons in vitro and in vivo. Brain Res 609:29–35

Korsching S (1993) The neurotrophic factor concept: a reexamination. J Neurosci 13:2739–2748

Kotani Y, Matsuda S, Wen TC, Sakanaka M, Tanaka J, Maeda N, Kondoh K, Ueno S, Sano A (1996) A hydrophilic peptide comprising 18 amino acid residues of the prosaposin sequence has neurotrophic activity in vitro and in vivo. J Neurochem 66:2197–2200

Krupinski J, Kumar P, Kumar S, Kaluza J (1996) Increased expression of TGF-beta 1 in brain tissue after ischemic stroke in humans. Stroke 27:852–857

Krupinski J (1997) A putative role for platelet-derived growth factor in angiogenesis and neuroprotection after ischemic stroke in humans. Stroke 28:564–573

Kumon Y, Sasaki S, Kadota O, et al. (1993) Transient increase in endogenous basic fibroblast growth factor in neurons of ischemic rat brains. Brain Res 605:169–174

Kumon Y, Sakaki S, Watanabe H, Nakano K, Ohta S, Matsuda S, Yoshimura H, Sakanaka M (1996) Ciliary neurotrophic factor attenuates spatial cognition impairment, cortical infarction and thalamic degeneration in spontaneously hypertensive rats with focal cerebral ischemia. Neurosci Lett 206:141–144

Lapchak PA, Araujo DM, Hefti F (1993) Cholinergic regulation of hippocampal brain-derived neurotrophic factor mRNA expression: evidence from lesion and chronic cholinergic drug treatment studies. Neuroscience 52:575–585

Lauterborn JC, Tran TM, Isackson PJ, Gall CM (1993) Nerve growth factor mRNA is expressed by GABAergic neurons in rat hippocampus. Neuroreport 13:273–276

Lee SH, Clemens JA, Bondy CA (1992) Insulin-like growth factors in the response to cerebral ischemia. Mol Cell Neurosci 3:36–43

Lee TH, Abe K, Aoki M, Nakamura M, Kogure K, Itoyama Y (1994) The protective effect of L–threo-3,4-dihydroxyphenylserine on ischemic hippocampal neuronal death in gerbils. Stroke 25:1425–1431

Leung DW, Cachianes G, Kuang WJ, Goeddel DV, Ferrara N (1989) Vascular endothelial growth factor is a secreted angiogenic mitogen. Science 246:1306–1309

Li YS, Milner PG, Chauhan AK et al. (1990) Cloning and expression of a developmentally regulated protein that induces mitogenic and neurite outgrowth activity. Science 250:1690–1694

Lim R, Miller JF, Zaheer A (1989) Purification and characterization of glia maturation factor beta: a growth regulator for neurons and glia. Proc Natl Acad Sci USA 86:3901–3905

Lin LFH, Mismer D, Lile JD et al. (1989) Purification, cloning, and expression of ciliary neurotrophic factor (CNTF). Science 246:1023–1025

Lin LF, Doherty DH, Lile JD, Bektesh S, Collins F (1993) GDNF: a glial cell line-derived neurotrophic factor for midbrain dopaminergic neurons. Science 260: 1130–1132

Lindefors N, Ernfors P, Falkenberg T, Persson H (1992) Septal cholinergic afferents regulate expression of brain-derived neurotrophic factor and beta-nerve growth factor mRNA in rat hippocampus. Exp Brain Res 88:78–90

Lindvall O, Ernfors P, Bengzon J, Kokaia Z, Smith ML, Siesjo BK, Persson H (1992) Differential regulation of mRNAs for nerve growth factor, brain-derived neurotrophic factor, and neurotrophin-3 in the adult rat brain following cerebral ischemia and hypoglycemic coma. Proc Natl Acad Sci USA 89:648–652

Lindvall O, Kokaia Z, Bengzon J, Elmér E, Kokaia M (1994) Neurotrophins and brain insults. Trends Neurosci. 17:490–496

Lippoldt A, Andbjer B, Rosen L, Richter E, Ganten D, Cao Y, Pettersson RF, Fuxe K (1993) Photochemically induced focal cerebral ischemia in rat: time dependent and global increase in expression of basic fibroblast growth factor mRNA. Brain Res 625:45–56

Lorez H, Keller F, Ruess G, Otten U (1989) Nerve growth factor increases in adult rat brain after hypoxic injury. Neurosci Lett 98:339–344

Lowenstein DH, Seren MS, Longo FM (1993) Prolonged increases in neurotrophic activity associated with kainate-induced hippocampal synaptic reorganization. Neuroscience 56:597–604

MacMillan V, Judge D, Wiseman A, Settles D, Swain J, Davis J (1993) Mice expressing a bovine basic fibroblast growth factor transgene in the brain show increased resistance to hypoxic-ischemic cerebral damage. Stroke 24:1735–1739

Maeda Y, Matsumoto M, Hori O, Kuwabara K, Ogawa S, Yan SD, Ohtsuki T, Kinoshita T, Kamada T, Stern DM (1994) Hypoxia/reoxygenation-mediated induction of astrocyte interleukin 6: a paracrine mechanism potentially enhancing neuron survival. J Exp Med 180:2297–2308

Maisonpierre PC, Suri C, Jones PF, Bartunkova S, Wiegand SJ, Radziejewski C, Compton D, McClain J, Aldrich TH, Papadopoulos N, Daly TJ, Davis S, Sato TN, Yancopoulos GD (1997) Angiopoietin-2, a natural antagonist for Tie2 that disrupts in vivo angiogenesis. Science 277:55–60

Marchionni MA, Goodearl, ADJ, Chen MS, et al. (1993) Glial growth factors are alternatively spliced erbB2 ligands expressed in the nervous system. Nature 362:312–316

Martinou JC, Dubois-Dauphin M, Staple JK, Rodriguez I, Frankowski H, Missotten M, Albertini P, Talabot D, Catsicas S, Pietra C (1994) Overexpression of BCL-2 in transgenic mice protects neurons from naturally occurring cell death and experimental ischemia. Neuron 13:1017–1030

Masumura M, Murayama N, Inoue T, Ohno T (1996) Selective induction of fibroblast growth factor receptor-1 mRNA after transient focal ischemia in the cerebral cortex of rats. Neurosci Lett 213:119–122

McNeill H, Williams CE, Guan J et al. (1994) Neuronal rescue with transforming growth factor-beta (1) after hypoxic-ischaemic brain injury. Neuroreport 5:901–904

Merenmies J, Rauvala H (1990) Molecular cloning of the 18-kDa growth-associated protein of developing brain. J Biol Chem 265:16721–16724

Merlio JP, Ernfors P, Jaber M, Persson H (1992) Molecular cloning of rat trkC and distribution of cells expressing messenger RNAs for members of the trk family in the rat central nervous system. Neuroscience 51:513–532

Merlio JP, Ernfors P, Kokaia Z, Middlemas DS, Bengzon J, Kokaia M, Smith ML, Siesjo BK, Hunter T, Lindvall O (1993) Increased production of the TrkB protein tyrosine kinase receptor after brain insults. Neuron 10:151–164

Morgan TE, Nichols NR, Pasinetti GM, Finch CE (1993) TGF-beta 1 mRNA increases in macrophage/microglial cells of the hippocampus in response to deafferentation and kainic acid-induced neurodegeneration. Exp Neurol 120:291–301

Nakata N, Kato H, Kogure K (1993) Protective effects of basic fibroblast growth factor against hippocampal neuronal damage following cerebral ischemia in the gerbil. Brain Res 605:354–356

Neeper SA, Gomez-Pinilla F, Choi J, Cotman CW (1996) Physical activity increases mRNA for brain-derived neurotrophic factor and nerve growth factor in rat brain. Brain Res 726:49–56

Nieto-Sampedro M, Berman MA (1987) Interleukin-1-like activity in rat brain: sources, targets and effects of injury. J Neurosci Res 17:214–219

Nitatori T, Sato N, Waguri S et al. (1995) Delayed neuronal death in the CA1 pyramidal cell layer of the gerbil hippocampus following transient ischemia is apoptosis. J Neurosci 15:1001–1011

Noble M, Wolswijk G, Wren D (1989) The complex relationship between cell division and the control of differentiation in oligodendrocyte-type-2 astrocyte progenitor cells isolated from perinatal and adult rat optic nerves. Prog Growth Factor Res 1:179–194

Nozaki K, Finklestein SP, Beal MF (1993a) Basic fibroblast growth factor protects against hypoxia/ischemia and NMDA neurotoxicity in neonatal rats. J Cereb Blood Flow Metab 13:221–228

Nozaki K, Finklestein SP, Beal MF (1993b) Delayed administration of basic fibroblast growth factor protects against N-methyl-D-aspartate neurotoxicity in neonatal rats. Eur J Pharmacol 232:295–297

Ogata N, Ogata K, Imhof HG, Yonekawa Y (1996) Effect of CNTF on ischaemic cell damage in rat hippocampus. Acta Neurochir (Wien)138:580–583

Pasinetti GM, Nichols NR, Rocco G, Morgan T, Laping N, Finch CE (1993) Transforming growth factor berta-1 (TGF-b1) and fibronectin mRNA in rat brain: responses to injury and cell type localization. Neuroscience 54:893–907

Patterson SL, Grover LM, Schwartzkroin PA, Bothwell M (1992) Neurotrophin expression in rat hippocampal slices: a stimulus paradigm inducing LTP in CA1 evokes increases in BDNF and NT-3 mRNAs. Neuron 9:1081–1088

Poulsen KT, Armanini MP, Klein RD, Hynes MA, Phillips HS, Rosenthal A (1994) TGF-b2 and TGF-b3 are potent survival factors for midbrain dopaminergic neurons. Neuron 13:1245–1252

Prehn JH, Backhauss C, Krieglstein J (1993) Transforming growth factor-beta 1 prevents glutamate neurotoxicity in rat neocortical cultures and protects mouse neocortex from ischemic injury in vivo. J Cereb Blood Flow Metab 13:521–525

Prehn JHM, Krieglstein J (1994) Opposing effects of transforming growth factor-beta 1 on glutamate neurotoxicity. Neurosci 60:7–10

Pringle AK, Sundstrom LE, Wilde GJ, Williams LR, Iannotti F (1996) Brain-derived neurotrophic factor, but not neurotrophin-3, prevents ischaemia-induced neuronal cell death in organotypic rat hippocampal slice cultures. Neurosci Lett 211:203–206

Recio-Pinto E, Rechler MM, Ishii DN (1986) Effects of insulin, insulin-like growth factor-II, and nerve growth factor on neurite formation and survival in cultured sympathetic and sensory neurons. J Neurosci 6:1211–1219

Ren JM, Finklestein SP (1997) Time window of infarct reduction by intravenous basic fibroblast growth factor in focal cerebral ischemia. Eur J Pharmacol 327:11–16

Rocamora N, Palacios JM, Mengod G (1992) Limbic seizures induce a differential regulation of the expression of nerve growth factor, brain-derived neurotrophic factor and neurotrophin-3 in the rat hippocampus. Brain Res Mol Brain Res 13:27–33

Sakaki T, Yamada K, Otsuki H, Yuguchi T, Kohmura E, Hayakawa T (1995) Brief exposure to hypoxia induces bFGF mRNA and protein and protects rat cortical neurons from prolonged hypoxic stress. Neurosci Res 23:289–296

Sasaki K, Oomura Y, Suzuki K, Hanai K, Yagi H (1992) Acidic fibroblast growth factor prevents death of hippocampal CA1 cells following ischemia. Neurochem Int 21:397–402

Sauer H, Rosenblad C, Bjorklund A (1995) Glial cell line-derived neurotrophic factor but not transforming growth factor beta 3 prevents delayed degeneration of nigral dopaminergic neurons following striatal 6-hydroxydopamine lesion. Proc Natl Acad Sci USA 92:8935–8939

Schabitz WR, Schwab S, Spranger M, Hacke W (1997) Intraventricular brain-derived neurotrophic factor reduces infarct size after focal cerebral ischemia in rats. J Cereb Blood Flow Metab 17:500–506

Schmidt-Kastner R, Tomac A, Hoffer B, Bektesh S, Rosenzweig B, Olson L (1994) Glial cell-line derived neurotrophic factor (GDNF) mRNA upregulation in striatum and cortical areas after pilocarpine-induced status epilepticus in rats. Brain Res Mol Brain Res 26:325–330

Schubert D, Kimura H, LaCorbiere M, Vaughn J, Karr D, Fischer WH (1990) Activin is a nerve cell survival molecule. Nature 344:868–870

Semkova I, Schilling M, Henrich-Noack P, Rami A, Krieglstein J (1996a) Clenbuterol protects mouse cerebral cortex and rat hippocampus from ischemic damage and attenuates glutamate neurotoxicity in cultured hippocampal neurons by induction of NGF. Brain Res 717:44–54

Semkova I, Wolz P, Schilling M, Krieglstein J (1996b) Selegiline enhances NGF synthesis and protects central nervous system neurons from excitotoxic and ischemic damage. Eur J Pharmacol 315:19–30

Shigeno T, Mima T, Takakura K, Graham DI, Kato G, Hashimoto Y, Furukawa S (1991) Amelioration of delayed neuronal death in the hippocampus by nerve growth factor. J Neurosci 11:2914–2919

Shozuhara H, Onodera H, Katoh-Semba R, Kato K, Yamasaki Y, Kogure K (1992) Temporal profiles of nerve growth factor b-subunit level in rat brain regions after transient ischemia. J Neurochem 59:175–180

Snider WD (1994) Functions of the neurotrophins during nervous system development: what the knockouts are teaching us. Cell 77:627–638

Speliotes EK, Caday CG, Do T, Weise J, Kowall NW, Finklestein (1996) Increased expression of basic fibroblast growth factor (bFGF) following focal cerebral infarction in the rat SP Brain Res Mol Brain Res 39:31–42

Suzuki F, Junier MP, Guilhem D, Sorensen JC, Onteniente B (1995) Morphogenetic effect of kainate on adult hippocampal neurons associated with a prolonged expression of brain-derived neurotrophic factor. Neuroscience 64:665–674

Suzumura A, Sawada M, Yamamoto H, Marunouchi T (1993) Transforming growth factor-beta suppresses activation and proliferation of microglia in vitro. J Immunol 151:69–76

Tagami M, Yamagata K, Nara Y, Fujino H, Kubota A, Numano F, Yamori Y (1997) Insulin-like growth factors prevent apoptosis in cortical neurons isolated from stroke-prone spontaneously hypertensive rats. Lab Invest 76:603–612

Takeda A, Onodera H, Sugimoto A, Kogure K, Obinata M, Shibahara S (1993) Coordinated expression of messenger RNAs for nerve growth factor, brain-derived neurotrophic factor and neurotrophin-3 in the rat hippocampus following transient forebrain ischemia. Neuroscience 55:23–31

Tanaka K, Tsukahara T, Hashimoto N, Ogata N, Yonekawa Y, Kimura T, Taniguchi T (1994) Effect of nerve growth factor on delayed neuronal death after cerebral ischaemia. Acta Neurochir (Wien) 129:64–71

Tenjin H, Anderson RE, Meyer FB (1995) Treatment with basic fibroblastic growth factor following focal cerebral ischemia does not prevent neuronal injury. J Neurol Sci 128:66–70

Tomac A, Lindqvist E, Lin LF, Ogren SO, Young D, Hoffer BJ, Olson L (1995) Protection and repair of the nigrostriatal dopaminergic system by GDNF in vivo. Nature, 373:335–339

Tomizawa Matsui H, Kondo E et al. (1995) Developmental alteration and neuron-specific expression of bone morphogenetic protein-6 (BMP-6) mRNA in rodent brain. Brain Res Mol Brain Res 28:122–128

Tsukahara T, Yonekawa Y, Tanaka K, Ohara O, Wantanabe S, Kimura T, Nishijima T, Taniguchi T (1994) The role of brain-derived neurotrophic factor in transient forebrain ischemia in the rat brain. Neurosurgery 34:323–331

Unoki K; LaVail MM (1994) Protection of the rat retina from ischemic injury by brain-derived neurotrophic factor, ciliary neurotrophic factor, and basic fibroblast growth factor. Invest Ophthalmol Vis Sci 35:907–915

Voll CL, Auer RN (1991) Insulin attenuates ischemic brain damage independent of its hypoglycemic effect. J Cereb Blood Flow Metab 11:1006–1014

Walicke P, Cowan WM, Ueno N, Baird A, Guillemin R (1986) Fibroblast growth factor promotes survival of dissociated hippocampal neurons and enhances neurite extension. Proc Natl Acad Sci USA 83:3012–3016

referWang X, Yue TL, White RF, Barone FC, Feuerstein GZ (1995) Transforming growth factor-beta 1 exhibits delayed gene expression following focal cerebral ischemia. Brain Res Bull 3635:607–609

Wang Y, Lin SZ, Chiou AL, Williams LR, Hoffer BJ (1997) Glial cell line-derived neurotrophic factor protects against ischemia-induced injury in the cerebral cortex. J Neurosci 17:4341–4348

Wen R, Song Y, Cheng T, Matthes MT, Yasumura D, LaVail MM, Steinberg RH (1995a) Injury-induced upregulation of bFGF and CNTF mRNAS in the rat retina. J Neurosci 15:7377–7385

Wen TC, Matsuda S, Yoshimura H, Kawabe T, Sakanaka M (1995b) Ciliary neurotrophic factor prevents ischemia-induced learning disability and neuronal loss in gerbils. Neurosci Lett 191:55–58

Yamada K, Kinoshita A, Kohmura E, Sakaguchi T, Taguchi J, Kataoka K, Hayakawa T (1991) Basic fibroblast growth factor prevents thalamic degeneration after cortical infarction. J Cereb Blood Flow Metab 11:472–478

Yamada K, Kinoshita A, Kohmura E et al. (1992) Detection and partial purification of ischaemia-related neurotrophic activity in the periinfarcted brain tissue. Neurol Res 3:267–72

Yamamoto S, Yoshimine T, Fujita T, Kuroda R, Irie T, Fujioka K, Hayakawa T (1992) Protective effect of NGF atelocollagen mini-pellet on the hippocampal delayed neuronal death in gerbils. Neurosci Lett 141:161–165

Yasuhara O, Muramatsu H, Kim SU, Maramatsu T, Maruta H, McGreer PL (1993) Midkine, a novel neurotrophic factor, is present in senile plaques of Alzheimer's disease. Biochem Biophys Res Commun 192:246–251

Yeh HJ, Ruit KG, Wang YX, Parks WC, Snider WD, Deuel TF (1991) PDGF A-chain gene is expressed by mammalian neurons during development and in maturity. Cell 64:209–216

Yoshida Y, Goto M, Tsutsui J et al. (1995) Midkine is present in the early stage of cerebral infarct. Brain Res 85:25–30

Zhang Y, Tatsuno T, Carney JM, Mattson MP (1993) Basic FGF, NGF and IGFs protect hippocampal and cortical neurons against iron-induced degeneration. J Cereb Blood Flow Metab 13:378–388

Zhu CZ, Auer RN (1994) Intraventricular administration of insulin and IGF-1 in transient forebrain ischemia. J Cereb Blood Flow Metab 14:237–242

CHAPTER 10

Strategies for Administering Neurotrophic Factors to the Central Nervous System

A.F. HOTTINGER and P. AEBISCHER

Abbreviations

6-OHDA	6-hydroxydopamine
AAV	adeno-associated virus
Ad	adenoviral
ALS	amyotrophic lateral sclerosis
BBB	blood–brain barrier
BHK	baby hamster kidney
CNS	central nervous system
CNTF	ciliary neurotrophic factor
GDNF	glial cell-derived neurotrophic factor
IGF-1	insulin-like growth factor-1
NF	neurotrophic factor
NGF	nerve growth factor
PD	Parkinson's disease
PNS	peripheral nervous system

A. Introduction

I. Characteristics of Neurotrophic Factors (NFs)

The study of neurotrophic factors (NFs) has become one of the most rapidly evolving and expanding fields in the contemporary neurosciences. NFs are growth factors that enhance the survival, maintenance, differentiation and repair of neural cells (LEVI-MONTALCINI 1987). NFs also increase neurite outgrowth and neurotransmitter production. The neurons derive neurotrophic support either by means of retrograde transport from the "target cells" they innervate or from anterograde trophic support of presynaptic terminals. Glial cells, like Schwann cells, astrocytes and oligodendrocytes do provide NFs as well.

The biological effects of these factors are mediated by specific binding to receptors present on the surface of the target neurons. Some neurons not only synthesize NFs, but also express their cognate receptors, allowing them to work in an autocrine fashion (ACHESON et al. 1995). Secreted NFs may also support adjacent neurons. For example, the survival of cerebellar granular cells appears to depend on Purkinje cells, which may mediate local actions of endogenous trophic substances on granular cells, an effect called paracrine secretion (SEGAL et al. 1992). A single NF can influence diverse types of neurons. NFs can also affect certain non-neuronal cells or neuronal precursor cells. Different NFs have an overlapping yet distinctive pattern of activities and can share receptor subunits. The interaction of different determinants achieves a high degree of specificity (KORSCHING 1993). The access of a particular neuronal type to a specific NF depends on the distinct anatomic location of the neuron, temporal factors, expression of specific receptors and activation of appropriate intracellular signaling cascades.

In the event of a nerve lesion, NF production is upregulated and regenerating axons are guided and stimulated by these trophic proteins (CURTIS et al. 1994).

II. Rationale for Using NFs in Clinical Paradigms

The potent effects of NFs have naturally sparkled interest for clinical applications. So far, very little is known about the physiopathology of most neurodegenerative diseases, for which only very few treatments are available. Nevertheless, different mechanisms might be implicated in the degenerative process and justify a therapeutic use of those factors. First, as suggested by YUEN and MOBLEY (1996), the degenerative process could be linked directly or indirectly to a particular NF. Second, a decrease of receptor density could decrease the effect of NF or, third, the disease could be linked to a metabolic process that is sensitive to NF. Fourth, a NF could induce compensatory mechanisms that would decrease the clinical effect of the disease. In the first case, physiological substitution of NF would be therapeutic. In the other cases, a pharmacological dose could increase the stimulation of the remaining receptors or improve neuronal viability by inducing metabolic changes. To date, none of the neurodegenerative diseases could be linked to the deficit of a particular NF and cannot, therefore, be aimed at as a substitution treatment.

B. Administration of NFs to the Central Nervous System

I. Delivery Issues

The administration of NFs to the brain is linked to several problems that can only be overcome by the selection of an adequate delivery mechanism. Until recently, the highly compartmentalized organization of the brain, the complexity of neuronal interactions, and the problems linked to the BBB rendered neurotrophic delivery to the CNS a seemingly impossible task. The brain is disconnected from all other tissues in the body by the BBB. This barrier ensures proper maintenance of intracerebral ion concentration, neurotransmitters and proteins. Moreover, the BBB protects the brain against surging fluctuations in ion concentrations. With the exception of molecules for which there are specific transporters, only small lipophilic molecules enter the brain. For instance, in PD, symptoms are reduced by the administration of l-DOPA, a dopamine precursor, which is transported by the neutral amino acid transporter into the brain, whereas dopamine itself is therapeutically ineffective because it is not transported. It results that, for most clinical applications of NFs, the delivery of the NF will have to bypass the BBB by one way or another, although some small passage of the BBB by NT-3, BDNF or CNTF has been described (Poduslo and Curran 1996). All in all, the high selectivity of the BBB makes the delivery of systemically administered NFs to the CNS a challenging task. Axons can project a considerable distance from the perikarya. Constructs injected into motor-innervation zones of muscles can be transported into perikarya of motoneurons, where they are transcribed and translated (Ghadge et al. 1995). Moreover NFs, such as GDNF, CNTF, BDNF, NT-3 or NGF, are themselves taken up at the terminal end of the axons and dendrites, and are retrogradely transported to the perikaryon (Curtis et al. 1993). Retrograde transport can be used advantageously, especially when considering the delivery of NFs to motoneurons as needed in ALS.

NFs are generally rather unstable proteins with short half-lives, although there are some exceptions, such as BDNF and NT-3 (Poduslo and Curran 1996). This fact complicates the delivery of these factors by classical pumps as the factors must remain stable over a prolonged period of time at physiological temperatures. Approaches to overcome this problem include the design of molecules that show enhanced stability, but retain the physiological activity of the NF, as for example Axokine (Anderson 1998). Attempts have also been made to increase the BBB permeability by derivatizing the therapeutic proteins with lipophilic molecules (Partridge et al. 1987) or by conjugating them with proteins, such as the transferrin receptors, to increase their passage across the BBB (Kordower et al. 1994). Another approach consists of de novo synthesis of NFs directly in the brain, thus bypassing the BBB; either by transducing neuronal or non-neuronal cells of the brain by different viral vectors, or by using non-cerebral cells that are engineered to release the desired NF. All of these approaches have been used in experimental models.

The advantages and disadvantages of the different delivery systems will be reviewed, using as examples three neurodegenerative diseases, i.e., ALS, PD and Huntington's disease (Table 1).

C. Delivery Methods

I. Delivery of NFs Using Mechanical-Release Devices

1. Systemic Delivery

As mentioned above, neurons are able to retrogradely transport NFs. Systemic delivery can, therefore, be considered a valid approach for diseases implying neurons that project to the PNS, such as motoneurons or sensory

Table 1. Delivery methods. *BBB* blood–brain barrier; *ALS* amyotrophic lateral sclerosis; *NF* neurotrophic factor

Delivery method	Advantages	Disadvantages
Mechanical methods:		
Systemic administration	– Simplicity of the delivery	– Bolus injections – No targeted delivery – Only for peripheral diseases such as neuropathies or ALS
Pumps	– Continuous programmable delivery – Release can be stopped in case of side effects – Appropriate for intracerebroventricular delivery	– Stability of NF issue – Need to be refilled – Risk of infection associated with refilling – Inadequate for parenchymal delivery
Polymer-release system	– Continuous delivery	– No control over release rate – Limited loading capacity – No re-loading
BBB permeabilizers	– Systemic administration	– High systemic doses are necessary – No localized brain delivery
In vivo gene delivery:		
Viral vectors		
Adenoviruses	– Infect non-dividing cells – No integration – High titers – Accommodate large inserts	– Issue of long-term expression – Immune response – No re-administration of Ad vectors – Cytotoxic in transduced cells
Adeno-associated viruses	– Infect non-dividing cells – Long-term expression – Non-pathogenic – Non-oncogenic – Repeated injections are possible	– Cannot accommodate inserts larger than 4.8 Kb – Difficult to produce
Oncoretroviruses	– Integration into host DNA	– Infect only dividing cells – Use limited to ex vivo gene therapy
Lentiviruses	– Infect non-dividing cells – No expression of viral proteins – Integration of vector – Accommodate large inserts	– Safety issue

Table 1. *Continued*

Delivery method	Advantages	Disadvantages
Non-viral vectors		
Liposomes	– Absence of viral components – No previous immune recognition	– Inefficient gene transfer – Lack of persistence of DNA – No tissue targeting
Ex vivo gene therapy:		
Cell grafts	– Selection of optimal cell line possible – Test for pathogenicity possible	– Immune rejection for non-syngeneic grafts – Tumorogenicity
Encapsulation of engineered cell lines	– No immune rejection – Possibility to use cell lines of either allo- or xenogeneic origin – Retrieval possible in case of adverse effects	– No integration into neural circuits – Complex technology

neurons. The systemic injection is certainly the easiest clinical approach to examine the efficacy of NFs in these diseases and has been widely used.

NFs hold great promise in the treatment of peripheral neuropathies, such as those induced by diabetes mellitus or certain anti-mitotic drugs, such as cisplatin or taxol. Based on the neurotrophic and neuroprotective activities of NGF, the systemic administration of NGF has been proposed as a treatment for several types of neuropathies. Results from recent pre-clinical studies indicate that NGF can be administered safely in clinical trials. Initial phase-I studies in humans indicate that NGF produces mild myalgias shortly following single intravenous or subcutaneous doses of 1 μg/kg. Patients suffering from diabetic neuropathy reported an improvement in clinical symptoms which correlated, in some cases, with improvements in neurological examinations (Rogers 1996). A large-scale phase-II clinical trial involving NGF in diabetic neuropathy was conducted by Genentech. Encouraging results have warranted the initiation of a phase-III trial. A similar study, evaluating the effects of NT-3 is being investigated by Regeneron Pharmaceuticals.

CNTF is a potent trophic factor for motoneurons (Arakawa et al. 1990). When applied to the distal stump of a transected rat neonatal facial nerve, CNTF can rescue 80% of facial motoneurons that normally degenerate after axotomy (Sendtner et al. 1990). CNTF was also able to delay clinical onset and death in the wobbler mouse, a model of ALS (Mitsumoto et al. 1994), making it a potential candidate for the treatment of patients suffering from this disease. Two phase-I/II trials were performed based on the subcutaneous injections, three times a week, and a maximum of 30 μg/kg recombinant human (rh) CNTF (ALS CNTF treatment study (ACTS) group 1996) or daily injections of 5 μg CNTF in the highest dose (Miller et al. 1996). However, survival and clinical scores were not different in either study between the treated and untreated groups. Moreover, severe adverse side effects, including weight loss, acute-phase response, fever and a dry cough, were noticed. These side effects were believed to be associated, for the most part, by the activation of CNTF receptors expressed in peripheral tissues (Fantuzzi et al. 1995) (Table 2).

IGF-I is another potential candidate for the treatment of ALS. In a phase-III study, patients were randomized into three dosage groups (0.05 mg/kg, 0.1 mg/kg and placebo) and received daily subcutaneous drug injections for 9 months. At these dosages, IGF-1 induced few side effects and the clinical scores used to quantify the evolution of the disease deteriorated less with higher dosages of IGF-1 (Lai et al. 1997). In another study, patients received injections of BDNF (BDNF study group 1998), but with no clinical improvements. As seen with CNTF, intravenous administration of NFs often leads to undesirable and unacceptable side effects. It is also not clear whether diseased motoneurons are capable of retrograde transport. These limitations have prompted the search of alternate delivery methods for the treatment of ALS that would release the therapeutic molecule directly into the CNS. The impossibility of delivering NF via the periphery for diseases such as PD or

Table 2. Clinical trials

Neurotrophic factor	Disease	Delivery method
CNTF	ALS	Subcutaneous injections
	ALS	Intrathecal delivery using a mechanical pump
	ALS	Intrathecal encapsulated BHK cells
IGF-1	ALS	Subcutaneous injections
NGF	Diabetic neuropathy	Systemic intravenous or subcutaneous injection
BDNF	ALS	Subcutaneous injection
	ALS	Intrathecal delivery with a pump
NT-3	Taxol and cisplatin sensory neuropathy	Systemic delivery
GDNF	ALS	Intracerebroventricular bolus injection
	PD	Intracerebroventricular bolus injection

ALS, amyotrophic lateral sclerosis; *PD*, Parkinson's disease; *CNTF*, ciliary neurotrophic factor; *IGF-1*, insulin-like growth factor-1; *NGF*, nerve growth factor; *BDNF*, brain-derived neurotrophic factor; *BHK*, baby hamster kidney; *NT-3*, neurotrophic factor-3; *GDNF*, glial cell-derived neurotrophic factor.

Huntington's disease also prompted the development of various alternate delivery systems (Table 1).

2. Pumps

Direct delivery of molecules to the CNS can theoretically be achieved with mechanical pumps. Numerous experiments have used osmotic pumps for the delivery of all kinds of molecules to the nervous system of rodents (MUFSON et al. 1996). For clinical use, mechanical pumps allowing the modulation of the delivery rate are being used. Usually the pump reservoir is implanted subcutaneously. Delivery to the CNS is obtained via a catheter attached to the implanted pump. These pumps are refillable by percutaneous injection of the bioactive molecule solution. These devices have been largely used in anesthesiology for the treatment of pain (LAMER 1994), but they have also found some neurological applications with the infusion of baclofen, a GABAergic drug for the treatment of spasticity (PENN 1988). Several limitations, however, prevent the widespread use of these devices. Although their use is well suited for delivery in the cerebrospinal fluid, delivery in the brain parenchyma can lead to cavitation and local inflammation in the target area (MAYER et al. 1993). In the parenchyma, a sharp decrease of the concentration of the therapeutic molecule is observed, since these pumps behave as a point-source delivery system (BJÖRKLUND 1991). This could be a limiting factor when large areas of the brain, such as the striatum, have to be treated. Moreover, Pumps need to be refilled on a regular basis. This procedure is associated with an increased risk of infection. Most NFs are unstable in solutions. CNTF, for example looses around 90% of its activity in less than 24 h when in solution (M. SENDTNER, personal communication).

Chronic intrathecal infusion of BDNF resulted in selective accumulation of BDNF in spinal cord motoneurons, forming a gradient along the whole axis of the spinal cord. There was no free accumulation of the NF in the spinal cord parenchyma, most likely resulting from the barrier formed by intact glial-limiting membrane. When the cannula releasing BDNF was implanted in the brain parenchyma, there was only limited diffusion of the factor within the tissue (MUFSON et al. 1994). Intracerebroventricular injection of NGF strongly labeled cholinergic neurons in the basal forebrain, whereas NT-3 was almost unable to cross the ependymal layer (YAN et al. 1994). This is linked to the presence of specific complete or truncated receptors for the different factors on the ependymal layer (KLEIN et al. 1990).

Based on these preliminary results, a clinical trial involving the intrathecal delivery of BDNF in ALS is currently being evaluated in a joint Amgen/Regeneron Pharmaceuticals effort. Penn et al. (1997) have evaluated the intrathecal delivery of CNTF by means of a mechanical pump in a phase-I clinical study. The NF was well distributed over the whole length of the spinal cord. The side effects noted with systemic delivery did not occur. Clinical evolution of these patients was, however, unmodified by this treatment.

GDNF is a member of the transforming growth factor b family and was found to have potent trophic activities on both dopaminergic neurons (LIN et al. 1993) and motoneurons (ZURN et al. 1994). This factor was shown to be expressed in limb buds, Schwann cells and cultured embryonic myotubes (HENDERSON et al. 1994). It is retrogradely transported to motoneuron perikarya. GDNF is also able to prevent the degeneration of motoneurons following facial nerve lesion (HENDERSON et al. 1994; YAN et al. 1995), suggesting that GDNF might be beneficial in ALS. This factor is being evaluated in those patients using intracerebroventricular delivery by a modified Omaya delivery system. Patients have received intraventricular boluses once a month with this device. The same approach is being investigated in a phase-I/II clinical trial for the delivery of GDNF in Parkinsonian patients (Table 2).

3. Slow Polymer-Release System

Slow release of NFs can be achieved by entrapment in polymer matrices (LANGER and FOLKMAN 1976). Materials such as resorbable polyesters (MCRAE-DEGUEURCE et al. 1988) or ethylene vinyl acetate copolymers (SABEL et al. 1990) have been used. The kinetics of release depend largely upon the hydrophobicity of the molecule. Unfortunately, most NFs are hydrophilic in nature and efficient release systems have been difficult to achieve. Development of slow-release systems requires methods to maintain stability during both the processing and release period. This approach has been investigated for the release of NGF, BDNF and NT-3 (HOFFMAN et al. 1990; VEJSADA et al. 1998). These polymers can be implanted into specific brain structures by standard stereotaxic procedures and are well tolerated by the host (WINN et al. 1989). They are, however, unsuited for applications longer than 1 month as they have a finite loading capacity. The implants would, therefore, have to be removed and replaced periodically, which is impractical in the brain. The technology could, however, be useful for the transitory release of trophic factors to improve for example the grafting of fetal neural cells.

HOFFMAN et al. (1990) have shown that the continuous delivery of NGF released from polymers can prevent the lesion-induced loss of choline acetyltransferase expression in septal neurons that degenerate following a fimbria-fornix axotomy. This model induces memory impairment and bears some validity for evaluating the survival of neurons afflicted in Alzheimer's disease. This principle was also studied in a model of acute motoneuron degeneration. Polymer rods chronically releasing BDNF were able to transiently prevent the degeneration of motoneurons in neonatal rats with a lesion of the sciatic nerve (VEJSADA et al. 1998).

II. Delivery of NFs Using Gene Therapy Approaches

Generally speaking, two distinct approaches can be considered for introducing genes of therapeutic interest into the CNS. The first method named "in vivo gene therapy" implies the direct introduction of the gene into the patient using specific vectors. The second, called "ex vivo gene therapy", implies that the genes of interest are transduced in cultivated cells and injected *ad secundum* into an appropriate site of the CNS.

1. In Vivo Gene Therapy

In vivo gene therapy requires the use of appropriate vectors. In the CNS, viral vectors are the most commonly used and the most efficacious for gene transfer. Other strategies involve direct injection of naked DNA, lipofection or the use of liposomes (Biewenga et al. 1997). However, the later strategies are characterized by low efficiency which currently precludes their utilization in the CNS. We, therefore, propose to review the advantages and drawbacks of the currently used viral vectors, as well as their applications in neurodegenerative diseases.

a) Viral Vectors

Due to their parasitic cycle of multiplication, viruses are natural vehicles for gene transfer, since they introduce their own genes into the cells they infect. It is not surprising that they are currently the most efficient tools for gene transfer, as they have evolved for millions of years to become efficient vesicles for transferring genetic material into cells.

Vectors used to synthesize NFs have been developed mainly from retroviruses, adenoviruses and adeno-associated viruses. More recently, vectors derived from herpes viruses have been developed for CNS applications (Bowers et al. 1997). In most cases, the virus is transformed into a vector by the removal of genes that are implicated in replication and pathogenicity of the virus and by replacing them with the therapeutic gene of interest. Using stereotaxic techniques, the modified viral vector can be injected into delimited areas of the CNS. However, since viral vectors can only diffuse over a few millimeters in the brain tissue, this strategy cannot be considered if large areas of the brain have to be treated. Retrograde axonal transport capabilities of adeno- and adeno-associated vectors can, however, be used to infect areas of the brain that are difficult to access.

b) Adenoviral Vectors

More than 40 different human serotypes of adenovirus have been identified. The more common serotypes (2 and 5) have been exploited for use in clinical trials for cystic fibrosis and cancer (Boucher 1996). Adenoviruses are, in general, responsible for only mild illnesses, such as upper-respiratory infections, and are non-oncogenic (Horellou et al. 1997).

Adenoviruses have two major advantages: they can infect non-dividing cells and allow transfer of large gene sequences. However the Ad genes (and therefore the therapeutic genes) are not integrated within the chromosomes of the host cell and induce, therefore, only a transient expression. Moreover, Ad vectors need the expression of viral proteins that induce an immune response leading to the elimination of the infected cells with time. This immune response also prevents re-infection (WOOD et al. 1996).

The adenoviruses are rendered incapable of replicating by deletion of the immediate early genes E1A and E1B, which encode proteins that regulate all the other viral functions. The therapeutic gene is, therefore, inserted at the place of the E1 genes. Larger inserts can be accommodated by also deleting the non-essential E3 gene. In order to propagate these recombinant vectors, human cell lines are engineered to express the Ad E1 genes. This first generation of vectors, used in pre-clinical rodent and non-human primate studies, have demonstrated that Ad vectors can efficiently transduce all types of cells with no particular cell specificity (PELTEKIAN et al. 1997). After adenovirus injection into the CSF, transduced cells can be found throughout the ependymal layer (OOBOSHI et al. 1995). However, intraparenchymal injection of adenovirus leads to neural cell transduction only within a restricted area of a few hundred microns. It has been suggested that this limited distribution is linked to the very high efficiency of transduction as well as natural boundaries formed by the astrocytic glia limitans and bundles of myelin fibers (PELTEKIAN et al. 1997). Outside the CNS, E1-deleted vectors induce a strong inflammation. The infected cells are eliminated within a few weeks by a robust host immune response mounted against the remnant level of viral gene expression that still occurs with E1-deleted vectors (CHRIST et al. 1997). This phenomenon prevents further re-administration of the vector (CHRIST et al. 1997).

In the brain, expression of the therapeutic gene has been shown to be transient, decreasing steadily and lasting from 2 weeks to 2 months, depending on the anatomic location and extent of myelinization (BYRNES et al. 1995). This loss of expression was accompanied by significant inflammation and cytotoxicity of neurons (BYRNES et al. 1996). The immune privilege of the brain is, however, not sufficient to prevent the observed decrease in expression. The injection of the Ad vector cannot be performed without a vascular breach and, therefore, some intrusion of immune cells remains a possibility. Moreover, microglial cells are rapidly induced to present antigens in an MHC-II environment when activated (GEHRMANN et al. 1995). In the brain, other mechanisms may also be involved, including direct toxicity of viral particles of the envelope and the very high multiplicity of infection (AKLI et al. 1993). These factors could potentially lead to an accumulation of debris around the transduced cells or toxicity of the transgene itself. In primates, significant morbidity was reported following intracerebral injection of high titers of Ad vectors containing the thymidine kinase (TK) gene. Pathological findings showed extensive coagulation necrosis, edema with mass effect and acute inflammation (FREESE et al. 1996).

These findings present a serious obstacle to the treatment of chronic diseases such as PD or ALS. Since repeated delivery of the therapeutic is impossible due to the immune response, alternatives are being investigated. Second generation Ad vectors have been designed with mutations in the E2 gene and deletions of larger regions of the E4, E2 and/or E3 genes. However, it was shown that vectors with very important deletions of viral genome show an even faster decline of reporter gene expression. It is speculated that low-level synthesis of early Ad DNA is needed to maintain Ad genomes in the infected cells. Alternatively, one can consider modulating the immune system of the recipient, either with cyclosporin A or FK 506, which is able to block both cellular and humoral immune responses (ILAN et al. 1997). These approaches are, however, unsuitable for long-term treatment of patients (CHRIST et al. 1997).

Nevertheless, a replication-defective Ad vector encoding human GDNF injected near the rat substantia nigra was found to protect DA neurons from the progressive degeneration induced by the neurotoxin 6-OHDA injected into the striatum. Ad GDNF gene therapy reduced loss of dopamine neurons approximately threefold, 6 weeks after 6-OHDA lesion. These results suggest that Ad vector-mediated GDNF gene therapy may slow the dopaminergic neuronal cell loss in humans with PD (CHOILUNDBERG et al. 1997). In a similar model, but injecting the GDNF expressing Ad vector in the striatum, BILANG-BLEUEL et al. (1997) were not only able to protect nigral dopaminergic neurons, but also to improve the drug-induced rotational behavior in those animals.

Using the ability of adenovirus to be retrogradely transported (GHADGE et al. 1995), BAUMGARTNER and SHINE (1997) were able to rescue a portion of motoneurons following facial nerve axotomy with Ad vectors expressing CNTF, BDNF or GDNF. When injected into the facial muscle, about 10% of the motoneurons were able to retrogradely transport the Ad vector and express the transgene.

In the *pmn-pmn* mouse model of ALS, characterized by a progressive motor neuronopathy (SCHMALBRUCH et al. 1991), HAASE et al. (1997) were able to show a 50% increase in the life span when they infected the mice intramuscularly with an Ad vector secreting NT-3. These Ad-NT-3-treated mice also showed a reduced loss of motor axons and improved neuromuscular function, as assessed by electromyography.

c) Adeno-Associated Viral Vectors

The AAV is a non-enveloped, single-stranded DNA parvovirus, that is dependent upon adenovirus for its replication. In AAV vectors, all viral coding sequences can be deleted and replaced by a therapeutic gene, as long as the 145-bp long minimum sequence that is required for transduction is preserved. The missing proteins are provided in *trans* by co-transfection of a helper plasmid. However, to obtain AAV vector, co-infection with an adenovirus is required. This leads to the formation of AAV vector and progeny adenovirus which will have to be separated (SAMULSKI et al. 1989). AAV can be purified and further concentrated on a cesium gradient, obtaining titers of approximately 5×10^{11}. It is stable in both a suspended and lyophilized form; an advantage for the preparation of viral vectors. AAV vectors allow the infection into the host-cell genome, but with a low efficiency, the vast majority of AAV genomes remaining episomal and non-integrated (KAPLITT et al. 1994b). Data suggest that the AAV genome is prone to rearrangement during integration, potentially jeopardizing the expression of the therapeutic gene (KREMER and PERRICAUDET 1995).

AAV vectors have several characteristics that make them attractive vectors for gene transfer: they have no known pathogenicity (DURING and LEONE 1995); they express a minimal number of viral antigens ensuring minimal immunogenicity; they are able to transduce post-mitotic cells; and show a broad host and cell range. In the brain, the vast majority of cells infected are neurons (KAPLITT et al. 1994b). There is no superinfection immunity for AAV vectors and repeated injections of the AAV vector are therefore possible (LEBKOWSKI et al. 1988). The efficiency of transduction observed might, however, depend on the presence of helper virus (AFIONE et al. 1996). The major limitations of these vectors is their small size, limiting the efficient packaging to about 4.8 Kb. This is, however, sufficient for most NFs, but will preclude the use of inducible promoter systems allowing gene dosing. For efficient transduction, the role of helper viruses needs to be further elucidated. In clinical trials, patients treated with recombinant viruses may be subsequently infected with helper viruses, and the interaction of the two is only poorly understood (BLÖMER et al. 1996). Moreover, purifying AAV from the helper adenovirus is very difficult (KREMER and PERRICAUDET 1995). To date, no packaging cell line is available for their preparation, implying batch to batch variations.

In experimental designs, injection of AAV vector expressing LacZ into several brain regions, showed that expression of the transgene is still present, although it is significantly decreased 6 months after injection (DURING and LEONE 1995). The expression can be traced as soon as 24 h after injection. The infected cells are spread several millimeters around the needle tract of the injection site and, as shown by double immunostaining for neurofilament and GFAP, the vast majority of transduced cells appear to be neurons even though some astrocytes are also marked. AAV is able to infect axon terminals and is retrogradely transported (DURING and LEONE 1995).

An AAV vector expressing mouse GDNF and injected into the striatum of 6-OHDA lesioned rats induced increased striatal dopamine content after 3 months. However, histological studies performed at 6 months did not show any significant difference in dopamine cell numbers or striatal TH-immunoreactivity between GDNF and control animals (DURING and LEONE 1995). It is unclear, so far, whether this observation is linked to a loss of transduced cells or a promoter that is shut off; a well described phenomenon for cytomegalovirus (CMV) and other viral promoters (DURING et al. 1994). In a similar short-term experiment with intranigral injection, MANDEL et al. (1997) were able to show that an AAV vector expressing GDNF was able to prevent the degeneration of nigral dopaminergic cells.

d) Retroviral Vectors

Retroviral viruses have several characteristics that make them strong candidates for gene therapy. They can package relatively large genes and, unlike Ad vectors, they integrate their genes permanently into the chromosomes of the infected cells. They do not code for any viral protein and should, therefore, not induce any immunological response.

First generation retroviruses were derived from oncoretroviruses such as murine leukemia viruses. These vectors have one major drawback: they can only transduce cells that are dividing, shortly after infection. This limitation is due to the voluminous protein complex surrounding the viral genome. It prevents its free diffusion to the nucleus of the cell, where the integration with the host genome takes place. For those viruses, the only period during which they can enter in contact with the host genome is when the nuclear membrane is disrupted during mitosis. However, in most organs, only a very limited number of cells is undergoing mitosis at any point in time. Moreover, most target cells of gene therapy, be it neurons, myocytes or hepatocytes, are terminally differentiated and do not divide anymore. Therefore, protocols aiming at infecting non-dividing cells require ex vivo manipulations, during which the cells are taken out from the body, stimulated for proliferation, infected and then re-introduced into the body.

Unlike oncoretroviruses, lentiviruses, a subgroup of retroviruses that includes the HIV virus, are able to infect and integrate their genes into the chromosomes of non-dividing cells. This property is linked to the karyophilic properties of the lentiviral pre-integration complex which govern recognition by the cell nuclear import machinery (Gallay et al. 1996). This complex is composed of the virion proteins, matrix, integrase and Vpr. Furthermore, HIV-based vectors can mediate efficient delivery, integration and sustained long-term expression of transgenes in adult post-mitotic cells such as neurons (Naldini et al. 1996).

The potential clinical use of these vectors raises a legitimate concern that the parental pathogenic virus might be reconstituted. Several groups addressed this issue by developing vectors with multiple deletions: the first line of defense is mounted by expressing the various components of the vector system from separate DNA units, so that only multiple rearrangement and recombination events could generate a replication competent virus. A second line of defense was adopted by deleting all accessory proteins that are required for replication and virulence in vivo (Trono 1995). Naldini et al. (1996) describe a three-plasmid expression system that is used to generate a HIV-derived retroviral vector. A packaging construct contains the human cytomegalovirus immediate early promoter, which drives the expression of all viral proteins required in *trans*. This plasmid is defective for the production of the viral envelope and the accessory proteins Vpu, vpr, nef and vif (Zufferey et al. 1997). The second plasmid codes for the G glycoprotein of the vesicular stomatitis virus (VSV G). This envelope offers the advantage of broadening the tropism of the vector. It also stabilizes the vector, allowing particle concentration by ultracentrifugation. The third plasmid is the transducing vector which contains *cis*-acting sequences of HIV required for packaging, reverse transcription and integration as well as the cDNA of the therapeutic gene of interest. The retroviral, replication-defective particles are generated by transient transfection of 293T human kidney cells with the three plasmids. This vector, unlike Moloney leukemia virus (MLV)-based vectors was shown to transduce G1-S- and G2-arrested Hela cells and proliferating cells. Infected neurons and astroglial cells were observed following the direct injection of the vector in the brain. Expression was maintained for at least 6 months (D. Trono, personal communication).

In summary, although viral vectors have entered the clinic for untreatable diseases, such as glioblastomas, and are an invaluable tool for testing the effects of NFs on all kinds of animal models, they do show limitations that will slow down their use in clinical protocols. The major problem of viral vectors is the relatively low efficacy of transduction. At most, a few thousand cells can be infected by a single injection. Even small brain nuclei would need large numbers of injections to achieve sufficient expression of the therapeutic gene. Moreover, possible recombination with wild-type viruses could form a widespread infection, malignant transformation of transduced cells and evolution into a brain tumor. Moreover, there are currently no possibilities to control the release of the therapeutic factor and no shut-down mechanisms in case of adverse effects of the transgene. For clinical applications, an inducible promoter system that would allow the controlled delivery of the therapeutic agent seems indispensable. These limitations currently restrict the clinical potential of these vectors. They do remain, however, invaluable tools for testing the effects of NFs on animal models of neurodegenerative diseases.

2. Ex Vivo Gene Therapy

The concept of ex vivo gene therapy is based on the idea that the transplantation of genetically modified cells could restore a normal function in the CNS by producing neurotransmitters, NFs or enzymes. This approach seems especially well suited for diseases that affect a specific neuronal circuit. Despite the complexity of the majority of human neurological disorders and the relative difficulty in accessing dysfunctional areas in the brain, intracerebral grafts of fetal- or adult-derived cells appear to be a useful alternative to somatic in vivo gene therapy. Cells of diverse origin survive transplantation into the brain and can provide trophic support or supplement deficient molecules.

a) Cell Grafting

The concept of cell grafting is based on the ability to genetically engineer primary cells or cell lines to produce large amounts of NF and to implant those cells into defined areas of the brain. The advantage of ex vivo gene therapy consists of the possibility to test and select cells for gene expression prior to transplantation (SUHR and GAGE 1993). The cultured cell lines used in ex vivo gene therapy can be either syngeneic, allogeneic or xenogeneic. A large variety of cell types have been used in experimental protocols and include fibroblasts (FISHER et al. 1991), neuroblastomas (HORELLOU et al. 1990), glioma-derived cells (UCHIDA et al. 1990) and neuroendocrine cells (HORELLOU et al. 1990). The choice of the optimal promoter is crucial to achieve long-term expression of the transgene. Viral promoters were chosen initially because of their high levels of expression in growing cells (HOCK et al. 1989). They may, however, be methylated and inactivated after grafting, when cells become quiescent (PALMER et al. 1991). Constitutive promoters, derived from housekeeping genes (SCHARFMANN et al. 1991) and tissue-specific promoters are able to maintain long-term expression (KAPLITT et al. 1994a). Current efforts are focusing on developing systems that combine promoters and enhancers from different genes to achieve stable and high-level expression (DAI et al. 1992).

The concept of transplanting genetically modified cells has been tested in various models of PD. LEVIVIER et al. (1995) showed that fibroblasts transduced with a vector expressing BDNF, are able to partially prevent the loss of nerve terminals and completely prevent the loss of cell bodies of the nigro–striatal pathway. Grafts consisting of allogeneic or xenogeneic immortalized cells show a very poor survival in the absence of immunosuppression. In contrast, syngeneic grafts are tolerated over an extended period of time (SUHR and GAGE 1993). However, cell-line derived grafts often lead to the formation of tumors, excluding this approach for clinical use (HORELLOU et al. 1990).

To minimize the problem of tumor formation and of immunological rejection, primary autologous cells are being evaluated (FREESE et al. 1996). Among these are primary skin fibroblasts (FISHER et al. 1991), Schwann cells (O'MALLEY and GELLER 1992) and astrocytes. YOSHIMOTO et al. (1995) transfected in vitro primary type-I astrocytes with a replication-deficient Moloney murine leukemia virus, carrying a human BDNF cDNA under the transcriptional control of the MoMuLV 5′ long terminal repeat promoter. This group showed that 6-OHDA lesioned rats would improve their amphetamine induced rotations if implanted with the BDNF secreting grafts. These primary transfected cultures have demonstrated long-term survival in vivo, but they cannot be retrieved in case of adverse side effects. A small but, nevertheless, possible risk of malignant transformation precludes their current use in clinical applications.

Immortalized neural progenitor cell lines derived from the developing CNS (SNYDER 1991) might minimize the above-mentioned limitations. HIB-5 cell lines are derived from E16 hippocampus and are conditionally immortalized by infection with a retroviral vector containing the temperature-sensitive double mutant of the SV 40 large T antigen. This cell line was shown to behave as multi-potent neural progenitors after transplantation in the developing brain. RENFRANZ et al. (1991) transduced this cell line in vitro with a Moloney

Murine leukemia virus vector containing the cDNA for mouse NGF. The axotomy-induced degeneration of septal cholinergic neurons could also be prevented using this cell line (MARTINEZ-SERRANO et al. 1995). Transplantation of this cell line overexpressing NGF was also able to protect striatal neurons from quinolinic acid excitotoxicity, a model of Huntington's disease (MARTINEZ-SERRANO and BJÖRKLUND 1996).

b) Encapsulation of Engineered Cell Lines

To avoid the problems of malignant transformation and immune rejection linked to the use of cell lines, our group has devised a method to physically separate the genetically engineered cells from the host brain tissue (AEBISCHER et al. 1991) (Fig. 1A). The use of encapsulated engineered cell lines offers several relevant advantages: (1) encapsulation allows the transplantation of xenogeneic cells in the absence of drug-induced host immunosuppression; (2) the capsule can be placed in almost any area in the brain, using standard stereotaxic procedures, thus, not only bypassing the BBB, but also ensuring a constant local delivery; and (3) in case of unwanted side effects, the device and therefore the transplanted cells can be retrieved. Although the mechanical characteristics of the implant make the inadvertent release of encapsulated cells unlikely, two additional safety mechanisms are incorporated to ensure the elimination of the implanted cells in case of capsule breakage. The immunogenicity of xenogeneic cells will lead to rejection even in immunoprivileged sites if they are not protected by an immunoisolating membrane. A suicide gene, such as the herpes simplex virus thymidine kinase gene is incorporated into the engineered cell lines. Cells can therefore be eliminated at any time following the per os intake of ganciclovir, an antimicrobial drug that will become selectively toxic for cells expressing thymidine kinase.

The immunoisolation is obtained by surrounding the cells with a physical barrier consisting of a permeable synthetic membrane with a controlled pore size. Molecular weight cut-off points in the range of 50 Kb are typically used, allowing the diffusion of oxygen, nutrients and bioactive cell secretions. However, cells of the host immune system, immunoglobulins and complement factors are excluded from the graft. Two different encapsulation systems have been developed. In macroencapsulation, the immunoisolating membrane is prepared from thermoplastics shaped as hollow fibers (AEBISCHER and LYSAGHT 1995; AEBISCHER et al. 1991). The diameter of these hollow fibers is in the range of 300–500 μm, with a wall thickness of approximately 100 μm, allowing the appropriate availability of nutrients to cells located in the middle of the device (Fig. 1B). In microencapsulation, cells are entrapped in approximately 500-μm microspheres formed from two oppositely charged polyelectrolytes, usually alginate and polylysine (LIM and SUN 1980; WINN et al. 1991). These capsules are, however, fragile and difficult to retrieve. Both types of membranes require optimal biocompatibility. This is obtained by fine tuning of chemical composition and surface morphology to minimize inflammatory

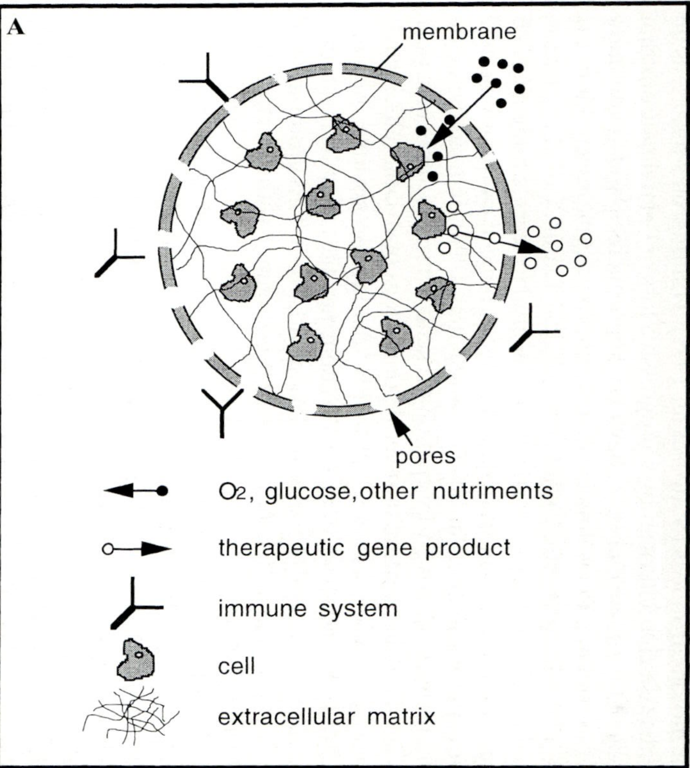

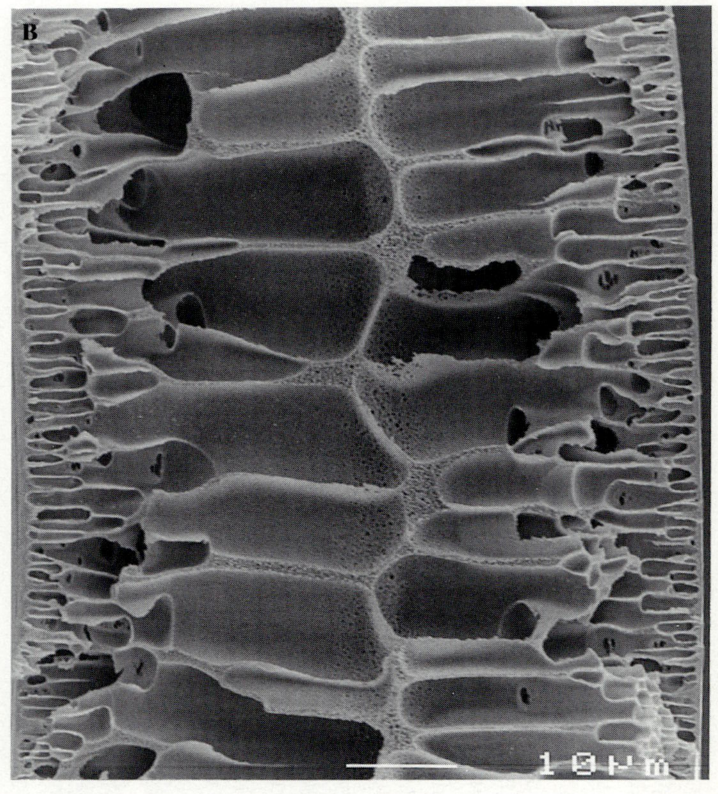

Fig. 1A,B. Principle of immunoisolation by encapsulation. **A** Cells genetically modified to secrete neurotrophic factors are embedded into a matrix. The pores of the membrane allow the diffusion of nutrients and bioactive cell products. The membrane provides protection from the xenogeneic molecules and cells of the host immune system. **B** Electron microscopic close-up view of a double-skin polyacrylonitrate–polyvinyl chloride (*PAN–PVC*)-type membrane used in clinical protocols

responses to the device. Depending upon the process of fabrication, the pores show a gaussian size distribution. Cells are typically embedded in hydrogel-based matrices. The identification of the optimal membrane and matrix composition depends widely on cell phenotype and growth characteristics and has to be adapted empirically for each cell line (Zielinski and Aebischer 1994).

Cell lines can be engineered by classical physical methods, cloned by limited dilution and selected for optimal parameters, including secretion of the desired NF, stability of secretion over time and in vitro and in vivo survival of the cell line. The absence of tumorigenicity can be assessed in different animal models using non-encapsulated cells.

Practically, clonal cells are amplified to generate master cell banks, which are, in turn, amplified for the constitution of working cell banks. These cell banks will ensure homogeneity and reproducibility in the preparation of the devices, ensuring that every patient will be implanted with an identical clonal line. These cell banks can then be checked for the presence of pathogens including bacteria, viruses, yeasts, fungi, mycoplasma and other bacteria (Aebischer et al. 1996a).

The feasibility of this approach has been shown in numerous models of neurodegenerative diseases. In *pmn-pmn* mice, a model for ALS, capsules containing BHK cells genetically engineered to secrete mouse CNTF were able to improve the mice's motor behavior and increase the survival of these animals by 40%. Histological counts of the myelinated axons of the phrenic nerve and of the motoneurons of the facial nucleus indicated a significant reduction of motoneuron loss (Sagot et al. 1995). Huntington's disease is an untreatable disease characterized by a progressive loss of striatal neurons that results in cognitive impairments, behavioral abnormalities and involuntary choreiform movements. Quinolinic acid, an excitotoxic drug injected into the striatum, is able to mimic clinical and histological features of this disease. Encapsulated BHK fibroblasts genetically engineered to secrete human CNTF were able to reduce the extent of striatal damage produced by quinolinic acid and improved motor functions in rats (Emerich et al. 1996). In a similar acute model, primates were lesioned by quinolinic acid. The same implants were able to prevent the degeneration of several populations of striatal cells, including GABAergic, cholinergic and NADPH diaphorase-positive neurons (Emerich et al. 1997). Mittoux et al. (1998) confirmed these results in another species of monkeys in a model of chronic lesion with NP-3. This group showed improved motor and cognitive functions that correlated with an important histological neuroprotection.

The transplantation of encapsulated cells releasing NFs has also been evaluated as a potential treatment of PD. Encapsulated cells releasing GDNF were also able to prevent the degeneration of dopaminergic cell bodies of the substantia nigra and lessened the drug-induced rotation behavior following a medial forebrain axotomy in a rodent model of PD (Tseng et al. 1997). In baboons chronically intoxicated with 1-methyl-4-phenyl-1,2,3,6-tetrahydropyridine (MPTP), the same encapsulated cell line was able to induce re-innervation of the striatum and was associated with significant behavioral improvements (PALFI et al. unpublished observations). Encapsulated fibroblasts producing NGF were able to prevent the lesion-induced loss of septal choline acetyltransferase expression of the medial septal cells following a fimbria-fornix lesion, a model bearing some validity for evaluating the survival of neurons afflicted in Alzheimer's disease (HOFFMAN et al. 1993).

Based on extensive animal experimentation, our group has performed a phase-I clinical trial, using 12 ALS patients, based on the intrathecal implantation of encapsulated BHK cells genetically engineered to secrete human CNTF (Fig. 2). This trial was initiated following the establishment of the ability to implant and retrieve them in various animal models and receiving the approval of the ethics committee of the Lausanne University Medical School and the Swiss Committee for Biological Safety. This study demonstrated the feasibility and safety of the encapsulated cell technology for the continuous intrathecal delivery of human CNTF (AEBISCHER et al. 1996b). Levels of CNTF in the order of nanograms could be detected in the cerebrospinal fluid of patients up to 60 weeks after transplantation (P. AEBISCHER, unpublished data), whereas no CNTF could be detected prior to implantation. All the implanted devices were intact and secreted CNTF at the time of explant (Fig. 2). No evidence of cell adherence to the external surface was observed, corroborating the excellent biocompatibility of the device. Simultaneous CSF lumbar and cervical measurements of CNTF showed that the cervical concentration was 14.6% of the lumbar level of CNTF, indicating that the whole spinal cord is exposed to the NF after lumbar subarachnoid implantation of the capsule. Clinically, although two phase-II trials administering CNTF systemically (SEEBURGER and SPRINGER 1993) had to be discontinued because of adverse side effects (BARINAGA 1994), the patients involved in our study did not suffer from any limiting side effects. The patients involved have been evaluated by clinical rating scales designed for ALS, including Norris, Tuft's quantitative neuromuscular evaluation (TQNE) and forced vital capacity (FVC) scores. Preliminary results indicate that the disease continues to progress; however, the small number of patients involved in the study does not allow assessment of a potential slowing down of the degenerative process.

D. Conclusion

The rapid advance in molecular biology and graft-transplant techniques have made possible the realization of a large number of approaches to deliver NFs to the CNS. Several in vivo and ex vivo approaches have been able to prevent or compensate for the cell loss of several models of neurodegenerative diseases. However, implementation of these results to clinical trials is slowed down by the problems of delivery. Different approaches are being investigated to circumvent the problem. The fast pace of new discoveries offers exciting hope for the delivery of NFs.

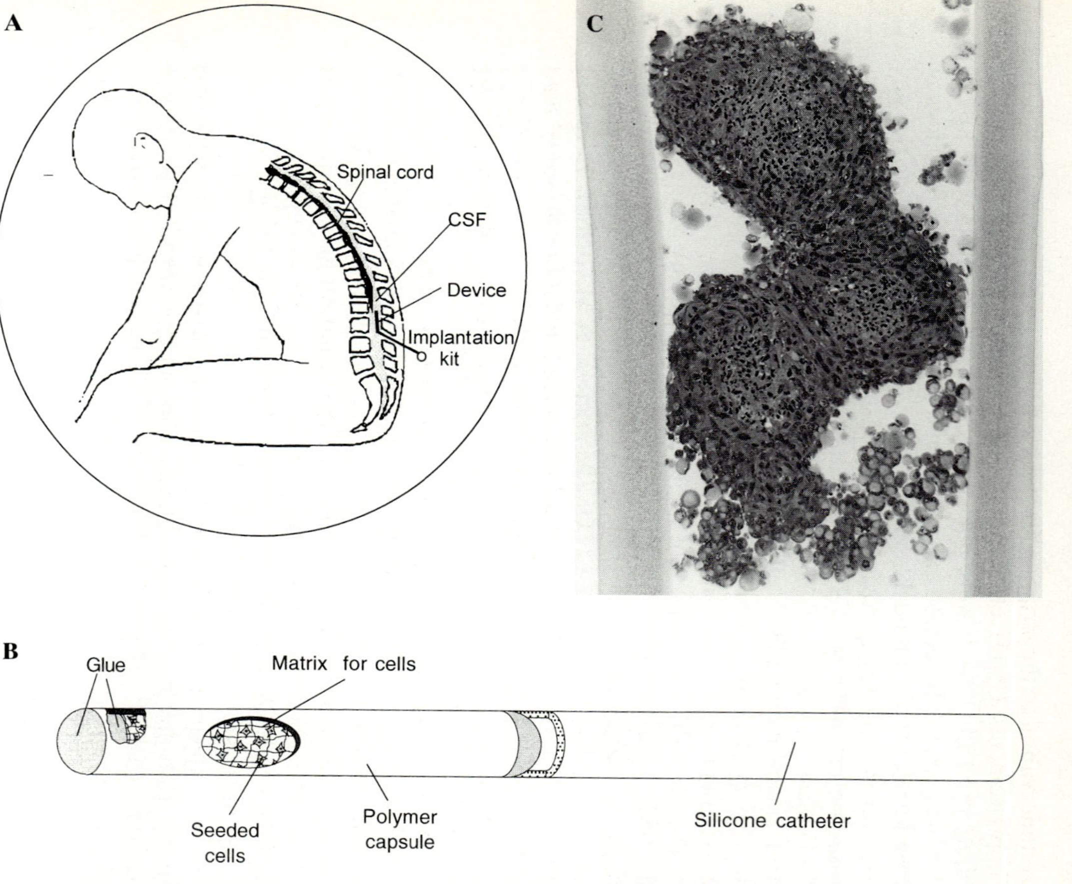

Fig. 2A–C. Clinical phase-I trial of genetically modified Baby-Hamster Kidney cells to secrete hCNTF in ALS patients. **A** Schematic representation of the implantation site. **B** Schematic drawing (not to scale) of the device employed in the clinical trial. **C** Longitudinal section of an explanted capsule from a patient 17 weeks post-implantation (hematoxylin and eosin). Printed with permission from Nature Medicine. *CSF* cerebrospinal fluid

Acknowledgements. The authors thank Nicole Déglon and Nicolas Bouche for their help and comments. A.F.H. is sponsored by a grant from the Roche Research Foundation MD-Ph.D. program.

References

Acheson A, Conover JC, Fandl JP, DeChiara TM, Russell M, Thadani A et al. (1995) A BDNF autocrine loop in adult sensory neurons prevents cell death. Nature 374:450–453

Aebischer P, Tresco PA, Winn SR, Greene LA, Jaeger CB (1991) Long-term cross-species brain transplantation of a polymer-encapsulated dopamine-secreting cell line. Exp Neurol 111:269–275

Aebischer P, Lysaght MJ (1995) Immunoisolation and cellular transplantation. Xeno 3: 43–48

Aebischer P, Pochon NA, Heyd B, Deglon N, Joseph JM, Zurn AD et al. (1996a) Gene therapy for amyotrophic lateral sclerosis (ALS) using a polymer encapsulated xenogenic cell line engineered to secrete hCNTF. Hum Gene Ther 7:851–860

Aebischer P, Schluep M, Deglon N, Joseph JM, Hirt L, Heyd B et al. (1996b) Intrathecal delivery of CNTF using encapsulated genetically modified xenogeneic cells in amyotrophic lateral sclerosis patients. Nature Med 2:696–699

Afione SA, Conrad CK, Kearns WG, Chunduru S, Adams R, Reynolds TC et al. (1996) In vivo model of adeno-associated virus vector persistence and rescue. J Virol 70:3235–3241

Akli S, Caillaud C, Vigne E, Stratford-Perricaudet LD, Poenaru L, Perricaudet M et al. (1993) Transfer of a foreign gene into the brain using adenovirus vectors. Nature Genet 3:224–228

ALS CNTF Treatment Study (ACTS) Group (1996) A double-blind placebo-controlled clinical trial of subcutaneous recombinant human ciliary neurotrophic factor (rHCNTF) in amyotrophic lateral sclerosis. Neurology 46:1244–1249

Anderson KD (1998) Effects of axokine in animal models of Huntington's disease. In: Peschanski M, Ollat H (eds) CNTF and associates: from gene to therapy. Paris, France, pp 58–60

Arakawa Y, Sendtner M, Thoenen H (1990) Survival effect of ciliary neurotrophic factor (CNTF) on chick embryonic motoneurons in culture: comparison with other neurotrophic factors and cytokines. J Neurosci 10:3507–3515

Barinaga M (1994) Neurotrophic factors enter the clinic. Science 264:772–774

Baumgartner BJ, Shine HD (1997) Targeted transduction of CNS neurons with adenoviral vectors carrying neurotrophic factor genes confers neuroprotection that exceeds the transduced population. J Neurosci 17:6504–6511

BDNF study group (1998) Recombinant methionyl human brain derived neurotrophic factor in the treatment of patients with amyotrophic lateral sclerosis. Ann Neurol (in press)

Biewenga JE, Destree OH, Schrama LH (1997) Plasmid-mediated gene transfer in neurons using the biolistics technique. J Neurosci Meth 71:67–75

Bilang-Bleuel A, Revah F, Colin P, Locquet I, Robert JJ, Mallet J et al. (1997) Intrastriatal injection of an adenoviral vector expressing glial-cell-line-derived neurotrophic factor prevents dopaminergic neuron degeneration and behavioral impairment in a rat model of Parkinson disease. Proc Natl Acad Sci USA 94: 8818–8823

Björklund A (1991) Neural transplantation – an experimental tool with clinical possibilities. Trends Neurosci 14:319–322

Blömer U, Naldini L, Verma IM, Trono D, Gage FH (1996) Applications of gene therapy to the CNS. Hum Mol Genet 5:1397–1404

Boucher RC (1996) Current status of CF gene therapy. Trends Genet 12:81–84

Bowers WJ, Howard DF, Federoff HJ (1997) Gene therapeutic strategies for neuroprotection – implications for Parkinson's disease. Exp Neurol 144:58–68

Byrnes AP, Rusby JE, Wood MJ, Charlton HM (1995) Adenovirus gene transfer causes inflammation in the brain. Neurosci 66:1015–1024

Byrnes AP, MacLaren RE, Charlton HM (1996) Immunological instability of persistent adenovirus vectors in the brain: peripheral exposure to vector leads to renewed inflammation, reduced gene expression, and demyelination. J Neurosci 16:3045–3055

Choilundberg DL, Lin Q, Chang YN, Chiang YL, Hay CM, Mohajeri H et al. (1997) Dopaminergic neurons protected from degeneration by GDNF gene therapy. Science 275:838–841

Christ M, Lusky M, Stoeckel F, Dreyer D, Dieterle A, Michou AI et al. (1997) Gene therapy with recombinant adenovirus vectors – evaluation of the host immune response. Immunol Lett 57:19–25

Curtis R, Adryan KM, Zhu Y, Harkness PJ, Lindsay RM, DiStefano PS (1993) Retrograde axonal transport of ciliary neurotrophic factor is increased by peripheral nerve injury. Nature 365:253–255

Curtis R, Scherer SS, Somogyi R, Adryan KM, Ip NY, Zhu Y et al. (1994) Retrograde axonal transport of LIF is increased by peripheral nerve injury: correlation with increased LIF expression in distal nerve. Neuron 12:191–204

Dai Y, Roman M, Naviaux RK, Verma IM (1992) Gene therapy via primary myoblasts: long-term expression of factor IX protein following transplantation in vivo. Proc Natl Acad Sci USA 89:10892–10895

During MJ, Naegele JR, KL OM, Geller AI (1994) Long-term behavioral recovery in parkinsonian rats by an HSV vector expressing tyrosine hydroxylase. Science 266:1399–1403

During MJ, Leone P (1995) Adeno-associated virus vectors for gene therapy of neurodegenerative disorders. Clin Neurosci 3:292–300

Emerich DF, Lindner MD, Winn SR, Chen EY, Frydel BR, Kordower JH (1996) Implants of encapsulated human CNTF-producing fibroblasts prevent behavioral deficits and striatal degeneration in a rodent model of Huntington's disease. J Neurosci 16:5168–5181

Emerich DF, Winn SR, Hantraye PM, Peschanski M, Chen EY, Chu YP et al. (1997) Protective effect of encapsulated cells producing neurotrophic factor CNTF in a monkey model of Huntington's disease. Nature 386:395–399

Fantuzzi G, Benigni F, Sironi M, Conni M, Carelli M, Cantoni L et al. (1995) Ciliary neurotrophic factor (CNTF) induces serum amyloid A, hypoglycaemia and anorexia, and potentiates IL-1 induced corticosterone and IL-6 production in mice. Cytokine 7:150–156

Fisher LJ, Jinnah HA, Kale LC, Higgins GA, Gage FH (1991) Survival and function of intrastriatally grafted primary fibroblasts genetically modified to produce L-dopa. Neuron 6:371–380

Freese A, Stern M, Kaplitt MG, WM OC, Abbey MV, MJ OC et al. (1996) Prospects for gene therapy in Parkinson's disease. Mov Disord 11:469–488

Gallay P, Stitt V, Mundy C, Oettinger M, Trono D (1996) Role of the karyopherin pathway in human immunodeficiency virus type 1 nuclear import. J Virol 70:1027–1032

Gehrmann J, Matsumoto Y, Kreutzberg GW (1995) Microglia: intrinsic immuneffector cell of the brain. Brain Res Brain Res Rev 20:269–287

Ghadge GD, Roos RP, Kang UJ, Wollmann R, Fishman PS, Kalynych AM et al. (1995) CNS gene delivery by retrograde transport of recombinant replication-defective adenoviruses. Gene Ther 2:132–137

Haase G, Kennel P, Vigne E, Akli S, Revah F, Schmalbruch H et al. (1997) Gene therapy of murine motor neuron disease using adenoviral vectors for neurotrophic factors. Nature Med 3:429–436

Henderson CE, Phillips HS, Pollock RA, Davies AM, Lemeulle C, Armanini M et al. (1994) GDNF: a potent survival factor for motoneurons present in peripheral nerve and muscle. Science 266:1062–1064

Hock RA, Miller AD, Osborne WR (1989) Expression of human adenosine deaminase from various strong promoters after gene transfer into human hematopoietic cell lines. Blood 74:876–881

Hoffman D, Wahlberg L, Aebischer P (1990) NGF released from a polymer matrix prevents loss of ChAT expression in basal forebrain neurons following a fimbria-fornix lesion. Exp Neurol 110:39–44

Hoffman D, Breakefield XO, Short MP, Aebischer P (1993) Transplantation of a polymer-encapsulated cell line genetically engineered to release NGF. Exp Neurol 122:100–106

Horellou P, Brundin P, Kalen P, Mallet J, Björklund A (1990) In vivo release of dopa and dopamine from genetically engineered cells grafted to the denervated rat striatum. Neuron 5:393–402

Horellou P, Sabate O, Buc-Caron MH, Mallet J (1997) Adenovirus-mediated gene transfer to the central nervous system for Parkinson's disease. Exp Neurol 144:131–138

Ilan Y, Jona VK, Sengupta K, Davidson A, Horwitz MS, Roychowdhury N et al. (1997) Transient immunosuppression with Fk506 permits long-term expression of therapeutic genes introduced into the liver using recombinant adenoviruses in the rat. Hepatology 26:949–956

Kaplitt MG, Kwong AD, Kleopoulos SP, Mobbs CV, Rabkin SD, Pfaff DW (1994a) Preproenkephalin promoter yields region-specific and long-term expression in adult brain after direct in vivo gene transfer via a defective herpes simplex viral vector. Proc Natl Acad Sci USA 91:8979–8983

Kaplitt MG, Leone P, Samulski RJ, Xiao X, Pfaff DW, KL OM et al. (1994b) Long-term gene expression and phenotypic correction using adeno-associated virus vectors in the mammalian brain. Nature Genet 8:148–154

Klein R, Conway D, Parada LF, Barbacid M (1990) The trkB tyrosine protein kinase gene codes for a second neurogenic receptor that lacks the catalytic kinase domain. Cell 61:647–656

Kordower JH, Charles V, Bayer R, Bartus RT, Putney S, Walus LR et al. (1994) Intravenous administration of a transferrin receptor antibody-nerve growth factor conjugate prevents the degeneration of cholinergic striatal neurons in a model of Huntington disease. Proc Natl Acad Sci USA 91:9077–9080

Korsching S (1993) The neurotrophic factor concept: a reexamination. J Neurosci 13:2739–2748

Kremer EJ, Perricaudet M (1995) Adenovirus and adeno-associated virus mediated gene transfer. Br Med Bull 51:31–44

Lai EC, Felice KJ, Festoff BW, Gawel MJ, Gelinas DF, Kratz R et al. (1997) Effect of recombinant human insulin-like growth factor-I on progression of ALS – a placebo-controlled study. Neurol 49:1621–1630

Lamer TJ (1994) Treatment of cancer-related pain: when orally administered medications fail. Mayo Clin Proc 69:473–480

Langer R, Folkman J (1976) Polymers for the sustained release of proteins and other macromolecules. Nature 263:797–800

Lebkowski JS, McNally MM, Okarma TB, Lerch LB (1988) Adeno-associated virus: a vector system for efficient introduction and integration of DNA into a variety of mammalian cell types. Mol Cell Biol 8:3988–3996

Levi-Montalcini R (1987) The nerve growth factor 35 years later. Science 237:1154–1162

Levivier M, Przedborski S, Bencsics C, Kang UJ (1995) Intrastriatal implantation of fibroblasts genetically engineered to produce brain-derived neurotrophic factor prevents degeneration of dopaminergic neurons in a rat model of Parkinson's disease. J Neurosci 15:7810–7820

Lim F, Sun AM (1980) Microencapsulated islets as bioartificial endocrine pancreas. Science 210:908–910

Lin LF, Doherty DH, Lile JD, Bektesh S, Collins F (1993) GDNF: a glial cell line-derived neurotrophic factor for midbrain dopaminergic neurons. Science 260:1130–1132

Mandel RJ, Spratt SK, Snyder RO, Leff SE (1997) Midbrain injection of recombinant adeno-associated virus encoding rat glial cell line-derived neurotrophic factor protects nigral neurons in a progressive 6-hydroxydopamine-induced degeneration model of Parkinson's disease in rats. Proc Natl Acad Sci USA 94:14083–14088

Martinez-Serrano A, Björklund A (1996) Protection of the neostriatum against excitotoxic damage by neurotrophin-producing, genetically modified neural stem cells. J Neurosci 16:4604–4616

Martinez-Serrano A, Lundberg C, Horellou P, Fischer W, Bentlage C, Campbell K et al. (1995) CNS-derived neural progenitor cells for gene transfer of nerve growth factor to the adult rat brain: complete rescue of axotomized cholinergic neurons after transplantation into the septum. J Neurosci 15:5668–5680

Mayer E, Fawcett JW, Dunnett SB (1993) Basic fibroblast growth factor promotes the survival of embryonic ventral mesencephalic dopaminergic neurons–II. Effects on nigral transplants in vivo. Neurosci 56:389–398

McRae-Degueurce A, Hjorth S, Dillon DL, Mason DW, Tice TR (1988) Implantable microencapsulated dopamine (DA): a new approach for slow-release DA delivery into brain tissue. Neurosci Lett 92:303–309

Miller RG, Petajan JH, Bryan WW, Armon C, Barohn RJ, Goodpasture JC et al. (1996) A placebo-controlled trial of recombinant human ciliary neurotrophic (rhCNTF) factor in amyotrophic lateral sclerosis. rhCNTF ALS Study Group. Ann Neurol 39:256–260

Mitsumoto H, Ikeda K, Klinkosz B, Cedarbaum JM, Wong V, Lindsay RM (1994) Arrest of motor neuron disease in wobbler mice cotreated with CNTF and BDNF. Science 265:1107–1110

Mittoux V, Joseph JM, Palfi S, Condé F, Zurn AD, Dautry C et al. (1998) Neuroprotective and behavioral effects of encapsulated CNTF-producing fibroblasts in a chronic primate model of Huntington's disease. In: Peschanski M, Ollat H (eds) CNTF and associates: from gene to therapy. Paris, France, pp 52–54

Mufson EJ, Kroin JS, Sobreviela T, Burke MA, Kordower JH, Penn RD et al. (1994) Intrastriatal infusions of brain-derived neurotrophic factor: retrograde transport and colocalization with dopamine containing substantia nigra neurons in rat. Exp Neurol 129:15–26

Mufson EJ, Kroin JS, Liu YT, Sobreviela T, Penn RD, Miller JA et al. (1996) Intrastriatal and intraventricular infusion of brain-derived neurotrophic factor in the cynomologous monkey: distribution, retrograde transport and co-localization with substantia nigra dopamine-containing neurons. Neurosci 71:179–191

Naldini L, Blömer U, Gallay P, Ory D, Mulligan R, Gage FH et al. (1996) In vivo gene delivery and stable transduction of nondividing cells by a lentiviral vector. Science 272:263–267

O'Malley K, Geller AI (1992) Gene therapy in neurology: potential application to Parkinson's disease. In: Vecsei L, Freese A, Swartz KJ, Beal MF (eds) Ellis Horwood, West Sussex

Ooboshi H, Welsh MJ, Rios CD, Davidson BL, Heistad DD (1995) Adenovirus-mediated gene transfer in vivo to cerebral blood vessels and perivascular tissue. Circ Res 77:7–13

Palmer TD, Rosman GJ, Osborne WR, Miller AD (1991) Genetically modified skin fibroblasts persist long after transplantation but gradually inactivate introduced genes. Proc Natl Acad Sci USA 88:1330–1334

Partridge WM, Kumagai AK, Eisenberg JB (1987) Chimeric peptides as a vehicle for peptide pharmaceutical delivery through the blood-brain-barrier. Biochem Biophys Res Commun 16:307–313

Peltekian E, Parrish E, Bouchard C, Peschanski M, Lisovoski F (1997) Adenovirus-mediated gene transfer to the brain: methodological assessment. J Neurosci Meth 71:77–84

Penn RD (1988) Intrathecal baclofen for severe spasticity. Ann NY Acad Sci 531:157–166

Penn RD, Kroin JS, York MM, Cedarbaum JM (1997) Intrathecal ciliary neurotrophic factor delivery for treatment of amyotrophic lateral sclerosis (phase I trial) Neurosurgery 40:94–99

Poduslo JF, Curran GL (1996) Permeability at the blood-brain and blood-nerve barriers of the neurotrophic factors: NGF, CNTF, NT-3, BDNF. Brain Res Dev Brain Res 36:280–286

Renfranz PJ, Cunningham MG, McKay RD (1991) Region-specific differentiation of the hippocampal stem cell line HiB5 upon implantation into the developing mammalian brain. Cell 66:713–729

Rogers BC (1996) Development of recombinant human nerve growth factor (RHNGF) as a treatment for peripheral neuropathic disease. Neurotoxicology 17:865–870

Sabel BA, Dominiak P, Hauser W, During MJ, Freese A (1990) Levodopa delivery from controlled-release polymer matrix: delivery of more than 600 days in vitro and 225 days of elevated plasma levels after subcutaneous implantation in rats. J Pharm Exp Ther 255:914–922

Sagot Y, Tan SA, Baetge E, Schmalbruch H, Kato AC, Aebischer P (1995) Polymer encapsulated cell lines genetically engineered to release ciliary neurotrophic factor can slow down progressive motor neuronopathy in the mouse. Eur J Neurosci 7:1313–1322

Samulski RJ, Chang LS, Shenk T (1989) Helper-free stocks of recombinant adeno-associated viruses: normal integration does not require viral gene expression. J Virol 63:3822–3828

Scharfmann R, Axelrod JH, Verma IM (1991) Long-term in vivo expression of retrovirus-mediated gene transfer in mouse fibroblast implants. Proc Natl Acad Sci USA 88:4626–4630

Schmalbruch H, Jensen HJ, Bjaerg M, Kamieniecka Z, Kurland L (1991) A new mouse mutant with progressive motor neuronopathy. J Neuropathol Exp Neurol 50:192–204

Seeburger JL, Springer JE (1993) Experimental rationale for the therapeutic use of neurotrophins in amyotrophic lateral sclerosis. Exp Neurol 124:64–72

Segal RA, Takahashi H, McKay RD (1992) Changes in neurotrophin responsiveness during the development of cerebellar granule neurons. Neuron 9:1041–1052

Sendtner M, Kreutzberg GW, Thoenen H (1990) Ciliary neurotrophic factor prevents the degeneration of motor neurons after axotomy. Nature 345:440–441

Snyder SH (1991) Parkinson's disease. Fresh factors to consider. Nature 350:195

Suhr ST, Gage FH (1993) Gene therapy for neurologic disease. Arch Neurol 50:1252–1268

Trono D (1995) HIV accessory proteins: leading roles for the supporting cast. Cell 82:189–192

Tseng JL, Baetge EE, Zurn AD, Aebischer P (1997) GDNF reduces drug-induced rotational behavior after medial forebrain bundle transection by a mechanism not involving striatal dopamine. J Neurosci 17:325–333

Uchida K, Ishii A, Kaneda N, Toya S, Nagatsu T, Kohsaka S (1990) Tetrahydrobiopterin-dependent production of L-dopa in NRK fibroblasts transfected with tyrosine hydroxylase cDNA: future use for intracerebral grafting. Neurosci Lett 109:282–286

Vejsada R, Tseng JL, Lindsay RM, Acheson A, Aebischer P, Kato AC (1998) Synergistic but transient rescue effects of BDNF and GDNF on axotomized neonatal motoneurons. Neurosci 84:129–139

Winn SR, Aebischer P, Galletti PM (1989) Brain tissue reaction to permselective polymer capsules. J Biomed Mat Res 23:31–44

Winn SR, Tresco, PA, Zielinski, B, Greene LA, Jaeger CB, Aebischer P (1991) Behavioral recovery following intrastriatal implantation of microencapsulated PC12 cells. Exp Neurol 113:322–329

Wood MJ, Charlton HM, Wood KJ, Kajiwara K, Byrnes AP (1996) Immune responses to adenovirus vectors in the nervous system. Trends Neurosci 19:497–501

Yan Q, Matheson C, Sun J, Radeke MJ, Feinstein SC, Miller JA (1994) Distribution of intracerebral ventricularly administered neurotrophins in rat brain and its correlation with trk receptor expression. Exp Neurol 127:23–36

Yan Q, Matheson C, Lopez OT (1995) In vivo neurotrophic effects of GDNF on neonatal and adult facial motor neurons. Nature 373:341–344

Yoshimoto Y, Lin Q, Collier TJ, Frim DM, Breakefield XO, Bohn MC (1995) Astrocytes retrovirally transduced with BDNF elicit behavioral improvement in a rat model of Parkinson's disease. Brain Res 691:25–36

Yuen EC, Mobley WC (1996) Therapeutic potential of neurotrophic factors for neurological disorders. Ann Neurol 40:346–354

Zielinski BA, Aebischer P (1994) Chitosan as a matrix for mammalian cell encapsulation. Biomaterials 15:1049–1056

Zufferey R, Nagy D, Mandel RJ, Naldini L, Trono D (1997) Multiply attenuated lentiviral vector achieves efficient gene delivery in vivo. Nature Biotech 15:871–875

Zurn AD, Baetge EE, Hammang JP, Tan SA, Aebischer P (1994) Glial cell line-derived neurotrophic factor (GDNF), a new neurotrophic factor for motoneurons. Neuroreport 6:113–118

CHAPTER 11

Neurotrophic Factor Mimetics

C. SWAIN, S. HARPER, S. POLLACK, R. SMITH, and F. HEFTI

A. Introduction

Preclinical and clinical data suggest that subcutaneous or intravenous administration of neurotrophic factors may be effective for the treatment of peripheral nervous system diseases. However, even though these proteins are natural products, they do present specific problems when used as therapeutic agents. They cannot be given by the oral route. They may elicit an immune response. Their pharmacokinetic behaviour is difficult to predict due to binding to other macromolecules and differential sensitivity to proteinases. Penetration into peripheral nerve sheets may be limited. Large scale production is labour and cost intensive. Small organic molecules as used in the "typical drugs" tend to be superior to protein therapeutics in most, if not all, of these aspects.

Neurotrophic factor treatment of central nervous system diseases presents an even more complex problem than treatment of peripheral neurons. Since the neurotrophic factors are not able to cross the blood–brain barrier, they must be given intracerebrally, or ways must be found to carry them across the barrier. As described in other chapters of this volume, there is an active search for alternative delivery strategies and many promising initial steps have been taken. However, for central nervous system diseases in particular the advantages of small molecule mimetics over proteins are evident. Small organic molecules can be modified to penetrate freely into the brain parenchyma and can be designed for oral administration. This chapter describes the strategies taken towards the development of small molecule mimetics for neurotrophic factors and the emerging drug candidates.

There are several possible approaches for replacing neurotrophic proteins with small molecule mimetics. For therapeutic use in the peripheral nervous system, neurotrophic proteins could be replaced by active peptide fragments with receptor binding properties similar to the mother proteins, but improved pharmacokinetic properties and perhaps lower production costs. In principle, it should be possible to replace the entire protein or a fully active peptide fragment by a non-peptidic molecule binding to the same receptor site. It may be possible to regulate neurotrophic factor receptor activity by allosterically acting molecules which influence the functional efficacy of the receptors. Understanding of the mechanisms regulating gene expression should provide opportunities to regulate synthesis of the neurotrophic factors. There is evidence for regulated release of neurotrophic factors, so that it might be possible to discover agents which selectively induce the release of such proteins. Finally, there is evidence that neurotrophic factor synthesis and release are influenced by the electrical activity of neurons, opening up the possibility of regulating them through ligands of neurotransmitter receptors.

B. Direct and Indirect Receptor Ligands

I. Peptide Mimetics

A small number of examples illustrate that it is possible to replace a protein growth factor with an active peptide fragment. Recently, a 14-amino acid peptide agonist was identified for the thrombopoietin receptor, mimicking the effects of the natural 332-amino acid ligand (CWIRLA et al. 1997). Dimers of the peptide were equipotent to thrombopoietin, probably reflecting the ability of these bi-functional peptides to induce dimerisation of the receptor. Earlier, a synthetic peptide analog of TGF-α (transforming growth factor-α) was shown to specifically inhibit EGF (epithelial growth factor) and TGF-α growth stimulatory actions on responsive cell lines (EPPSTEIN et al. 1989), and fragments of IGF-I (insulin-like growth factor) and -II were reported to be biologically active (KONISHI et al. 1989). For several years, attempts have been made to generate fragments of neurotrophic factors which retain activity, however a clear success has so far been elusive. LONGO et al. (1997) reported the production of peptide fragments which inhibit biological actions of NGF (nerve growth factor), but effective concentrations of the active peptides were much higher than those of the native proteins.

For uses directed to the peripheral nervous system, peptidic neurotrophic factor mimetics or modified neurotrophic factors could have advantages over natural proteins if their potency or pharmacokinetic properties are superior. In the case of CNTF (ciliary neurotrophic factor), it was possible to generate variants with increased biological potency by introducing a small number of amino acid mutations (SAGGIO et al. 1995). In the case of the neurotrophin (NT) family, it was possible to generate heterodimers which retain functional activity for both receptors; e.g., heterodimers composed of NGF and NT-4/5 subunits stimulated both Trk A and Trk B receptors (TREANOR et al. 1995). Such heterodimers thus represent artificial neurotrophins with different receptor subtype selectivity and they might become therapeutically useful if combinations of neurotrophins show maximal therapeutic benefit. Immunogenicity is likely to represent a significant problem with chronic use of proteins with amino acid alterations. Single amino acid exchanges, as well as novel interfaces in heterodimers can form neoepitopes which might elicit an immune response.

Besides potentially leading to therapeutically useful compounds, studies with peptide fragments and modified peptides are attractive, since they might provide a basis for molecular modelling studies attempting to replace peptides with non-peptide effectors. The theoretical feasibility of the approach is based on neuropeptides, as illustrated by the example of endorphins and morphine which act on the same receptors, and by the discovery of non-peptide ligands for other peptide receptors, such as those for substance P (SNIDER et al. 1991; LONGMORE et al. 1994). Alternatively, it may be possible to produce compounds mimicking receptor-binding sites of growth factors based on the tertiary structure of the proteins. In the case of neurotrophins the amino acids have been identified which interact with the receptors (URFER et al. 1994; IBANEZ 1994; BARBACID 1995). The fact that heterodimers retain functional activity (TREANOR et al. 1995) suggests that a single binding site might be sufficient to elicit a response, offering an opportunity for structural modelling of the active site. Indeed, two recent studies have shown that neurotrophin binding to Trk receptors appears to require only the so-called immunoglobulin-like extracellular domains of Trk, also supporting the view that the neurotrophin-Trk interaction is spatially limited (URFER et al. 1995; HOLDEN et al. 1997). In one of these studies, the interaction was narrowed down to a single immunoglobulin-like domain, which, when expressed as a fusion with the kinase domain, resulted in functional neurotrophin-dependent activation (URFER et al. 1995). In both studies, similar affinities for the neurotrophins were obtained with the receptors containing only the immunoglobulin-like extracellular domains, compared to wild-type receptors. However, other studies using synthetic peptides (WINDISCH et al. 1995a, 1995b) and naturally-occurring TrkB variants (NINKINA et al. 1997) have shown that the leucine-rich motifs of the extracellular domain are responsible for the affinity and specificity of neurotrophin binding to Trk receptors. It may be that the discrepancies among these studies are due to different experimental approaches. More work will be required to fully understand the functional importance of Trk domains in neurotrophin binding and receptor dimerisation, and it is likely that more than one domain is involved. However, even in that case, it is clear from these studies that interactions with one domain may be sufficient to mimic a neurotrophin response.

II. K-252a and Related Compounds that Modulate Trk Receptor Signalling

Peptide or non-peptide analogues of neurotrophic factors are designed to mimic the conformation of the natural protein ligand and interact with the same binding site on the neurotrophin receptor. Besides these direct ligands, it may be possible to find compounds that affect neurotrophin receptor function by binding to regions different from those interacting with the neurotrophins, as allosteric regulators of receptor activation. This situation would be in analogy to the benzodiazepine modification of GABA-A (γ-aminobutyric acid) receptor function. Such compounds could act on their own or could potentiate the action of neurotrophins. The latter mechanism is more conceivable for small molecules if receptor dimerisation is a prerequisite to activation.

A different starting point to such a strategy would be provided by compounds that selectively modify a function of Trk neurotrophin receptors. The activation of receptors by neurotrophins triggers an array of cellular signalling responses. Receptor activation involves extracellular ligand-induced dimerisation, followed by transphosphorylation of the intracellular region of the receptor by its kinase domain (Greene and Kaplan 1995; Fig. 1). The phosphorylation of particular tyrosine residues on this intracellular region follows a precise sequence of events as the receptor kinase itself is activated. Signalling molecules, including PI (phosphatidylinositol)-3-kinase, shc (src homologous and collagen protein) (Ras/MAP kinase pathway), PLC-γ (phospholipase C) and SNT (suc-associated neurotrophic factor), bind to specific phosphotyrosine-containing recognition sequences and become phosphory-

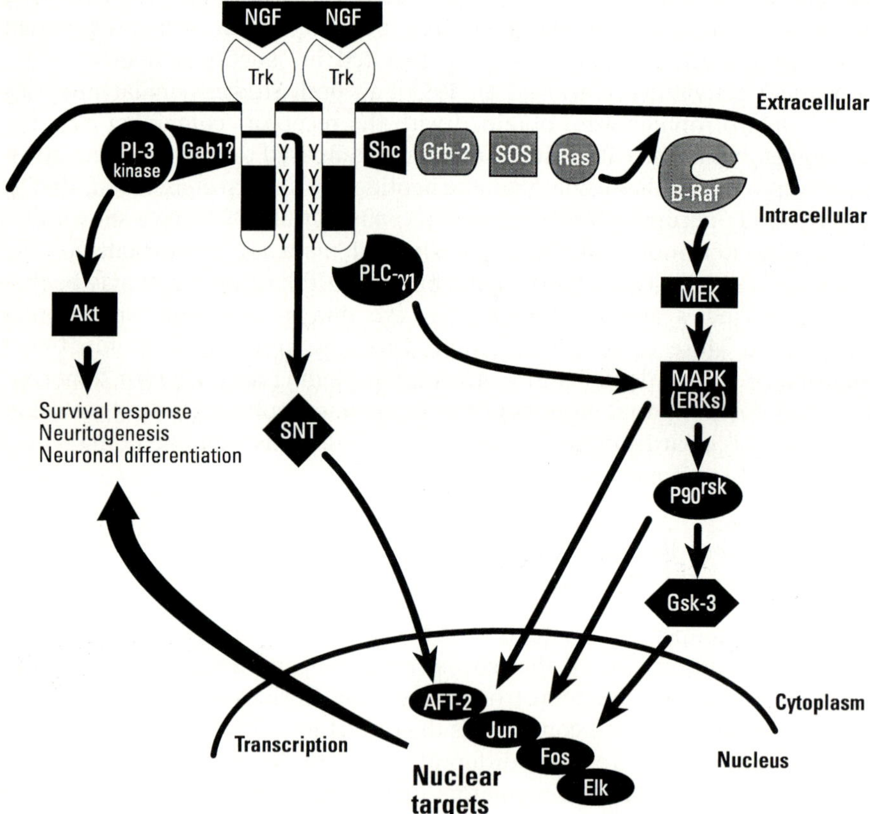

Fig. 1. Signalling of neurotrophins and subsequent intracellular actions. Binding of neurotrophic factors to Trk receptors (Trk) triggers activation of the Ras/MAP kinase signalling pathways which serve to stimulate transcription of specific target genes, leading to a range of cellular responses. NGF, nerve growth factor; SNT, suc-associated neurotrophic factor; Y, tyrosine residues

lated themselves through the tyrosine kinase activity of the Trk receptor. The activated signalling molecules then trigger effects on gene transcription and regulation of cytoskeletal machinery, leading to cell survival (mainly PI-3-kinase-mediated) and differentiation (mainly MAP kinase-mediated) responses. Overlap and cross-talk among signalling pathways complicates an understanding of which components are responsible for which effect, and it would probably be undesirable to interfere with only one branch of a neurotrophin-mediated signalling pathway. The most faithful neurotrophin mimetic would act early on to trigger the entire cascade of signalling events.

p75 is a second neurotrophin receptor that binds all the known neurotrophins and appears to interact with Trk to modulate its neurotrophin binding affinity and kinetics (Greene and Kaplan 1995). For example, p75 appears to contribute to the proportion of high affinity binding sites present on neurons. p75 also modulates the binding specificity of TrkA, preventing neurotrophin 3 (NT-3) from binding as an alternative ligand to NGF, whereas both ligands can bind in its absence. Finally, p75 has a Trk-independent role in cell death signalling that is just beginning to be elucidated (Carter and Lewin 1997; Bredesen and Rabizadeh 1997). In specific subpopulations of neurons (developmental and TrkA-expressing CNS (central nervous system) neurons, e.g. Stucky and Koltzenburg 1997; Ryden et al. 1997) the role of p75 as a Trk modulator is essential to keep in mind in evaluating the effects of potential neurotrophin mimetics.

The K-252 class of compounds provides the most well-characterised example of molecules with an early modulatory role in Trk signalling. K-252a and K-252b are related low molecular weight alkaloids of microbial origin that have been known for years to interfere with protein kinase activities in cell free systems (Fig. 2). They are related to staurosporin, a protein kinase inhibitor from *Streptomyces*. At nanomolar concentrations, compounds of the K-252 class act as competitive inhibitors at the intracellular ATP binding site of the

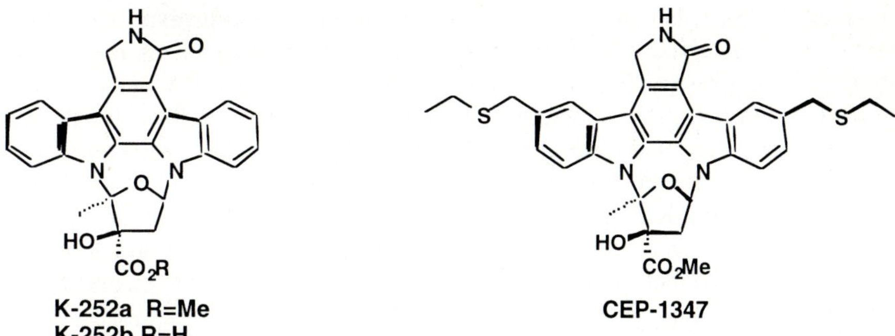

Fig. 2. K-252a and related compounds

Trk kinase (Berg et al. 1992; Nye et al. 1992; Ohmichi and Decker 1992). These compounds prevent the NGF-induced morphological transformation of proliferating PC12 cells into neuron-like cells, and inhibit the NGF-stimulated, but not the bFGF (basic fibroblast growth factor)- or EGF-stimulated phosphorylation of selected proteins (Koizumi et al. 1988; Matsuda and Fukuda 1988). K-252a and K-252b selectively inhibit neurotrophic actions on cholinergic neurons of the basal forebrain and dopaminergic neurons of the mesencephalon without interfering with the trophic actions of bFGF, insulin or IGF-1 (Knüsel and Hefti 1992; Knüsel et al. 1992). Of the two, K-252b, which differs from K-252a only in the presence of a free carboxylate in place of an ester, is effective over a wider range of concentrations and lacks general cytotoxicity. These inhibitory actions reflect a direct inhibition of Trk receptors, since the effects were shown to occur with immunopurified Trk protein (Berg et al. 1992). In intact cells, K-252a and K-252b only affect Trk receptors, without interfering with the function of EGF, PDGF (platelet-derived growth factor) or IGF–1 receptors, but this selectivity is lost in cell homogenates (Knüsel and Hefti 1992; Nye et al. 1992; Ohmichi et al. 1992; Tapley and Lamballe 1992).

In addition to inhibiting Trk phosphorylation, K-252b potentiates the stimulatory effect of NT-3 on cholinergic differentiation, peripheral sensory neuron survival, and TrkA phosphorylation and neurite outgrowth in PC12 cells, at lower concentrations than those producing measurable inhibitory effects (Knüsel et al. 1992). The NT-3 response in the presence of K-252b is equivalent to an optimal NGF response and leads to the full signalling cascade observed with TrkA activation by NGF (Knüsel et al. 1992; Isono et al. 1994). When assayed by [^{3}H]thymidine incorporation, the potentiation effect appeared specific for NT-3 acting at TrkA, since no effect with NGF (at submaximal doses), BDNF (brain-derived neurotrophic factor) or NT-4/5 was observed (Maroney et al. 1997), and only TrkA (not TrkB or TrkC) responded to K-252b/NT-3. Since K-252b, unlike K-252a, has been claimed not to cross the cell membrane except at relatively high concentrations (Ross et al. 1995), this potentiation effect may be due to an extracellular interaction with Trk, NT-3 or another protein. It has recently been established that p75 is not involved in this effect since it was observed in NIH3T3 cells expressing only TrkA in the absence of p75 (Maroney et al. 1997). In fact, as mentioned above, p75 expression has the opposite effect, limiting TrkA activation to NGF. It is interesting to speculate on an interaction of K-252b with Trk at a similar site to that of the putative p75 interaction, but with a different functional outcome. In any event, the potentiating effect of K-252b on TrkA receptor activation is unlikely to relate to its inhibitory effect on Trk kinase, since the latter effect requires long incubations with higher compound concentrations to achieve cell penetration and kinase inhibition (Knüsel and Hefti 1992; Ross et al. 1995; Maroney et al. 1997).

K-252 compounds also have clearly non-Trk-related neurotrophic effects. For instance, at relatively high concentrations, K-252a, but not K-252b, enhanced MAP kinase activity and neurite outgrowth induced by EGF or bFGF in PC12 cells, although receptor autophosphorylation was not affected (ISONO et al. 1994; WU and ZHANG 1993). In addition, MARONEY and co-workers (1995) have shown that K-252a induces tyrosine phosphorylation of focal adhesion kinase and neurite outgrowth in human neuroblastoma SH-SY5Y cells. All of these phenomena occurred independently of Trk and protein kinase C effects. Finally, K-252a was shown to promote survival and choline acetyltransferase activity in primary cultures of striatal neurons, dorsal root ganglion and ciliary ganglion neurons, and spinal cord- and basal forebrain-derived neurons (BORASIO 1990; GLICKSMAN et al. 1993; GLICKSMAN et al. 1995). Although K-252 derivatives clearly are not pharmacologically clean compounds, it may be possible to dissect effects on Trk receptors from these other activities by examining related structures. Together, the findings with K-252b point to the possibility of developing compounds able to distinguish among the different Trk receptors and to inhibit or potentiate actions of neurotrophins selectively.

In another approach, KANEKO et al. (1997) evaluated various analogues of K-252a and were able to identify molecules that retain the ability to stimulate neuronal survival without affecting Trk phosphorylation or protein kinase C activity. One of these molecules, CEP-1347, was shown to rescue forebrain cholinergic neurons from a neurotoxic insult in the adult rat brain (KANEKO et al. 1997). CEP-1347 also increased survival of cultured spinal motor neurons, dorsal root ganglia, and striatal GABAergic neurons. The molecular target of CEP-1347 seems to be downstream of Trk, since Trk phosphorylation is not affected. It is now thought to involve inhibition of the c-Jun kinase-mediated cell death pathway (KANEKO et al. 1997).

III. Immunophilin Ligands

Another group of compounds claimed to have neuritogenic and or neurotrophic actions are the immunophilin ligands, including cyclosporin A, FK506 (Tacrolimus) and rapamycin. Cyclosporin A (CsA), a cyclic peptide of 11 amino acids, was introduced in the 1980s to overcome the problem of rejection of organ transplants. The discovery of the compound led to a large amount of work on the mechanisms whereby CsA suppresses T cell function and to the identification of cyclophilin A (HANDSCHUMACHER et al. 1984), an 18 kDa soluble protein that binds to CsA. There are now known to be 6 cyclophilins, Cyp A, Cyp B, Cyp C, Cyp D, CypNK and Cyp-40; (BRAM et al. 1993; KAY 1996), although the immunosuppressive actions are largely attributable to cyclophilins A and B. A second immunosuppressive drug, FK506, was introduced in the mid 1980s and has similar immunosuppressive actions to CsA, but at much lower doses (OCHIAI et al. 1987). FK506 has a completely different structure from CsA in that it is a member of a macrolide family of antibiotics. Subsequent studies showed that FK506 acts through a distinct receptor protein, termed FK506 binding protein (FKBP), and there are now known to be a number of such binding proteins (KAY 1996) including FKBP12, FKBP12A, FKBP13, and FKBP25, which has low affinity for FK506 but high affinity for rapamycin and FKBP52, which forms part of the glucocorticoid receptor complex. The immunosuppressant actions are largely mediated by FKBP12.

Both cyclophilins and immunophilins possess peptidyl prolyl isomerase (rotamase) activity which is thought to play a role in folding of proteins. CsA and FK506 inhibit the rotamase activity of cyclophilin A and FKBP12, respectively. Cyclophilin A catalyses the in vitro folding of a number of proteins including type I collagen (STEINMANN et al. 1991), transferrin (LODISH and KONG 1991) and carbonic anhydrase (FRESKGARD et al. 1992). Initially it was assumed that the immunosuppressive actions of FK506 and CsA were related to the inhibition of the rotamase activity, and thus inhibition of folding of a protein crucial for the functioning of the immune system. However, it became clear that concentrations required to inhibit T cell activation were tenfold lower than concentrations required to inhibit the rotamase activity. In addition, other FK506 derivatives such as 506BD and L-685,818 bind to FKBP12 and inhibit its rotamase activity but are not immunosuppressive (BIERER et al. 1990b; DUMONT et al. 1992).

Immunosuppressive effects of FK506 are mediated through binding to FKBP12 and the calcium and calmodulin-dependent protein phosphatase calcineurin. FK506 and CsA when bound to FKBP12 or cyclophilin A inhibit calcineurin activity. Immunosuppressive actions correlate with inhibition of calcineurin and FK506 derivatives such as L-685,818 and 506BD, which lack immunosuppressive activity, fail to inhibit calcineurin. In the immune system, treatment with FK506 prevents the de-phosphorylation and translocation of the transcription factor nuclear factor of activated T cells (NF-AT) to the nucleus, thereby preventing interleukin-2 gene expression and T cell activation. Other events downstream of calcineurin whose phosphorylation states are enhanced by FK506 or CsA include nitric oxide synthase (NOS) (DAWSON et al. 1993). FK506 prevents the calcineurin-mediated de-phosphorylation of NOS, thereby reducing the enzyme's catalytic activity and thus reducing the amount of NO formed. Another calcineurin target whose phosphorylation is enhanced by FK506 is growth associated protein-43 (GAP-43) or neuromodulin (LUI and STORM 1989), which is involved in neuronal process formation.

Rapamycin has a different mechanism of action. It binds to FKBP12, but rather than interacting with calcineurin it binds to a recently identified target RAFT (rapamycin and FKBP12 target) or FRAP (FKBP-rapamycin-associated protein) (SABATINI et al. 1994; BROWN et al. 1994), blocking the action of IL-2 rather than its expression (BIERER et al. 1990a) and inhibiting downstream targets such as p70s6, p34cdc2 and cdk2 kinases.

The early work in the immunophilin field was aimed at elucidating the function of these proteins in the immune system. However, it has recently become evident that immunophilins may play a role in the nervous system.

Patients treated with FK506 and CsA show neurological side effects including hand tremor, apraxia of speech, nightmares and acute psychosis (ATKINSON et al. 1984; WIJDICKS et al. 1994), all of which disappear on cessation of treatment. FKBP mRNA is expressed in a variety of tissues including the brain (MAKI et al. 1990) and [^{3}H]FK506 binding reveals 10 times higher levels of FKBPs in the brain than in the immune system (STEINER et al. 1992) and co-localisation with calcineurin. Substantial amounts of FKBPs are seen in the anterior olfactory nucleus and nearby cortex and high levels are seen in the caudate putamen, accumbens nucleus and the olfactory tubercle. High levels are also seen in CA1 of the hippocampus with lower levels in the CA3 region and in the molecular layer of the cerebellum (DAWSON et al. 1994). Cyclophilin A is also present in higher concentrations in the brain than any other tissue (RYFFEL et al. 1991). Highest levels of expression are seen in the granule cell layer of the cerebellum and the pyramidal and granule cell layer of the hippocampus. Other areas of high expression include the motor nuclei (oculomotor, facial and spinal cord) (GOLDNER and PATRICK 1996). Recently cyclophilins A, B and C have all been shown to have sequence homology to NUC18, a nuclease isolated from apoptotic thymocytes (MONTAGUE et al. 1997). In addition, denatured cyclophilins are capable of degrading DNA, suggesting a potential role in the apoptotic process. Other proposed roles for cyclophilins include acting as chaperones (FRESKGARD et al. 1992; BAKER et al. 1994), chemotactic agents (XU et al. 1992) and stress response proteins (SYKES et al. 1993; MARIVET et al. 1994). Cyclophilin A is required for insertion of a heterologously expressed neurotransmitter-gated ion channel into the membrane of Xenopus oocytes, suggesting a possible role in maturation of neuron specific membrane proteins (HELEKAR et al. 1994).

In vitro evidence for a possible neurological role for immunophilins comes from studies in PC12 cells and cultured embryonic dorsal root ganglion (DRG) neurons treated with immunophilin ligands. In PC12 cells a variety of immunophilin ligands, such as FK506, L-685,818, rapamycin and CsA all enhance the effects of low concentrations of NGF in promoting neurite outgrowth (LYONS et al. 1994; STEINER et al. 1997b). None of the compounds have any neurotrophic effect on PC12 cells in the absence of NGF. In chick DRG explants, neurotrophic effects are seen in the absence of added NGF and all of the above compounds are claimed to increase both the number of neurites emanating from the ganglia and the length of these neurites (STEINER et al. 1997b). In vivo, regeneration following a crush injury causes an up-regulation of FKBP-12 mRNA in the facial nucleus following facial nerve crush and in the lumbar motor neurons and DRG following a sciatic nerve crush (LYONS et al. 1995) in a time course that parallels GAP-43 mRNA expression. In addition, FK506 and L-685,818 enhance regeneration following sciatic nerve crush (GOLD et al. 1995; STEINER et al. 1997b).

FK506 and cyclosporin inhibit the neurotoxicity of N-methyl-D-aspartate (NMDA) in primary cortical neurons (DAWSON et al. 1993). As NMDA toxicity is mediated in part by NO, it is likely that the mechanism of neuroprotection, in this instance, is by phosphorylation of NOS, inhibiting the catalytic activity of the enzyme and therefore reducing the amount of NO generated. In vivo, FK506 has been demonstrated to be neuroprotective in a rat middle cerebral artery occlusion model of ischaemia (SHARKEY and BUTCHER 1994) whereas, CsA and rapamycin have no effect. The mechanism of action of FK506 in this model is not clear, but is unlikely to be due to inhibition of the peptidyl prolyl isomerase activity of FKBP12 in view of the lack of effect of CsA and rapamycin.

The neurotrophic and neuroprotective effects seen with immunophilin ligands both in vitro and in vivo have led to modifications of the FK506 molecule in an attempt to produce compounds that will have the neurotrophic effects but lack the undesirable immunosuppressive effects. FK506 possesses two binding domains. One part of the molecule binds at the prolyl isomerase site of FKBP12 while the remainder of the molecule forms part of the calcineurin binding (effector) domain of the FKBP12/FK506 complex. Compounds lacking this effector domain would possess the neurotrophic activity, bind to and inhibit FKBK12 but would not inhibit calcineurin or suppress T cell proliferation and would thus be devoid of the immunosuppressive actions.

In a recent paper, STEINER et al. (1997a) report a compound, GPI-1046, with these qualities (Fig. 3). GPI-1046, 3-(3-pyridyl)-1-propyl (2S)-1-(3,3-dimethyl-1,2-dioxopentyl)-2-pyrrolidinecarboxylate, is reported to be neurotrophic both in vitro and in several in vivo models of neuronal degeneration. GPI-1046 promotes neurite outgrowth from chick sensory ganglia explants. In the sciatic nerve crush model, GPI-1046 increased the diameter and cross-sectional area of regenerating fibres and also increased myelin levels distal to the crush site. GPI-1046 is also neuroprotective in a number of central degenerative models including the PCA (para-chloro-amphetamine) lesion, the MPTP (1-methyl-4-phenyl-1,2,3,6-tetrahydropyridine) mouse model of

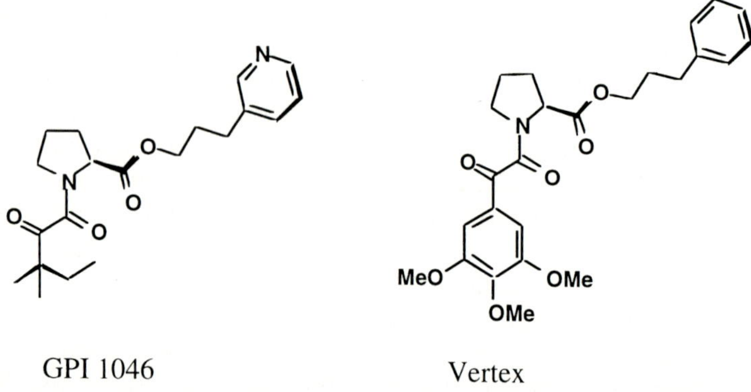

Fig. 3. FK-506 derivatives

Parkinson's disease and the 6-hydroxydopamine lesion in the rat. Our own studies with GPI-1046 in a sciatic nerve crush model have shown an increase in motor and sensory fibre regeneration, as shown with an electrophysiological measure of regeneration distance (manuscript in preparation). After 3 days treatment with GPI-1046, the increase in axon regeneration was equivalent to that seen previously with acidic fibroblast growth factor ($3\mu g$/kg per day; LAIRD et al. 1995). However, neurofilament staining of the nerve indicated there was no increase in the number of regenerating fibres at any point along the nerve and therefore the mechanism behind the increase in axon regeneration is not obvious.

The mechanism of action of GPI-1046 is not clear. Since it does not bind to calcineurin, it is unlikely to have effects due to phosphorylation of either GAP-43 or NOS. However, FKBP12 is directly associated with a number of receptors. FKBP12 associates with and is able to modulate the ryanodine receptor calcium release channel in skeletal muscle (JAYARAMAN et al. 1992) and the inositol 1,4,5 triphosphate receptor (CAMERON et al. 1995). In both cases FK506 displaces FKBP12 at the receptor and causes a change in the conductance of the channel. Given the importance of intracellular calcium levels for neuronal survival, changes in receptor conductance could plausibly affect neuronal survival in a variety of neurodegenerative models. Recently FKBP12 has been found to interact with the TGFβ family type I receptor (WANG et al. 1994). In the presence of ligand, the type II receptor phosphorylates the type I receptor leading to the release of FKBP12 from the type I receptor. Blocking the FKBP12/TGFβRI interaction with FK506 enhances ligand activity suggesting that the binding of FKBP12 to TGFbRI is inhibitory for signal transduction (WANG et al. 1996). In this way FKBP12 ligands could enhance TGFβ or other growth factor signal transduction. Further work is required in the area of immunophilin ligands in order to elucidate the mechanisms of 'neurotrophic' actions.

IV. Others

Besides the K-252a analogues and the immunophilin ligands several other chemicals have been reported to mimic actions of neurotrophins or to have direct neurotrophic activity (Fig. 4). Among them is SR 57746A, 1-[2(naphth-2-yl)ethyl]-4-(3-trifluoromethylphenyl)-1,2,5,6-tetrahydropyridine, which was identified as a neurotrophic agent in cell culture assays and later found to be a high affinity ligand for 5-HT_{1A} receptor (FOURNIER et al. 1992; PRADINES et al. 1995). Biochemical and behavioural effects in vivo were described which are compatible with the 5-HT receptor activity (BACHY et al. 1993). In neurodegeneration models, SR 57746A was found to attenuate ischaemia-induced cell loss as well as to promote regeneration of peripheral nerves following injury (FOURNIER et al. 1993). The mechanism underlying these claimed neuroprotective actions remains to be established. It is not clear whether any of the actions could reflect an indirect response following 5-HT receptor

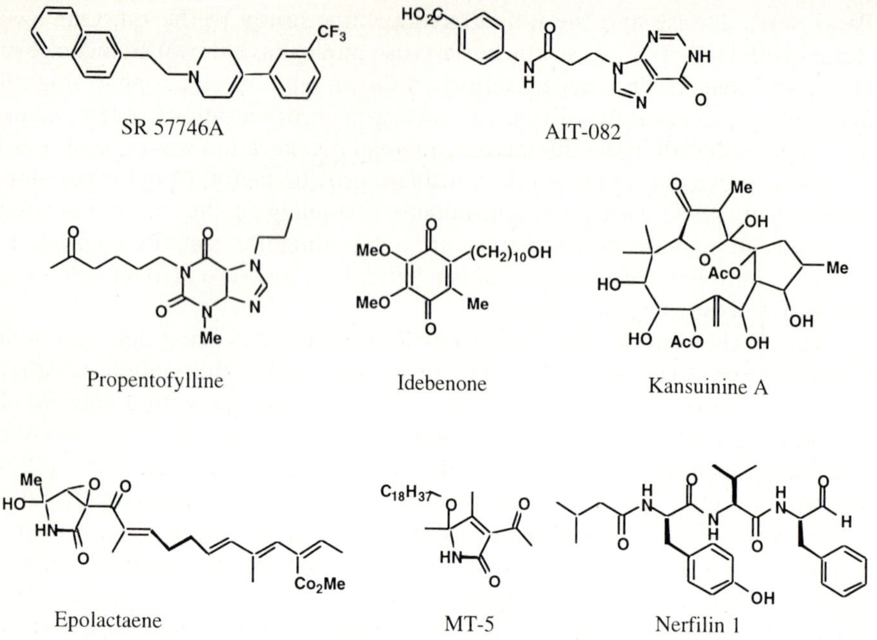

SR 57746A AIT-082

Propentofylline Idebenone Kansuinine A

Epolactaene MT-5 Nerfilin 1

Fig. 4. Compounds with reported neurotrophic properties

stimulation. Several analogues with neuroprotective properties have been identified (e.g. WO 97/01536).

AIT-082, a purine derivative, has been reported to enhance NGF-mediated neurite outgrowth from PC12 cells and to improve cognitive performance in rodents (MIDDLEMISS et al. 1995; GLASKY et al. 1994). While the compound appears to have attractive pharmacokinetic properties, the experimental evidence is rather weak in support of neurotrophic factor-enhancing properties. Direct neurotrophic actions were described for long-chain fatty acids which support survival of cultured neurons (BORG and TOAZARA 1987) and promote survival of septal cholinergic neurons after fimbria-fornix transections (BORG 1991). 1,1,3-Tricyano-2-amino-1-propene (triap) mimics the actions of NGF in cell culture assays and promotes the differentiation of NGF-sensitive cholinergic neurons in vivo after systemic administration (PAUL et al. 1990; PAUL and DAVANZO 1992). Other compounds with neurotrophic activities in cell culture assays were isolated from a variety of sources, including sesquiterpene-neoligans (FUKUYAMA et al. 1989, 1990; FUKUYAMA and ASAKAWA 1991; FUKUYAMA and OTOSHI 1992; DOI et al. 1993; KAWAGISHI and SHIMADA 1994) and diterpenoids such as kansuinin A (YAMAGUCHI et al. 1994). Epolactaene isolated from *Penicillium* sp. 1689-P and analogues of this compound induce neurite outgrowth in some human neuroblastoma cells (KAKEYA et al. 1997). Several other compounds, among them Nerfilin 1 (HIRAO et al. 1995), have been reported in the patent literature to have neurite growth-enhancing effects or to increase neurotrophic factor synthesis. The mechanisms of action of these compounds are presently not understood and the specificity of their actions for neurotrophic factors remains to be established. Nevertheless, they may serve as lead compounds for the development of potent and selective stimulators of neurotrophic factor synthesis.

C. Regulators of Neurotrophic Factor Synthesis or Release

As an alternative approach to regulating signal transduction steps of neurotrophic factors, it is feasible to influence neurotrophic actions by specifically manipulating any step in the synthesis, release and transduction mechanisms of endogenous neurotrophic factors. Ongoing characterisation of the regulatory sequences of neurotrophins (D'MELLO and HEINRICH 1991; PSHENICHKIN et al. 1994; SOHRABJI et al. 1995; HAYES et al. 1997) and other neurotrophic proteins may reveal possibilities for direct pharmacological manipulation of gene expression. Some of the hormonal effects discussed below may reflect direct influences on transcriptional control elements.

Neurotrophin gene expression appears to be regulated by specific neurotransmitter receptors, thus opening opportunities for pharmacological manipulation. While earlier findings suggested that neurotrophin synthesis is a direct reflection of the electrical activity of individual neurons (THOENEN 1995), more recent data suggest more complex, transmitter-specific regulatory processes. Neurotrophin mRNA expression in the brain is affected by an agonist of metabotropic glutamate receptors (MURRAY et al. 1996). Lesion studies and pharmacological experiments indicate that the expression of BDNF in the hippocampus is influenced by the septal cholinergic afferents acting through muscarinic receptors (LAPCHAK et al. 1993a). Yohimbine (STONE et al. 1994) was reported to affect neurotrophin expression. However, extensive studies on the noradrenergic input from the locus coeruleus failed to reveal any influence by these adrenergic afferents (REEBEN et al. 1996). A mixed 5-$HT_{2A/2C}$ receptor agonist was found to differentially regulate BDNF mRNA expression in various brain areas (VAIDYA et al. 1997). Interleukin-1β, given systemically is able to regulate neurotrophin expression in the brain (LAPCHAK et al. 1993b).

In recent years, it has become clear that neurotrophic factors have a more dynamic function than that predicted by the original concepts which saw them as nurturing proteins regulating cell survival. At least the neurotrophins are involved in the short-term regulation of synaptic plasticity as illustrated by the involvement of BDNF in long-term plasticity in the hippocampus (PATTERSON et al. 1996; KORTE et al. 1996). It appears that the release of neurotrophins can be regulated locally in short time intervals, perhaps comparable to that of neurotransmitters (Blochl and Thoenen 1996; Goodman et al. 1996). The regulatory mechanisms are poorly understood and some of the findings are controversial. A more fruitful area of pharmacological investigation would be opened if mechanisms regulating neurotrophin release turned out to be highly specific and different from those of other transmitters and secreted proteins. Recent discoveries indicate that these thoughts are not entirely speculative. The best example is provided by the discovery of molecules which selectively stimulate the release of growth hormone from pituitary cells. The discovery of these 'growth hormone secretagogues' is summarised at the end of this chapter since it serves as perhaps the best example of a successful effort to find a highly specific releasing agent for a protein growth factor.

I. Hormonal Regulation of Neurotrophin or Neurotrophin Receptor Expression

There is strong evidence that the synthesis of neurotrophic factors and their receptors can be regulated by non-protein hormones. Glucocorticoids prevent the elevation of NGF gene transcription following injury of peripheral nerves (Lindholm et al. 1990) but elevate NGF expression in the brain (Saporito and Brown 1994). Brain levels of NGF are affected by testosterone (Katoh-Semba et al. 1990). The expression of the CNTFR-α receptor protein is influenced by a member of the steroid receptor superfamily (Young et al. 1997). Influences of thyroid hormones on NGF mechanisms have been known for several years (Walker et al. 1979, 1981) and have been extended to the other members of the neurotrophin family (Calza et al. 1997).

Of particular interest are the interactions between oestrogen and neurotrophin mechanism in relationship to menopausal changes and Alzheimer's disease. The work by Torran-Allerand and collaborators revealed that oestrogen receptor mRNA is co-localised with that coding for neurotrophins and their Trk receptors (Toran-Allerand 1996). At least in tissues of the peripheral nervous system, oestrogen administration has been shown to up-regulate the expression of NGF receptor mRNA, suggesting the possibility that oestrogen regulates neurotrophin receptor expression in the brain (Miranda and Sohrabji 1994). There is tentative evidence that oestrogen therapy has a preventative and therapeutic effect on Alzheimer's disease (Paganinihill and Henderson 1996; Henderson 1997; Birge 1997). These findings prompt the speculation that oestrogen stimulates neurotrophin mechanisms in the brain and thus increases its morphological plasticity and ability to cope with degenerative events. More specifically, one can speculate that oestrogen stimulates the synthesis of NGF or NGF receptors in the cholinergic pathway of the basal forebrain, thus representing an indirect NGF therapy of the disease. Basal forebrain cholinergic neurons contain receptors for oestrogen (Toran-Allerand and Miranda 1992) and oestrogen regulates the expression of TrkA receptors and, indirectly, that of choline acetyltransferase (McMillan et al. 1996). While oestrogen has been reported to downregulate the expression of p75 NGFR in cholinergic cells (GIBBS and PFAFF 1992), this effect may be of little consequence since the neuroprotective actions of NGF on cholinergic neurons seem to be mediated by the TrkA receptors (LUCIDI-PHILLIPI et al. 1996). It has to be pointed out that, while attractive, these thoughts are highly speculative and that oestrogen's beneficial effects may be mediated by mechanisms different from those of the neurotrophins.

II. Compounds Regulating Neurotrophin Synthesis

Catechol derivatives, including 1,4-benzoquinone and 4-methylcatechol, stimulate synthesis and secretion of NGF from cultured astrocytes or fibroblast cell lines (FURUKAWA et al. 1989, 1993; TAKEUCHI et al. 1990; CARSWELL et al. 1992) (Fig. 5). Beneficial effects were reported for 4-methylcatechol in an experimental animal model of diabetic neuropathy (HANAOKA and OHI 1994). To improve brain penetration of effective catechols, a dihydropyridine-pyridinium moiety was integrated and this pro-drug was shown to convey delivery of active catechols into the brain (KOUROUNAKIS et al. 1996). The therapeutic usefulness of catechols and derivatives remains to be demonstrated. Effective concentrations are high and a variety of toxic effects have to be expected from these highly reactive chemicals.

Hericones, complex phenols isolated from mushrooms, stimulated NGF production by astrocytes (KAWAGISHI et al. 1991; KAWAGISHI and SHIMADA 1994). Similarly, pyrroloquinoline quinone and its derivatives were reported to stimulate NGF synthesis in a cell line as well as in the rat brain (YAMAGUCHI and SASANO 1993). Idebenone and propentofylline were reported to induce NGF synthesis in the rat brain and to improve behavioural performance of rats with cognitive impairment (NITTA and HASEGAWA 1993; YAMADA et al. 1997). Idebenone has been reported to produce mild beneficial effects in Alzheimer patients (BERGAMASCO et al. 1994; GILLIS et al. 1994). In preliminary reports, RS-66252 increased NGF synthesis and release in human glioblastoma cells and, in vivo, in the hippocampus of aged rats (EMMETT et al. 1996).

D. Examples of Growth Hormone Secretagogues

While not strictly a neurotrophic factor, growth hormone (GH) can serve as an example of a protein growth factor for which a small molecule mimetic was developed. In this case an indirect strategy was adopted, because as a 22 kDa peptide, GH itself is not a good template for the design of a small molecule mimetic. Moreover, although GH deficiency is treated by bolus injections of the recombinant protein, the resulting profiles of GH in the blood do not resemble those of a normal subject. A more natural approach for treating GH deficiency would be to use a drug that initiates and amplifies endogenous GH pulsatility. Ideally, such a drug should have the convenience of once daily oral

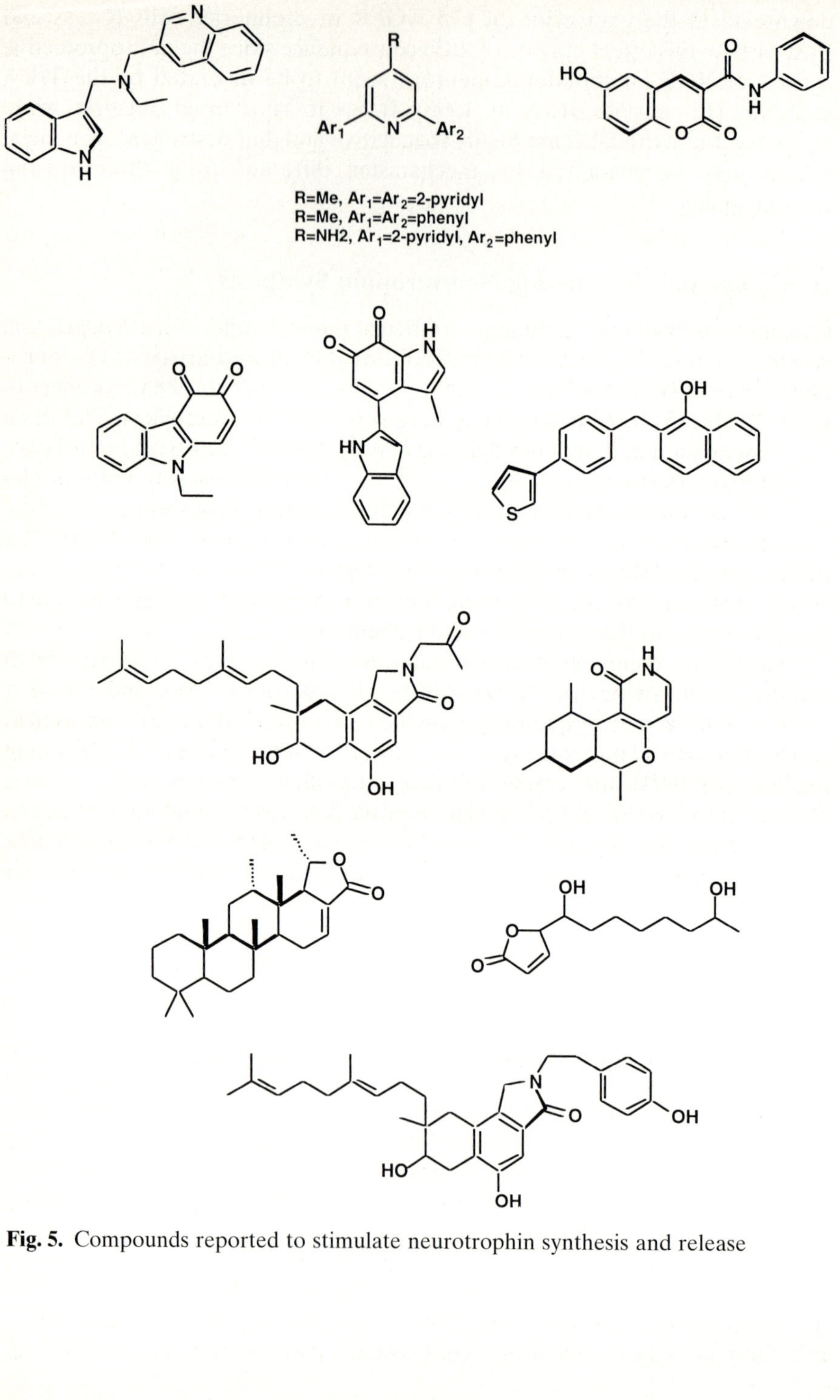

R=Me, Ar_1=Ar_2=2-pyridyl
R=Me, Ar_1=Ar_2=phenyl
R=NH2, Ar_1=2-pyridyl, Ar_2=phenyl

Fig. 5. Compounds reported to stimulate neurotrophin synthesis and release

administration. Identifying such a molecule required a heterodox approach since the specific drug target that controls pulsatility was unknown. By using functional assays, small molecules capable of selectively stimulating GH release in vitro were discovered. In vivo, these compounds were shown to stimulate and amplify GH pulsatility. Based on reverse pharmacology, a novel physiological pathway controlling pulsatile GH release was characterised and the receptor that regulated this pathway was cloned.

Identification of new GH secretagogues was aided by investigating the molecular mechanisms governing GH release at the level of the CNS and the anterior pituitary gland. Two hypothalamic hormones, growth hormone releasing hormone (GHRH) and somatostatin are known regulators of GH release from the pituitary gland. GHRH stimulates GH secretion, and somatostatin is involved in negative feedback (BERTHERAT et al. 1995; CONWAY et al. 1985; FROHMAN et al. 1992). His-DTrp-Ala-Trp-DPhe-LysNH2 (GHRP-6), and related synthetic peptides are also selective GH secretagogues (MOMANY et al. 1984; BOWERS et al. 1984; GUILLEMIN et al. 1982). For development of a drug that is suitable for once daily oral administration, a nonpeptide structure is preferred since it provides more flexibility than conventional peptides for optimising pharmacokinetic properties. GHRP-6, because of its small size, was an obvious template for the design of a nonpeptide mimetic. However, little was known about how GHRP-6 stimulated GH release. Therefore, before undertaking a discovery program based on GHRP-6, it was necessary to elucidate its mechanism of action. It was also important to determine whether GHRP-6 interacted with the pathways regulated by GHRH and somatostatin. GHRP-6 was shown to transduce its signal through phospholipase C (SMITH et al. 1996). GHRP-6 also amplified the stimulatory effects of GHRH on GH release and behaved as a functional antagonist of somatostatin (SMITH et al. 1996). Understanding how GHRP-6 functioned made it intuitively obvious that GHRP-6 had ideal properties for increasing the amplitude of GH pulsatility.

I. Discovery of L-692,429 and MK-0677

Incorporating random high volume screening to seek a GHRP-6 mimetic was impractical because the GHRP-6 receptor was unknown and the search for cell lines responsive to GHRP-6 proved fruitless. Therefore, potential lead candidates were rationally selected based on structural features of GHRP-6 and the suggestion that GHRP-6 activated a G-protein coupled receptor. The selected compounds were added to primary rat pituitary cell cultures to identify those that selectively caused GH release (SMITH et al. 1993). The signal transduction pathway through which each active compound stimulated GH release was elucidated. In vivo selectivity and efficacy were evaluated in rats and dogs.

Based on the structure of GHRP-6, approximately 120 compounds were selected and tested for their ability to stimulate GH release in vitro. A

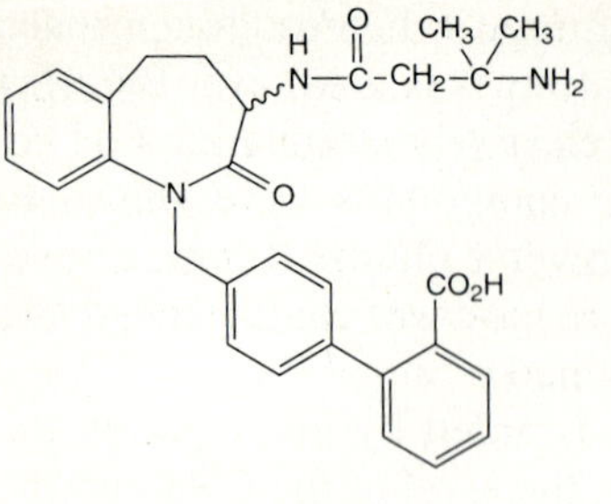

1

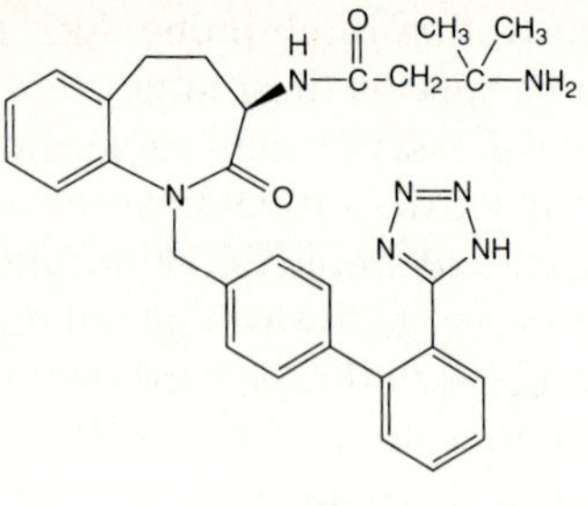

2

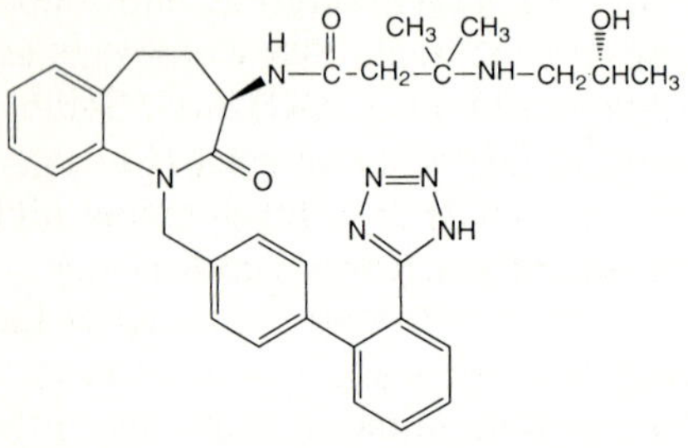

3

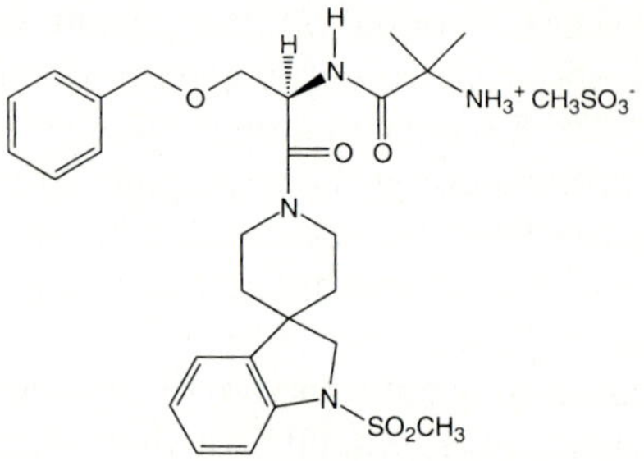

4 (MK-0677)

Fig. 6. Growth hormone secretagogues. 1, benzolactam; 2, L-692,429; 3, L-692,585, a 2-(*R*)-hydroxypropyl analog; 4, MK-0677

benzolactam (Fig. 6, compound 1) was identified having an EC_{50} of 3000 nM for GH release in the rat pituitary cell assay. Replacement of the carboxylic acid moiety with a tetrazole and resolution of the enantiomers furnished L-692,429 (Fig. 6, compound 2) with an EC_{50} of 60 nM (SMITH et al. 1993; SCHOEN et al. 1994a; SCHOEN et al. 1993; CHENG et al. 1993). L-692,429 was the first example of a potent nonpeptide GH secretagogue. L-692,428 the *S* enantiomer of L-692,429 was inactive, demonstrating the stereoselectivity of the stimulatory effect on GH secretion. The activity of L-692,429 was blocked by both peptide and nonpeptide antagonists of GHRP-6, but not by an antagonist of GHRH, consistent with the notion that L-692,429 was a peptidomimetic of GHRP-6 (SMITH et al. 1993). Attempts to improve the efficacy of L-692,429 by systematic investigation of the dimethyl-b-alanine side chain led to the identification of L-692,585, a 2-(*R*)-hydroxypropyl analog (Fig. 6, compound 3), which was more potent than L-692,429 in vitro and in vivo (SCHOEN et al. 1994b; OK et al. 1994). However, despite much improved potency and highly reproducible oral activity, the oral bioavailability of L-692,585 was considered too low (ca. 4%) for clinical development.

Another structural class of GH secretagogues was discovered by screening derivatized "privileged structures". The terminology "privileged structures" refers to structural units that are commonly found in receptor ligands. Derivatization of these structures is a useful way to prepare receptor agonists and antagonists (EVANS et al. 1988). A spiroindanylpiperidine core was selected for elaborating ligands that would stimulate GH release and have favourable pharmacokinetics. This approach provided MK-0677 (Fig. 6, compound 4), a highly orally bioavailable (ca. 60%), potent and specific GH secretagogue. MK-0677 subsequently entered clinical studies.

II. The MK-0677 Receptor

The highly specific effects of MK-0677 on GH secretion indicated that this molecule binds to a selective receptor. Radiolabelled MK-0677 was synthesised to identify the corresponding binding site, which was found to exist in porcine and rat pituitary and hypothalamic membranes. An expression cloning strategy was then developed for the MK-0677 receptor based on the knowledge that this receptor transduced its signal through phospholipase C (SMITH et al. 1996). The receptor was cloned from a pig pituitary cDNA library by expression in *Xenopus* oocytes (HOWARD et al. 1996). The nucleotide sequence of the MK-0677 receptor cDNA clone predicted a protein of 366-amino acids with 7 transmembrane (7-TM) spanning domains, 3 intra- and extra-cellular loops and a G-protein coupled receptor triplet signature sequence (HOWARD et al. 1996). Because the GHRP-6 class of GH secretagogues also bind and activate the MK-0677 receptor, the receptor was designated the growth hormone secretagogue receptor (GHS-R). In situ hybridisation studies were used to localise expression of the receptor in the pituitary gland and brain. Expression was detected in the anterior but not the posterior lobe of the pituitary. GHS-R expression was seen in the arcuate nucleus, consistent with the electrical excitation and c-*fos* induction in arcuate neurons that occurs following injection of MK-0677 into rats and mice. Expression was also detected in other brain areas, suggesting involvement of the GHS-R in functions other than the regulation of GH secretion (GUAN et al. 1997).

III. Clinical Use

In humans, MK-0677 increases the amplitude of GH pulses following single daily oral dosing (PATCHETT et al. 1995; LEUNG et al. 1996). MK-0677 was generally well tolerated and once daily oral administration was sufficient to increase serum concentrations of both GH and IGF-1. In elderly subjects treated with MK-0677, GH and IGF-1 levels similar to those of healthy young adults were attained (CHAPMAN et al. 1996).

In summary, based on a rational approach, a class of orally active small molecules was identified as mimetics of the synthetic peptide GH secretagogue, GHRP-6. Importantly, MK-0677 is the first GH secretagogue to provide a sustained increase in pulsatile GH release and an increase in IGF-1 levels following a single oral dose (JACKS et al. 1996; SMITH et al. 1996; HICKEY et al. 1997). The identification of small synthetic molecules capable of amplifying episodic GH release led to the characterisation of a new physiologically relevant regulatory pathway. The receptor regulating this pathway was cloned and shown to be distinct from known families of G-protein coupled receptors (Howard et al. 1996). The remarkable conservation of the GHS-R across species attests to the importance of this receptor and suggests that its unknown natural ligand plays an important physiological role in the control of pulsatile GH release.

E. Conclusions

Small molecule mimetics are likely able to solve the problems which hamper the clinical use of protein growth factors. The discovery and clinical development of the growth hormone secretagogue best illustrates this point. While many molecules have neurotrophic factor mimetic properties, their precise mechanisms of action remain to be established and considerable work will be necessary to bring them to a clinically useful stage. Direct stimulants of tyrosine kinase receptors are yet to be discovered, which are desired to mimic neurotrophin actions on Trk receptors.

References

Atkinson K, Biggs J, Darveniza P, Concannon A, Dodds A (1984) Cyclosporine associated central nervous system toxicity after allogenic bone marrow transplants. N Engl J Med 310:527

Bachy A, Steinberg R, Santucci V, Fournier M, Landi M, Hamon M, Manara L, Keane PE, Soubrie P, Le Fur G (1993) Biochemical and electrophysiological properties of SR 57746A, a new potent 5-HT1A receptor agonist. Fundam Clin Pharmacol 7(9):487–497

Baker EK, Colley NJ, Zuker CS (1994) The cyclophilin homologue ninaA functions as a chaperone forming a stable complex in vivo with its protein target rhodopsin. EMBO J 13:4886–4895

Barbacid M (1995) Neurotrophic factors and their receptors. Curr Opin Cell Biol 7(2):148–155

Berg MM, Sternberg DW, Parada LF, Chao MV (1992) K-252a inhibits nerve growth factor-induced Trk proto-oncogene tyrosine phosphorylation and kinase activity. J Biol Chem 267:13–16

Bergamasco B, Scarzella L, La Commare P (1994) Idebenone, a new drug in the treatment of cognitive impairment in patients with dementia of the Alzheimer type. Funct Neurol 9:161–168

Bertherat J, Bluet-Pajot MT, Epelbaum J (1995) Neuroendocrine regulation of growth hormone. Eur J Endocrinol 132:12–24

Bierer BE, Mattila PS, Standaert RF, Herzenberg L Al, Burakoff SJ, Crabtree G, Schreiber SL (1990a) Two distinct signal transmission pathways in T-lymphocytes are inhibited by complexes formed between an immunophilin and either FK506 or rapamycin. Proc Natl Acad Sci USA 87:9231–9235

Bierer BE, Somers PK, Wandless TJ, Burakoff SJ, Schreiber SL (1990b) Probing immunosuppressive action with a nonnatural immunophilin ligand. Science 250:556–559

Birge SJ (1997) The role of estrogen in the treatment of Alzheimer's Disease. Neurology 48(5):S36–S41

Blochl A, Thoenen H (1996) Localization of cellular storage compartments and sites of constitutive and activity-dependent release of nerve growth factor (NGF) in primary cultures of hippocampal neurons. Mol Cell Neurosci 7(3):173–190

Borasio GD (1990) Differential effects of the protein kinase inhibitor K-252a on the in vitro survival of chick embryonic neurons. Neurosci Lett 108:207–212

Borg J (1991) The neurotrophic factor, n-hexacosanol, reduces the neuronal damage induced by the neurotoxin, kainic acid. J Neurosci Res 29:62–67

Borg J, Toazara J (1987) Neurotrophic effect of naturally occurring long-chain fatty alcohols on cultured CNS neurons. FEBS Lett 213:406–410

Bowers CY, Momany FA, Reynolds GA, Hong A (1984) On the in vitro and in vivo activity of a new synthetic hexapeptide that acts on the pituitary to specifically release growth hormone. Endocrinology 114:1537–1545

Bram RJ, Hung DT, Martin PK, Shreiber SL, Crabtree GR (1993) Identification of the immunophilins capable of mediating inhibition of signal transduction by cyclosporin A and FK506: roles of calcineurin binding and cellular location. Mol Cell Biol 13:4760–4769

Bredesen DE, Rabizadeh S (1997) P75 (NTR) and apoptosis – Trk-dependent and Trk-independent effects. Trends Neurosci 20(7):287–290

Brown EJ, Albers MW, Shin TB, Ichikawa K, Keith CT, Lane WS, Schreiber SL (1994) A mammalian protein targeted by G1 arresting rapamycin-receptor complex. Nature 369:756–758

Calza L, Giardino L, Aloe L (1997) Thyroid hormone regulates NGF content and P75 (LNGFR) expression in the basal forebrain of adult rats. Exp Neurol 143(2):196–206

Cameron AM, Steiner JP, Roskams AJ, Ali SM, Ronnett GV, Snider SH (1995) Calcineurin associated with the inositol 1,4,5 triphosphate receptor-FKBP12 complex modulates Ca^{2+} flux. Cell 83:463–472

Carswell S, Hoffman EK, Clopton Hartpence K, Wilcox HM, Lewis ME (1992) Induction of NGF by isoproterenol, 4-methylcatechol and serum occurs by three distinct mechanisms. Brain Res Mol Brain Res 15:145–150

Carter BD, Lewin GR (1997) Neurotrophins live or let die – does P75 (NTR) decide? Neuron 18(2):187–190

Chapman IM, Bach MA, Van Cauter E, Farmer M, Krupa DA, Taylor AM, Schilling LM, Cole KY, Skiles EH, Pezzoli SS, Hartman ML, Veldhuis JD, Gormley GJ, Thorner MO (1996) Stimulation of the growth hormone (GH)-insulin-like growth factor-I axis by daily oral administration of a GH secretagogue (MK-0677) in healthy elderly subjects. J Clin Endocrinol Metab 81:4249–4257

Cheng K, Chan WW-S, Butler BS, Wei L, Schoen WR, Wyvratt MJ Jr, Fisher MH, Smith RG (1993) Stimulation of growth hormone release from rat pituitary cells by L-692,429, a novel non-peptidyl GH secretagogue. Endocrinology 260:1640–1643

Conway S, McCann SM, Krulich L (1985) On the mechanism of growth hormone autofeedback regulation: possible role of somatostatin and growth hormone-releasing factor. Endocrinology 117:2284–2292

Cwirla SE, Balasubramanian P, Duffin DJ, Wagstrom CR, Gates CM, Singer SC, Davis AM, Tansik RL, Mattheakis LC, Boytos CM, Schatz PJ, Baccanari DP, Wrighton NC, Barrett RW, Dower WJ (1997) Peptide agonist of the thrombopoietin receptor as potent as the natural cytokine. Science 276(5319):1696–1699

Dawson TM, Steiner JP, Dawson VL, Dinerman JL, Uhl GR, Snider SH (1993) Immunosuppressant FK506 enhances phosphorylation of nitric oxide synthase and protects against glutamate neurotoxicity. Proc Natl Acad Sci USA 90:9808–9812

Dawson TM, Steiner JP, Lyons WE, Fotuhi M, Blue M, Snider SH (1994) The immunophilins, FK506 and cyclophilin are discretely localized in the brain: relationship to calcineurin. Neuroscience 62:569–580

D'Mello SR, Heinrich G (1991) Structural and functional identification of regulatory regions and cis elements surrounding the nerve growth factor gene promotor. Brain Res Mol Brain Res 11:255–264

Doi Y, Shigemori H, Ishibashi M, Mizobe F, Kawashima A, Nakaike S, Kobayashi J (1993) New sesterterpenes with nerve growth factor synthesis-stimulating activity from the Okinawan marine sponge Hyritos sp. Chem Pharm Bull 41(12):2190–2191

Dumont FJ, Staruch MJ, Koprak SL, Siekierka JJ, Lin CS, Harrison R, Sewell T, Kindt VM, Beattie TR, Wyvratt M, Sigal NH (1992) The immunosuppressive and toxic effects of FK506 are mechanistically related: pharmacology of a novel antagonist of FK506 and rapamycin. J Exp Med 176:751–760

Emmett CJ, Haraguchi M, Baecker PA, Chang T, Eglen RM, Johnson RM (1996) Characterization of nerve growth factor release by RS-66252. Proc Soc Neurosci 22:2124

Eppstein DA, Marsh YV, Schryver BB, Bertics PJ (1989) Inhibition of epidermal growth factor/transforming growth factor-alpha-stimulated cell growth by a synthetic peptide. J Cell Physiol 141:420–430

Evans BE, Rittle KE, Bock MG, DiPardo RM, Freidinger RM, Whitter WL, Lundell GF, Veber DF, Anderson PS, Chang RSL, Lotti VJ, Cerino DJ, Chen TB, Kling PJ, Kunkel KA, Springer JP, Hirshfield J (1988) Methods for drug discovery: development of potent, selective orally effective cholecystokinin antagonists. J Med Chem 31:2235–2246

Fournier J, Gauthier T, Keane PE, Coudé FK, Guzzi U, Soubrié P, Le Fur G (1992) Neurotrophic effects of SR 57746A, a new non-peptide compound in in vitro studies. Br J Pharmacol 106:120

Fournier J, Steinberg R, Gauthier T, Keane PE, Guzzi U, Coude FX, Bougault I, Maffrand JP, Soubrie P, Le Fur G (1993) Protective effects of SR 57746A in central and peripheral models of neurodegenerative disorders in rodents and primates. Neuroscience 55(3):629–641

Freskgard PO, Bergenhem N, Jonsson BH, Svensson M, Carlsson U (1992) Isomerase and chaperone activity of prolyl isomerase in the folding of carbonic anhydrase. Science 258:466–468

Frohman LA, Downs TR, Chomczynski P (1992) Regulation of growth-hormone secretion. Front Neuroendocrinol 13:344–405

Fukuyama Y, Asakawa Y (1991) Neurotrophic secoaromadendrane-type sesquiterpenes from the liverwort *plagiochila fruticosa*. Phytochemistry 30(12): 4061–4065

Fukuyama Y, Otoshi Y (1992) Neurotrophic sesquiterpene-neolignans from Magnolia obovata: structure and neurotrophic activity. Tetrahedron 48:377–392

Fukuyama Y, Otoshi Y, Kodama M (1989) Novel neurotrophic sesquiterpene-neolignans from *magnolia obovata*. Tetrahedron Lett 30(43):5907–5910

Fukuyama Y, Otoshi Y, Kodama M (1990) Structure of clovanemagnolol, a novel neurotrophic sesquiterpene-neolignan from *magnolia obovata*. Tetrahedron Lett 31(31):4477–4480

Furukawa Y, Tomioka N, Sato W, Satoyoshi E, Hayashi K, Furukawa S (1989) Catecholamines increase nerve growth factor mRNA content in both mouse astroglial cells and fibroblast cells. FEBS Lett 247(2):463–467

Furukawa Y, Furukawa S, Omae F, Awatsuji H, Hayashi K (1993) Alkylcatechols regulate NGF gene expression in astroglial cells via both protein kinase C- and cAMP-independent mechanisms. J Neurosci Res 35:522–529

Gibbs RB, Pfaff DW (1992) Effects of estrogen and fimbria/fornix transection on p75NGFR and ChAT expression in the medial septum and diagonal band of Broca. Exp Neurol 116:23–39

Gillis JC, Benefield P, McTavish D (1994) Idebenone: a review of its pharmacodynamic and pharmacokinetic properties, and therapeutic use in age-related cognitive disorders. Drugs Aging 5:133–152

Glasky AJ, Melchior CL, Pirzadeh B, Heydari N, Ritzmann RF (1994) Effect of AIT-082, a purine analog, on working memory in normal and aged mice. Pharmacol Biochem Behav 47(2):325–329

Glicksman MA, Prantner JE, Meyer SL, Forbes ME, Dasgupta M, Lewis ME, Neff NT (1993) K-252a and staurosporine promote choline acetyltransferase activity in rat spinal cord cultures. J Neurochem 61:210–221

Glicksman MA, Forbes ME, Prantner JE, Neff NT (1995) K-252a promotes survival and choline acetyltransferase activity in striatal and basal forebrain neuronal cultures. J Neurochem 64:1502–1512

Gold BG, Katoh K, Storm-Dickerson T (1995) The immunosuppressant FK506 increases the rate of axonal regeneration in rat sciatic nerve. J Neurosci 15:7509–7516

Goldner FM, Patrick JW (1996) Neuronal localization of the cyclophilin A protein in the adult rat brain. J Comp Neurol 372:283–293

Goodman LJ, Valverde J, Lim F, Geschwind MD, Federoff HJ, Geller AI, Hefti F (1996) Regulated release and polarized localization of brain-derived neurotrophic factor in hippocampal neurons. Mol Cell Neurosci 7:222–238

Greene LA, Kaplan DR (1995) Early events in neurotrophin signalling via Trk and p75 receptors. Curr Opin Neurobiol 5:579–587

Guan X-M, Yu H, Palyha OC, McKee KK, Feighner SD, Sirinathsinghji DJS, Smith RG, Van der Ploeg LHT, Howard AD (1997) Distribution of mRNA encoding the growth hormone secretagogue receptor in brain and peripheral tissues. Brain Res Mol Brain Res 48:23–29

Guillemin R, Brazeau P, Bohlen P, Esch F, Ling N, Wehrenberg WB (1982) Growth hormone-releasing factor from a human pancreatic tumor that caused acromegaly. Science 218:585–587

Hanaoka Y, Ohi T (1994) The therapeutic effects of 4-methylcatechol, a stimulator of endogenous nerve growth factor synthesis, on experimental diabetic neuropathy in rats. J Neurol Sci 122:28–32

Handschumacher RE, Harding MW, Rice J, Drugge RJ, Speicer DW (1984) Cyclophilin: a specific cytosolic binding protein for cyclosporin A. Science 226:544–547

Hayes VY, Towner MD, Isackson PJ (1997) Organization, sequence and functional analysis of a mouse BDNF promoter. Brain Res Mol Brain Res 45(2):189–198

Helekar SA, Char D, Neff S, Patrick J (1994) Prolyl isomerase requirement for the expression of functional homo-oligomeric ligand gated ion channels. Neuron 12:179–189

Henderson VW (1997) The epidemiology of estrogen replacement therapy and Alzheimer's disease. Neurology 48(7):S27–S35

Hickey GJ, Jacks TM, Schleim K, Frazier E, Chen HY, Krupa DA, Feeney WP, Nargund RP, Patchett AA, Smith RG (1997) Repeat administration of the growth hormone secretagogue MK-0677 increases and maintains elevated IGF-1 levels in beagles. J Endocrinol 152:183–192

Hirao T (1995) Nerfilin I, a novel microbial metabolite inducing neurite outgrowth of PC12 cells. J Antibiot 48(12):1494–1496

Holden PH, Asopa V, Robertson AGS, Clarke AR, Tyler S, Bennett GS, Brain SD, Wilcock GK, Allen SJ, Smith SKF, Dawbarn D (1997) Immunoglobulin-like domains define the nerve growth factor binding site of the TrkA receptor. Nat Biotechnol 15(7):668

Howard AD, Feighner SD, Cully DF, Arena JP, Liberator PA, Rosenblum CI, Hamelin M, Hreniuk DL, Palyha OC, Anderson J, Paress PS, Diaz C, Chou M, Liu KK, McKee KK, Pong S-S, Chaung L-YP, Elbrecht A, Dashkevicz M, Heavens R, Rigby M, Sirinathsinghji DJS, Dean DC, Melillo DG, Patchett AA, Nargund RP, Griffin PR, DeMartino JA, Gupta SK, Schaeffer JM, Smith RG, Van der Ploeg LHT (1996) A receptor in pituitary and hypothalamus that functions in growth hormone release. Science 273:974–977

Ibanez CF (1994) Structure-function relationships in the neurotrophin family. J Neurobiol 25(11):1349–1361

Isono F, Widmer HR, Hefti F, Knüsel B (1994) EGF induces PC12 cell differentiation in presence of the protein kinase inhibitor K-252a. J Neurochem 63:1235–1245

Jacks TM, Smith RG, Judith F, Schleim K, Frazier E, Chen HY, Krupa DA, Hora DH Jr, Nargund RP, Patchett AA, Hickey GJ (1996) MK-0677, a potent, novel orally-active growth hormone (GH) secretagogue: GH, IGF-1 and other hormonal responses in beagles. Endocrinology 137:5284–5289

Jayaraman T, Brillantes AM, Timerman AP, Fleischer S, Erdjument-Bromage H, Tempst P, Marks AR (1992) FK506 binding protein associated with the calcium release channel (ryanodine receptor). J Biol Chem, 267:9474–9477

Kakeya H, Onozawa C, Sato M, Arai K, Osada H (1997) Neuritogenic effect of epolactaene derivatives on human neuroblastoma cells which lack high-affinity nerve growth factor receptors. J Med Chem 40(4):391–394

Kaneko M, Saito Y, Saito H, Matsumoto T, Matsuda Y, Vaught JL, Dionne CA, Angeles TS, Glicksman MA, Neff NT, Rotella DP, Kauer JC, Mallamo JP, Hudkins RL, Murakata C (1997) Neurotrophic 3,9-BIS[(alkylthio)methyl]- and BIS(alkoxymethyl)-K-252a derivatives. JMed Chem 40(2):1863–1869

Katoh-Semba R, Semba R, Kashiwamata S, Kato K (1990) Influences of neonatal and adult exposures to testosterone on the levels of the beta-subunit of nerve growth factor in the neural tissues of mice. Brain Res 522:112–117

Kawagishi H, Shimada A (1994) Erinacines A, B and C, strong stimulators of nerve growth factor (NGF) synthesis, from the mycelia of Hericium erinaceum. Tetrahedron Lett 35(10):1569–1572

Kawagishi H, Ando M, Sakamato H, Yoshida S, Ojima F, Ishiguro Y, Ukai N, Furokawa S (1991) Hericenones C, D and E, stimulators of nerve-growth factor (NGF) synthesis, from the mushroom Hericium erinaceum. Tetrahedron 32:4561–4564

Kay JE (1996) Structure-function relationships in the FK506-binding protein family of peptidylprolyl cis-trans isomerases. Biochem J 314:361–385

Knüsel B, Hefti FF (1992) K-252 compounds: modulators of neurotrophin signal transduction. J Neurochem 59:1987–1996

Knüsel B, Kaplan DR, Winslow JW, Rosenthal A, Burton LE, Beck KD, Rabin S, Nikolics K, Hefti FF (1992) K-252b selectively potentiates cellular actions and Trk tyrosine phosphorylation mediated by neurotrophin-3. J Neurochem 59:715–722

Koizumi S, Contreras ML, Matsuda Y, Hama T, Lazarovici P, Guroff G (1988) K-252a: a specific inhibitor of the action of nerve growth factor on PC12 cells. J Neurosci 8:715–721

Konishi Y, Kotts CE, Bullock LD, Tou JS, Johnson DA (1989) Fragments of bovine insulin-like growth factors I and II stimulate proliferation of rat L6 myoblast cells. Biochemistry 28:8872–8877

Korte M, Staiger V, Griesbeck O, Thoenen H, Bonhoeffer T (1996) The involvement of brain-derived neurotrophic factor in hippocampal long-term potentiation revealed by gene targeting experiments. J Physiol Paris 90(3–4):157–164

Kourounakis A, Bodor N, Simpkins J (1996) Synthesis and evaluation of a brain-targeted catechol derivative as a potential NGF-inducer. International Journal of Pharmaceutics 141(1–2):239–250

Laird JMA, Mason GS, Thomas KA, Hargreaves RJ, Hill RG (1995) Acidic fibroblast growth factor stimulates motor and sensory axon regeneration after sciatic nerve crush in the rat. Neuroscience 65(1):209–216

Lapchak PA, Araujo DM, Hefti F (1993a) Cholinergic regulation of hippocampal brain-derived neurotrophic factor mRNA expression: Evidence from lesion and chronic cholinergic drug treatment studies. Neuroscience 5:575–585

Lapchak PA, Araujo DM, Hefti F (1993b) Systemic interleukin-1 beta decreases brain-derived neurotrophic factor messenger RNA expression in the rat hippocampal formation. Neuroscience 53(2):297–301

Leung KH, Miller RR, Cohn DA, Colletti A, McGowan E, Feeney WP, Nargund RP, Rosegay A, Wallace A (1996) Pharmacokinetics and disposition of MK-0677, a novel growth hormone secretagogue. Proceedings of the International Society for the Study of Xenobiotics 7th International Meeting, San Diego, CA, October 20–24,10:277 (Abstract)

Lindholm D, Hengerer B, Heumann R, Carroll P, Thoenen H (1990) Glucocorticoid hormones negatively regulate nerve growth factor expression in vivo and in cultured rat fibroblasts. Eur J Neurosci 2:795–801

Lodish HF, Kong N (1991) Cyclosporin A inhibits an initial step in the folding of transferrin within the endoplasmic reticulum. J Biol Chem, 266:14835–14838

Longmore J, Razzaque Z, Shaw D, Hill RG (1994) Differences in the effects of NK1 receptor antagonists (+/-)-CP96,345 and CP99,994 on agonist-induced responses in guinea-pig trachea. Br J Pharmacol 112(1):176–178

Longo FM, Manthorpe M, Xie YM, Varon S (1997) Synthetic NGF peptide derivatives prevent neuronal death via a P75 receptor-dependent mechanism. Jl Neurosci Res 48(1):1–17

Lucidi-Phillipi CA, Clary DO, Reichardt LF, Gage FH (1996) TrkA activation is sufficient to rescue axotomized cholinergic neurons. Neuron 16(3):653–663

Lui Y, Storm DR (1989) Dephosphorylation of neuromodulin by calcineurin. J Biol Chem, 264:12800–12804

Lyons WE, George EB, Dawson TM, Steiner JP, Snider SH (1994) Immunosuppressant FK506 promotes neurite outgrowth in cultures of PC12 cells and sensory ganglia. Proc Natl Acad Sci USA 91:3191–3195

Lyons WE, Steiner JP, Snider SH, Dawson TM (1995) Neuronal regeneration enhances the expression of the immunophilin FKBP-12. J Neurosci 15:2985

Maki N, Sekiguchi F, Nishimaki J, Miwa K, Hayano T, Takashi N, Suzuki M (1990) Complementary DNA encoding the human T cell FK506-binding protein, a peptidylprolyl cis-trans isomerase distinct from cyclophilin. Proc Natl Acad Sci USA 87:5440–5443

Marivet J, Margis-Pinheiro M, Frendo P, Burkard G (1994) Bean cyclophilin gene expression during plant development and stress conditions. Plant Mol Biol 26:1181–1189

Maroney AC, Lipfert L, Forbes ME, Glicksman MA, Neff NT, Siman R, Dionne CA (1995) K-252a induces tyrosine phosphorylation of the focal adhesion kinase and neurite outgrowth in human neuroblastoma SH-SY5Y cells. J Neurochem 64:540–549

Maroney AC, Sanders C, Neff NT, Dionne CA (1997) K-252b potentiation of neurotrophin-3 is TrkA specific in cells lacking P75 (NTR). J Neurochem 68(1):88–94

Matsuda Y, Fukuda J (1988) Inhibition by K-252a, a new inhibitor of protein kinase, of nerve growth factor-induced neurite outgrowth of chick embryo dorsal root ganglion cells. Neurosci Lett 87:295–301

McMillan PJ, Singer CA, Dorsa DM (1996) The effects of ovariectomy and estrogen replacement on TrkA and choline acetyltransferase mRNA expression in the basal forebrain of the adult female Sprague-Dawley rat. J Neuroscie 16(5):1860

Middlemiss PJ, Glasky AJ, Rathbone MP, Werstuik E, Hindley S, Gysbers J (1995) AIT-082, a unique purine derivative, enhances nerve growth factor mediated neurite outgrowth from PC12 cells. Neurosci Lett 199(2):131–134

Miranda RC, Sohrabji F (1994) Interactions of estrogen with the neurotrophins and their receptors during neural development. Horm Behav 28:367–375

Momany FA, Bowers CY, Reynolds GA, Hong A, Newlander K (1984) Conformational energy studies and in vitro and in vivo activity data on growth hormone-releasing peptides. Endocrinology 114:1531–1536

Montague JW, Hughes Jnr FM, Cidlowski JA (1997) Native recombinant cyclophilins A, B and C degrade DNA independently of peptidyl cis trans isomerase activity. J Biol Chem, 272:6677–6684

Murray KD, Wood PL, Rosasco C, Isackson PJ (1996) A metabotropic glutamate receptor agonist regulates neurotrophin messenger RNA in rat forebrain. Neuroscience 70(3):617–630

Ninkina N, Grashchuck M, Buchman VL, Davies AM (1997) TrkB variants with deletions in the leucine-rich motifs of the extracellular domain. J Biol Chem 272(20):13019–13025

Nitta A, Hasegawa T (1993) Oral administration of idebenone, a stimulator of NGF synthesis, recovers reduced NGF content in aged rat brain. Neurosci Lett 163:219–222

Nye SH, Squinto SP, Glass DJ, Stitt TN, Hantzopoulos P, Macchi MJ, Lindsay NS, Ip NY, Yancopoulos GD (1992) K-252a and staurosporine selectively block autophosphorylation of neurotrophin receptors and neurotrophin-mediated responses. Mol Biol Cell 3:677–686

Ochiai T, Nakajima K, Nagat M (1987) Effect of a new immunosuppressive agent, FK506, on heterotopic cardiac allotransplantation in the rat. Transplant Proc 19:1284–1286

Ohmichi M, Decker SJ (1992) Inhibition of the cellular actions of nerve growth factor by staurosporine and K-252a results from the attenuation of the activity of the Trk tyrosine kinase. Biochemistry 31:4034–4039

Ok D, Schoen WR, Hodges P, DeVita RJ, Brown JE, Chang K, Chan WW-S, Butler BS, Smith RG, Fisher MH, Wyvratt MJ Jr (1994) Structure activity relationships of the non-peptidyl growth hormone secretagogue L-692,429. Bioorg Med Chem Lett 4:2709–2714

Paganini-Hill A, Henderson VW (1996) Estrogen replacement therapy and risk of Alzheimer disease. Arch Intern Med 156(19):2213–2217

Patchett AA, Nargund RP, Tata JR, Chen M-H, Barakat KJ, Johnston DBR, Cheng K, Chan WW-S, Butler BS, Hickey GJ, Jacks TM, Scleim K, Pong S-S, Chaung L-YP, Chen HY, Frazier E, Leung KH, Chui S-HL, Smith RG (1995) The design and biological activities of L-163,191 (MK-0677): a potent orally active growth hormone secretagogue. Proc Natl Acad Sci USA 92:7001–7005

Patterson SL, Abel T, Deuel TAS, Martin KC, Rose JC, Kandel ER (1996) Recombinant BDNF rescues deficits in basal synaptic transmission and hippocampal LTP in BDNF knockout mice. Neuron 16:1137–1145

Paul JW, DaVanzo JP (1992) 1,1,3 Tricyano-2-amino-1-propene (Triap) stimulates choline acetyltransferase activity in vitro and in vivo. Brain Res Dev Brain Res 67:113–120

Paul JW, Quach TT, Duchemin A-M, Schrier BK, DaVanzo JP (1990) 1,1,3 Tricyano-2-amino-1-propene (Triap): a small molecule which mimics or potentiates nerve growth factor. Brain Res Dev Brain Res 55:21–27

Pradines A, Magazin M, Schiltz P, Lefur G, Caput D, Ferrara P (1995) Evidence for nerve growth factor-potentiating activities of the non-peptidic compound SR 57746A in PC12 cells. J Neurochem 64(5):1954–1964

Pshenichkin SP, Szekely AM, Wise BC (1994) Transcriptional and posttranscriptional mechanisms involved in the interleukin-1, steroid, and protein kinase C regulation of nerve growth factor in cortical astrocytes. J Neurochem 63:419–428

Reeben M, Arbatova J, Palgi J, Miettinen R, Halmekyto M, Alhonen L, Janne J, Riekkinen P, Saarma M (1996) Induced expression of neurotrophins in transgenic mice overexpressing ornithine decarboxylase and overproducing putrescine. J Neurosci Res 45(5):542–548

Ross AH, McKinnon CA, Daou M-C, Ratliff K, Wolf DE (1995) Differential biological effects of K252 kinase inhibitors are related to membrane solubility but not to permeability. J Neurochem 65:2748–2756

Ryden M, Hempstead B, Ibanez CF (1997) Differential modulation of neuron survival during development by nerve growth factor binding to the P75 neurotrophin receptor. J Biol Chem 272(26):16322–16328

Ryffel B, Woerly G, Greiner B, Haendler B, Mihatsck MJ, Foxwell BMJ (1991) Distribution of the cyclosporine binding protein cyclophilin in human tissues. Immunology 72:399–404

Sabatini DM, Erdjument-Bromage H, Lui M, Tempst P, Snyder SH (1994) RAFT1: a mammalian protein that binds to FKBP12 in a rapamycin-dependent fashion and is homologous to yeast TORs. Cell 78:35–43

Saggio I, Gloaguen I, Poiana G, Laufer R (1995) CNTF variants with increased biological potency and receptor selectivity define a functional site of receptor interaction. EMBO J 14(13):3045–3054

Saporito MS, Brown ER (1994) Systemic dexamethasone administration increases septal Trk autophosphorylation in adult rats via an induction of nerve growth factor. Mol Pharmacol 45:395–401

Schoen WR, Wyvratt MJ Jr, Smith RG (1993) Growth hormone secretagogues. Ann Reports Med Chem 28:177–186

Schoen WR, Ok D, DeVita RJ, Pisano JM, Hodges P, Cheng K, Chan WW-S, Butler BS, Smith RG, Wyvratt MJ Jr, Fisher MH (1994a) Structure-activity relationships in the amino acid sidechain of L-692,429. Bioorg Med Chem Lett 4:1117–1122

Schoen WR, Pisano JM, Wyvratt MJ Jr, Fisher MH, Prendergast K, Cheng K, Chan WW-S, Butler BS, Smith RG, Ball RG (1994b) A novel 3-substituted benzazepinone growth hormone secretagogue (L-692,429). J Med Chem 37:897–906

Sharkey J, Butcher SP (1994) Immunophilins mediate the neuroprotective effects of FK506 in focal cerebral ischaemia. Nature 371:336–339

Smith RG, Cheng K, Schoen WR, Pong S-S, Hickey GJ, Jacks TM, Butler BS, Chan WW-S, Chaung L-YP, Judith F, Taylor AM, Wyvratt MJ Jr, Fisher MH (1993) A nonpeptidyl growth hormone secretagogue. Science 260:1640–1643

Smith RG, Pong S-S, Hickey GJ, Jacks TM, Cheng K, Leonard RJ, Cohen CJ, Arena JP, Chang CH, Drisko JE, Wyvratt MJ Jr, Fisher MH, Nargund RP, Patchett AA (1996) Modulation of pulsatile GH release through a novel receptor in hypothalamus and pituitary gland. Recent Prog Horm Res 51:261–286

Snider RM, Constantine JW, Lowe JA 3rd, Longo KP, Lebel WS, Woody HA, Drozda SE, Desai MC, Vinick FJ, Spencer RW (1991) A potent nonpeptide antagonist of the substance P (NNK1) receptor. Science 251(4992):435–437

Sohrabji F, Miranda RCG, Toranallerand CD (1995) Identification of a putative estrogen response element in the gene encoding brain-derived neurotrophic factor. Proc Natl Acad Sci USA 92(24):11110–11114

Steiner JP, Dawson TM, Fotuhi M, Glatt CE, Snowman AM, Cohen N, Snyder SH (1992) High brain densities of the immunophilin FKBP co-localized with calcineurin. Nature 358:584–587

Steiner JP, Hamilton GS, Ross DT, Valentine HL, Guo H, Connolly MA, Liang S, Ramsey C, Li J-H J, Huang W, Howorth P, Soni R, Fuller M, Sauer H, Nowotnik AC, Suzdak PD (1997a) Neurotrophic immunophilin ligands stimulate structural and functional recovery in neurodegenerative animal models. Proc Natl Acad Sci USA 94:2019–2024

Steiner JP, Connolly MA, Valentine HL, Hamilton GS, Dawson TM, Hester L, Snyder SH (1997b) Neurotrophic actions of nonimmunosuppressive analogues of immunosuppressive drugs FK506, rapamycin and cyclosporin A. Nat Med 3:421–428

Steinmann B, Bruckner P, Superti-Furga A (1991) Cyclosporin A slows collagen triple helix formation in vivo: indirect evidence for a physiologic role of peptidyl-prolyl cis-trans isomerase. J Biol Chem 266:1299–1303

Stone EA, Manavalan JS, Basham DA, Bing G (1994) Effect of yohimbine on nerve growth factor mRNA and protein levels in rat hippocampus. Neurosci Lett 167:11–13

Stucky CL, Koltzenburg M (1997) The low-affinity neurotrophin receptor P75 regulates the function but not the selective survival of specific subpopulations of sensory neurons. J Neurosci 17(11):4398–4405

Sykes K, Gething MJ, Sambrooke J (1993) Proline isomerases function during heat shock. Proc Natl Acad Sci USA 90:5853–5857

Takeuchi R, Murase K, Furukawa Y, Furukawa S, Hayashi K (1990) Stimulation of nerve growth factor synthesis/secretion by 1,4-benzoquinone and its derivatives in cultured mouse astroglial cells. FEBS Lett 261:63–66

Tapley P, Lamballe F, (1992) K252a is a selective inhibitor of the tyrosine protein kinase activity of the Trk family of oncogenes and neurotrophin receptors. Oncogene 7:371–381

Thoenen H (1995) Neurotrophins and neuronal plasticity. Science 270(5236):593–598

Toran-Allerand CD (1996) The estrogen/neurotrophin connection during neural development – Is co-localization of estrogen receptors with the neurotrophins and their receptors biologically relevant? Dev Neurosci 18(1–2):36–48

Toran-Allerand CD, Miranda RC (1992) Estrogen receptors co-localize with low-affinity nerve growth factor receptors in cholinergic neurons of the basal forebrain. Proc Natl Acad Sci USA 89:4668–4672

Treanor JJS, Schmelzer C, Knusel B, Winslow JW, Shelton DL, Hefti F, Nikolics K, Burton LE (1995) Heterodimeric neurotrophins induce phosphorylation of Trk receptors and promote neuronal differentiation in PC12 cells. J Biol Chem 270(39):23104–23110

Urfer R, Tsoulfas P, Soppet D, Escandon E, Parada LF, Presta LG (1994) The binding epitopes of neurotrophin-3 to its receptors TrkC and GP75 and the design of a multifunctional human neurotrophin. EMBO J 13(24):5896–5909

Urfer R, Tsoulfas P, O'Connell L, Shelton DL, Parada LF, Presta LG (1995) An immunoglobulin-like domain determines the specificity of neurotrophin receptors. EMBO J 14(12):2795–2805

Vaidya VA, Marek GJ, Aghajanian GK, Duman RS (1997) 5-HT2A receptor-mediated regulation of brain-derived neurotrophic factor mRNA in the hippocampus and the neocortex. J Neurosci 17(8):2785–2795

Walker P, Weichsel ME, Fischer DA, Guo SM, Fischer DA (1979) Thyroxine increases nerve growth factor concentration in adult mouse brain. Science 204:427–429

Walker P, Wil ML, Weichsel ME, Fischer DA (1981) Effect of thyroxine on nerve growth factor concentration in adult mouse brain. Science 204:1777–1787

Wang T, Donahoe PK, Zervos AS (1994) Specific interaction of Type I receptors of the TGF-b family with the immunophilin FKBP-12. Science 265:674–676

Wang T, Li B-Y, Danielson PD, Shah P, Rockwell S, Manganaro T, Donahoe PK (1996) The immunophilin FKBP12 functions as a common inhibitor of the TGFb family type I receptor. Cell 86:435–444

Wijdicks EFM, Wiesner RH, Dahlke LJ, Krom RAF (1994) FK506-induced neurotoxicity in liver transplantation. Ann Neurol 35:498–501

Windisch JM, Marksteiner R, Schneider R (1995a) Nerve growth factor binding site on TrkA mapped to a single 24-amino acid leucine-rich motif. J Biol Chem 270(47):28133–28138

Windisch JM, Bernhard A, Marksteiner R, Lang ME, Schneider R (1995b) Specific neurotrophin binding to leucine-rich motif peptides of TrkA and TrkB. FEBS Lett 374:125–129

Wu C-F, Zhang M (1993) K252a potentiates epidermal growth factor-induced differentiation of PC12 cells. J Neurosci Res 36:539–550

Xu Q, Leiva MC, Fischkoff SA, Handschumacher RE, Lyttle CR (1992) Leukocyte chemotactic activity of cyclophilin. J Biol Chem, 267:11968–11971

Yamada K, Nitta A, Hasegawa T, Fuji K, Hiramatsu M, Kameyama T, Furukawa Y, Hayashi K, Nabeshima T (1997) Orally active NGF synthesis stimulators: potential therapeutic agents in Alzheimer's disease. Behav Brain Res 83:117–122

Yamaguchi K, Sasano A (1993) Stimulation of nerve growth factor production by pyrroloquinoline quinone and its derivatives in vitro and in vivo. Biosci Biotech Biochem 57(7):1231–1233

Yamaguchi K, Uemura D, Tsuji T, Kondo K (1994) Stimulation of nerve growth factor production by diterpenoids isolated from plants of *Euphorbia* species. Biosci Biotech Biochem 58:1749–1751

Young WJ, Smith SM, Chang CS (1997) Induction of the intronic enhancer of the human ciliary neurotrophic factor receptor (CNTFR-alpha) gene by the TR4 orphan receptor – A member of steroid receptor superfamily. J Biol Chem 272(5):3109–3116

Subject Index

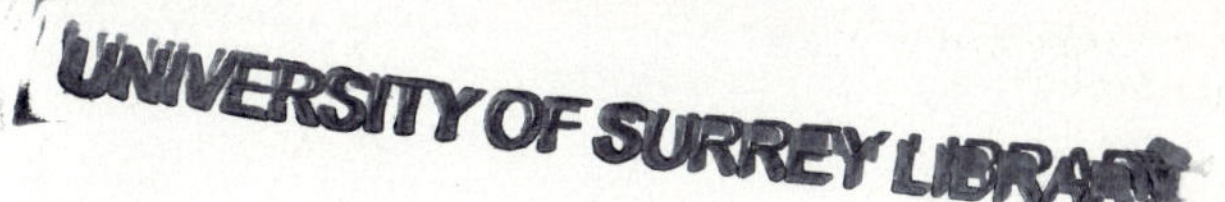

Printing: Saladruck, Berlin
Binding: Buchbinderei Lüderitz & Bauer, Berlin